Birthing a Mother

Birthing a Mother

The Surrogate Body and the Pregnant Self

Elly Teman

UNIVERSITY OF CALIFORNIA PRESS
Berkeley · Los Angeles · London

University of California Press, one of the most distin-
guished university presses in the United States, enriches
lives around the world by advancing scholarship in the
humanities, social sciences, and natural sciences. Its
activities are supported by the UC Press Foundation
and by philanthropic contributions from individuals
and institutions. For more information, visit www
.ucpress.edu.

University of California Press
Berkeley and Los Angeles, California

University of California Press, Ltd.
London, England

Library of Congress Cataloging-in-Publication Data

Teman, Elly.
  Birthing a mother : the surrogate body and the preg-
nant self / Elly Teman.
      p.   cm.
  Includes bibliographical references and index.
  ISBN 978-0-520-25963-8 (cloth : alk. paper)
  ISBN 978-0-520-25964-5 (pbk. : alk. paper)
  1. Surrogate mothers—Israel.   2. Mothers—Israel.
3. Pregnancy—Israel.   4. Judaism.   I. Title.
HQ759.5.T46   2010
306.874'3—dc22   2009019426

Manufactured in the United States of America

19 18 17 16 15 14 13 12
10 9 8 7 6 5 4 3 2

This book is printed on Cascades Enviro 100, a 100%
post-consumer waste, recycled, de-inked fiber. FSC recycled certified and processed chlorine free. It is acid free,
Ecologo certified, and manufactured by BioGas energy.

This book is dedicated to my one-of-a-kind mother, Rhisa Teman—adoptive mother to many generations of students, but the only mother for me. And it is dedicated to the memory of my beautiful grandmother, Ruth Ellen Erlich, whom we knew as Sasi.

And that's why I say, I didn't just give birth to a baby,
I gave birth to a mother.

Tamar, surrogate

I always say, my mother gave birth to me the first
time, she gave me life. But my surrogate gave me life
the second time.

Shlomit, intended mother

You are not just giving birth to children; you are
giving birth to new mothers and to new and happy
families.

Mali, intended mother

Let your Mother and Father be glad; let she who bore
you rejoice.

Proverbs 23:25

Contents

PART FOUR · *Redefining*

Illustrations

Acknowledgments

This book could never have come to completion without generous funding from various sources. Fieldwork and early writing of the manuscript were enabled by generous scholarships from the Canadian Friends of the Hebrew University, the Golda Meir Foundation, and the Social Sciences Faculty Rector's Prize of the Hebrew University. I also thank the Hadassah Brandeis Institute, the Israeli Association of Academic Women, and the Lafer Center for Gender Studies for research awards in support of this project. Postdoctoral fellowships from the Yad Hanadiv-Rothschild Foundation and from the Morris Ginsberg Foundation enabled me to spend a full academic year at the University of California, Berkeley, to further my training and to complete this book. The Beatrice M. Bain Research Group and the Science, Technology, and Society Center at UC Berkeley gave me a stimulating intellectual environment in which to write. This book came to completion while I was a postdoctoral research scholar at the Penn Center for the Integration of Healthcare Technologies (Penn CIGHT) at the University of Pennsylvania. I am grateful to the center and its staff for supporting my completion of this project.

A number of articles based on this research have been published in journals and in edited volumes. Part of the prologue appeared in 2006 in Gardner and Hoffman's *Dispatches from the Field: Neophyte Ethnographers in a Changing World* (Long Grove, IL: Waveland Press). Part of part 1 appeared in 2001 in *Women's Studies Quarterly* 31 (3&4): 11–34 and in 2003 in *Medical Anthropology Quarterly* 17 (1): 78–98.

Part of part 2 appeared in 2003 in a chapter in Cook, Sclater, and Kaganas's *Surrogate Motherhood: International Perspectives* (Oxford, UK: Hart Publishing, pp. 261–280) and is forthcoming in *Body and Society* 15 (3). Finally, part of the conclusion was published in *Social Science & Medicine* 67 (7): 1104–1112. I am grateful to the editors and anonymous reviewers of these publications for their suggestions and feedback. The illustrations in this book have been reproduced with the generous permissions of the following Israeli illustrators: Ruth Gwily, Gila Kaplan, Rutu Modan, Naama Peleg-Segal, David Polonsky, Danna Shamir, and Rhisa Teman.

Over the years, a number of scholars have provided invaluable guidance and support. I especially want to thank Eyal Ben-Ari, my dissertation advisor. He has an unmatchable ability to take the jumble of theory, ethnography, and random thoughts presented to him and help one shape it into a coherent outline. I am grateful for this opportunity to formally acknowledge his peerless mentorship. Meira Weiss has been an important mentor from the time I began my M.A. studies at Hebrew University. Meira's continuous support and encouragement during my fieldwork and her influential perspective on the anthropology of the body are in evidence throughout my work. She encouraged me to publish my work even at its early stages and introduced me to some of the top scholars in my field; to me, this exemplifies feminist mentorship in its truest form.

During the course of this project at Hebrew University, I had the good fortune to receive guidance from several people who informally included me as one of their own mentees. Don Seeman helped me formulate my very first thoughts on surrogacy as my final paper in the medical anthropology course he taught; his close readings and comments on various drafts of this manuscript were important to my thinking throughout this project. Tamar Rapoport and Edna Lomsky-Feder generously included me in a reading and research group they mentored for several years with their graduate students. I learned valuable lessons about theory and critical analysis from them and benefited greatly from the support and comments on my writing from the members of the group.

My fellow graduate students and the faculty of the department of sociology and anthropology at Hebrew University provided a collegial network during this research. I especially want to thank those who closely read various chapters or drafts of this study, many of whom are also good friends: Svetta Roberman, Lydia Ginzberg, Adi Kuntsman, Limor Darash, Michal Lester, Lauren Erdreich, Omi Leisner, Tali Berner, Tzvia Birman, Danny Kaplan, Tamar El-Or, Nurit Stadler, and Daphna

Birenbaum-Carmeli. I am especially grateful to Noa Aploig for reading through the full manuscript. Tsipy Ivry and I were midwives of one
another's studies; in the lonely world of the "via doctoroza," it is rare that
one finds co-mentorship like ours. I hope that people will read our books
in tandem for what they reveal about the anthropology of pregnancy.

Several North American scholars have been extremely helpful to me
and my work. This book would never have come to fruition without the
unwavering enthusiasm, guidance, and belief in me shown by the amazing Robbie Davis-Floyd. The influence of her path-breaking scholarship
in the anthropology of reproduction is central to the conceptual toolkit
used in this analysis. Meeting Susan Martha Kahn through our mutual
interest in reproductive technologies in Israel has been one of the greatest
perks of this project. She has been an inspiration to me with her scholarship, a wise guide in this study, and a great friend. Charis Thompson was
the kindest host a postdoc in a strange land could ask for. Her input into
my thinking about reproductive technologies and her comments on this
book have been invaluable. Diane L. Wolf read through several drafts of
these pages and offered important comments and encouragement. She
encouraged me to "go out on a limb" with the conclusion, and I hope
that my efforts follow her call. Heather Paxson, Michelle Pridmore-
Brown and D. Kelly Weisberg also gave detailed and crucial comments
on the full manuscript. A writing group at Berkeley, including Kalindi
Vora, Neda Antonosky, and Kimberly Tallbear provided a great support
system as well. Special thanks to Susan Markens and Simon Bronner for
important advice along this journey. The amazing editing work of Linda
Forman is evident throughout this manuscript; her work impressed me
so much it led me to seek her out five years after working with her on
a journal article. I am also grateful to Tzipporah Avraham and Jennifer
Morgan for their edits on other versions of the manuscript. Heartfelt
thanks to Stan Holwitz, my editor at UC Press, for giving my book a
chance and for his true kindness. I also thank the production staff at UC
Press, especially Caroline Knapp and Nick Arrivo.

Many friends and family are also present behind the scenes of the
fieldwork and writing experiences out of which this dissertation grew.
My husband Avi Solomon read through many drafts and made incisive
comments and editorial corrections. He has always believed in me more
than I did in myself, with patience, grace and love. My parents, Rhisa
and Nissan Teman, have been the greatest support team I could ask for,
holding my hand in times of crisis and celebrating my achievements;
my mom also spent many hours editing my grammar and babysitting

my children so I could finish this book, while my dad helped me search for the artists whose work is included in these pages. My godfather David B. Sherman read and commented on papers and drafts, hosted me on my way to conferences, and kept me updated with carefully collected news clippings on important news relevant to my research. He and Roberto Benitez bought me my first business suit for my first international anthropology conference. I am also grateful for the love and support of my beloved grandparents, Ruth (in blessed memory) and Robert Erlich; my brother Adi Teman; and my aunts, uncles, in-laws, and cousins. My aunt Barbara Erlich was especially supportive of my efforts towards this book. My precious children, Uriel Moshe Solomon and Rachela Tilly Solomon, have brought us all so much joy and awarded me an insider's perspective on becoming a mother. And I could not have made it through the years of this research without other good friends not mentioned above, among them Danna Harari, Liat Ventura, Naama Shay-Catrieli, Rinat Zohar Menachem, Itsik Nachum, Helene Goldberg, Lisa Carlsson, Gretty Shweizer, and Aliza Haas.

Finally, it goes without saying in a text such as this that I am deeply indebted to all of those who have opened their lives, homes, and hearts to me in the course of my fieldwork. To preserve their anonymity, I cannot thank them by their full real names, but Ruti, whose courage paved the way for Israeli intended mothers; Michal, who led me into this field; Merav, who opened the doors for me and for so many others; and Sylvie, Sigal, Tami, Chagit and everyone else who welcomed me into their lives and became my friends along the way—I hope that you will be pleased with the result of my research. To all of the wonderful people involved in the Tapuz surrogacy web forum and to the couples, surrogates, and director, Merav Levy, of the Pundekaut Hoveket [Embracing Surrogacy] agency, I hope you will find this an appropriate representation of the surrogacy experience.

Prologue: Yael

This work took me into the lives of surrogates and intended mothers alike, forging close anthropologist-informant relationships with each, yet the person who seeped into my consciousness the most was my first informant, Yael, an intended mother. Perhaps this is because she faced so many obstacles on her route to motherhood; perhaps it is because hers was the first surrogacy story I was exposed to. What is clear to me now is that Yael's story initiated me into the frame of mind necessary to undertake this study—a frame of mind in which I was conscious of the mental, physical, and emotional challenges faced by the women I came to know, both surrogates and intended mothers.

I met Yael for our first interview in a coffee shop in Haifa on a Sunday afternoon. I was a newly minted graduate student in anthropology—unmarried, but hoping to become a mother "someday." She had been married for fifteen years, and her life was completely focused on having her own genetic child, created from an egg harvested from her ovaries and gestated in another woman's womb. After telling me about the long process she had been through to find a surrogate, she told me about the pregnancy in a whisper that communicated, "If I say it out loud, it might disappear." Leaning forward, I immediately became a partner in her conspiracy. I, too, whispered each time I mentioned the pregnancy.

That first interview began simply. "Tell me your story," I said, "from wherever it begins." Instinctively, she began with the day that the army doctor, on examining her physical health for the mandatory Israeli draft, told her that she had been born without a womb. "Imagine," she said, "finding out that you could never have children when you were only eighteen years old."

That was the beginning—the day everything changed, the day that her story began. Each of her days since then had been devoted to having a child. "I had planned on going to university," she told me, "but somehow my life became so wrapped up in having a child that the years just slipped by." And "it wasn't easy," she repeated twice, even though she spoke with a smile. It wasn't easy at all.

Thinking about adoption, choosing surrogacy. The ups and downs of finding the "right" surrogate. The worry, the wait. The changes she and her husband had to incorporate into their lives. "It was strange," she said, "giving up part of our personal life as a couple and letting a third person in." Learning to stop living as two, beginning to live life as three. "In some ways," I suggested, "it was preparation for parenthood." "But different," she replied.

Tali was the fourth potential surrogate Yael and her husband had proposed to the state committee in charge of approving surrogacy arrangements; the first three women had not been approved for various reasons. Yael recalled the day they met and the joyful day that the pregnancy test was positive. "We didn't know then what lay ahead," Yael said. "Now I know not to get excited at least until the first months have passed." Tali miscarried five months into the first pregnancy.

After the miscarriage, another IVF embryo transfer was attempted, and Tali became pregnant with twins. Three months into the pregnancy, the doctors were keeping a close watch to prevent another loss. Yael showed me the ultrasound photos that documented the twins' existence. She passed the small square photos showing white fuzz on a black background across the table to me. I touched them. Three photos, none of them clear. "Do you see them?" she asked me. I didn't see a thing. "Wow," I answered, pretending I did. "I try not to look at them too much," she told me. "I don't want to believe it yet. Just in case."

I passed the photos back across the table to her, and she retrieved them with a careful hand. "Are you going to frame those" I asked her, "or put them in an album?" "No," she answered, "I keep them here," and she put them back into her bag, in an envelope. I watched the way she inserted the photos into their package. It was like she was putting them to sleep. She held the envelope gently but firmly, securely tucking the photos into her bag. Her babies. They were with her all the time. It occurred to me that she was almost really pregnant. Her babies in a bag, which she carried near her belly. Those little bleeps on the ultrasound monitor.

I felt apprehensive calling Yael to find out how the pregnancy was progressing. On the one hand, her experience was data for my study. On the other hand, her life was her own, and I identified with her hopes that this time it would be okay. I crossed my fingers for her. But when I returned to Israel after spending the summer abroad, I found out that Yael's surrogate had miscarried again. My heart dropped. She had lost the twins.

What if a live baby never came? I felt the fear and expectation of the wait. I was pregnant with Yael. Yael was pregnant with her surrogate. I wondered if all of Yael's friends were pregnant with her, too—in spirit, in heart, in the wait.

I called Yael on Rosh Hashanah, the Jewish New Year. We exchanged small talk, but the real conversation occurred beneath the surface of our words. It was the loud silence behind the empty words that I heard most clearly. She felt it as strongly as I did. I could tell because there was a tension on the line that was uncomfortable, even painful. "My heart is with yours," I told her, and I meant every word. She replied with a simple, but fully aware, "I know." She did not tell me that Tali was already pregnant again. Two weeks later, she called me to tell me the news. They had just had an ultrasound. It was a boy.

In December, I called Yael. She told me that the pregnancy had become complicated. Tali had decided to stop working and stay home. They had run to the hospital a few nights before because Tali was bleeding heavily. "We almost lost the baby. And of all nights, when Miki [Yael's husband] was in reserve duty and had taken the car. We got to the hospital in a taxi, just in time." She had taken out her book of Psalms and prayed and prayed, she said. This time it had to work. And then Yael told me that, just that night, Tali, who was of Iraqi heritage, had called her with a craving for a certain type of soup that Moroccans make. Yael's mother made her a pot, telling Yael that it was like she was making it for her own daughter, because Yael's son was the one responsible for Tali's cravings.

I came home at nine o'clock one night several months later and listened to my messages on the answering machine. The third message took a minute to register, so I pressed the button and listened to it again. I hadn't misheard it. It was Yael: "Hi, Elly. Our son was born an hour ago at eleven o'clock this morning. We are here at the hospital. Tali is feeling well. Bye." I danced around the room and sang a little tune.

Some see surrogacy as the ultimate form of exploitation. Others have called it a "brave new world." For the women I write about in this book, surrogacy is an emotional roller coaster ride in which one mother, through strategy and sacrifice, helps another woman to also become a mother. For the anthropologist, it is about bodies, boundaries, maternities, and meanings. For Yael's son, who turns ten as this book goes to press, it is the story of how he was born.

Introduction

In early 2008, surrogacy became the hot topic of the moment, grabbing cover stories in *The New York Times* and *Newsweek*.[1] Though it would seem that this relatively rare mode of reproduction has become the latest trend in reproduction, it is not new. In fact, the roots of surrogacy can be traced to the book of Genesis.[2] Despite the media frenzy that accompanied the heatedly debated Baby M case two decades ago,[3] the practice of surrogacy has quietly continued, staying out of the limelight until its recent resurgence in the headlines. Indeed, since the late 1970s, tens of thousands of women have given birth through surrogacy, and an estimated 1,500 babies are born through this practice each year in the United States.[4] The practice's current high profile may perhaps be explained by a slew of celebrities creating families through surrogacy and a surge in surrogacy births in the United States over the past five years.[5] As women today increasingly delay childbearing, infertility levels rise, and single persons and same-sex couples pursue more family-building options, the use of surrogacy is not just gaining momentum but is likely to increase exponentially.

There has been an abundance of interdisciplinary academic inquiry into surrogacy arrangements, generating a complex and nuanced critical debate about the ethical, religious, legal, and broad social issues that these arrangements bring into focus. In general, much of this scholarship has displayed a sense of uneasiness with respect to surrogacy, raising concerns about the commodification of women and children, class and gender-based exploitation of women's bodies, the distortion of nature, and the devaluing of human life and of women's reproductive labor.[6] Yet, despite the huge attention surrogacy has received in scholarly circles, most explorations of the subject are primarily theoretical and only vaguely based on the actual experiences of those involved in these arrangements: the surrogates and intended parents who come together to bring new humans and new kin relations into the world. Particularly odd, despite the wealth of anthropological attention to many diverse aspects of reproductive technologies,[7] is the dearth of ethnographic inquiry into surrogacy. Although the character of surrogacy has evolved over the past decade to privilege the use of gestational surrogacy, no full ethnography of the phenomenon has been attempted since the publication of Helena Ragoné's study of traditional surrogacy arrangements more than a decade and a half ago.[8]

Like many of these scholarly conversations, popular accounts of the practice have implied some discomfort with surrogacy, insinuating, for instance, that it might be merely another way for the economically privileged to exploit the lower classes by "renting" poor women's wombs. This tone of accusation carries over into the current media depictions of celebrities becoming parents with the aid of invisible "gestational carriers" and reports of "outsourcing" surrogacy to India.[9] Misrepresented in these generalizations are the majority of women contracting with surrogates; they are not choosing this option lightheartedly because of a fear of stretch marks, nor are they following a fad. When married or heterosexually partnered couples choose to pursue surrogacy, it is usually after long struggles with infertility, pregnancy loss, or other medical conditions.[10] For other individuals, such as those for whom the law prevents adoption because they are too old, single, or in a same-sex partnership, surrogacy may provide the only option for becoming parents. The stories behind their decisions to pursue surrogacy and their experiences of the process are far more complex than are implied by one-sided depictions of technological and commercial exploitation.

Also left untold in the academic and popular coverage of surrogacy are the stories of the women behind the wombs—the women who have contractually agreed to carry a baby to term. On television, in film, and in popular journalism, they are portrayed in ways that suggest that their decision to voluntarily relinquish a child of their womb to relative strangers in exchange for money can be neatly explained by comparison to the cherished notion of the "good mother." Indeed, an analysis of the media portrayals suggests an attempt to show that only unnatural or abnormal women would make this nonnormative choice; surrogates are, in fact, depicted as financially desperate, greedy, emotionally unstable, or overly altruistic to the degree of psychological impairment.[11] Women in India who become surrogates are portrayed as desperately poor and in need of rehabilitation, while American military wives who give birth for others are accused of profiting dishonestly at the expense of the military health insurance that covers their surrogate pregnancies.[12]

The scarce empirical research that exists on surrogacy, primarily psychosocial in nature, also commonly implies surrogates are deviant by hypothesizing their difference from the majority of the population in terms of personality characteristics, morals, and/or psychological history.[13] In spite of such a priori assumptions, nearly all of these studies have concluded that surrogates are not markedly different by any measure and that most are within what the researchers consider to be "the normal range" of psychological stability, intelligence, and moral standards.[14] There also exists widespread discomfort with the surrogate's contracted commitment to relinquish the baby, resulting from the belief that the surrogate ought to bond with the baby she carries and that relinquishment therefore ought to be a traumatic event for her. This idea, based on the widespread attention accorded the Baby M case, has little foundation in reality. Indeed, it is estimated that over 99 percent of surrogates have willingly relinquished the child and that less than one-tenth of 1 percent of surrogacy cases in the United States end up in court battles.[15] The majority of surrogates actually report high satisfaction with the process and report no psychological problems as a result of relinquishment. Longitudinal studies show that these positive attitudes remain stable over time, and most surrogates express their interest in being surrogates again.[16]

It is here that the work of the anthropologist is needed to think against the grain of what we believe ought to be true. In *Birthing a Mother*, I am not concerned with making an argument for or against surrogacy or entering into the debate over whether it is right or wrong. Instead, I take a fresh look at surrogacy and attempt to completely rethink what we know about this reproductive practice by taking the experiences of persons immediately involved in it at face value and trying to understand what surrogacy means to them, in their own words. This book is first and foremost an in-depth ethnography of the complex "ontological choreography" of surrogacy arrangements, a metaphor Thompson formulated to describe the "materiality, structural constraint, performativity, discipline, co-dependence of setting and performers, and movement" involved in assisted reproduction.[17] It is also an anthropological intervention into wider debates about motherhood, kinship, embodiment, and the natural. My interpretive approach employs a cross-cultural perspective, contrasting comparative insights with ethnographic data gleaned from an in-depth ethnographic study of surrogacy participants in Israel; as I show, Israel provides an exceptionally advantageous cultural, national, religious, and political context for thinking about these issues.

Many different actors are potentially involved in this production; at the very least, it includes doctors, lawyers, intended parents, surrogates, and the state. In addition, an increasing percentage of surrogacy arrangements involve intended parents who are same-sex couples and single persons. The focus of *Birthing a Mother* is on what still constitutes, in the first decade of the twenty-first century, the majority of surrogacy arrangements, those in which the surrogate is contracted by a married or legally paired heterosexual couple. I analyze the stories surrogates and intended parents tell of the journey they begin from the moment they enter into the world of third-party reproduction and confront the difficult task of making sense of previously taken-for-granted understandings of kinship and maternity. This journey entails navigating an entirely new kind of relationship that creates intimate links between individuals who might otherwise never interact, and it necessitates complex negotiations of personal boundaries and of kin relations. An intricate and delicate balance is required of surrogates and couples as they manage this relationship, which is riddled with risks, miscommunications, and exhilarating moments.

My ethnography concentrates on gestational surrogacy arrangements, in which the surrogate conceives using in vitro fertilization (IVF) technology: the egg of the intended mother or of a donor is fertilized in a Petri dish with the sperm of the intended father or of a donor, and the embryo is "implanted" in the surrogate's uterus. In particular, I explore the avenues through which surrogates and intended mothers navigate the emergent questions they face in relation to motherhood, family, the body, and interpersonal boundaries. I pay particular attention to the social relationship that develops between the two women involved in the process; the intended father's secondary role is a reflection of his distance from the women's relationship in most surrogacy arrangements observed in this study.

The stakes are high for each of these women in their cooperative but by no means uncomplicated endeavor. Surrogates run the risk of taking part in a process that can easily be constructed as deviant and unnatural when viewed against the cultural expectation that women should raise the children they bear. An intended mother faces the reality that another woman is carrying her baby; this other woman potentially has a privileged claim to social recognition as the baby's mother. Both women straddle a delicate position vis-à-vis one another in terms of control: each has reason to feel loss of control during the process, just as each has reason to blame the other party for misusing her power. My study follows surrogates as they continuously abdicate, through language and embodied practice, the title of mother to the babies they carry; they cognitively partition their bodies and "natures" to ensure that their own maternity remains devoted to their own biological children, while the processes of gestation they embody actually facilitate the maternity of their intended mothers. The study also follows intended mothers as they make concentrated efforts to claim the maternal title for themselves and to bridge their embodied distance from the pregnancy by "carrying" the weight of pregnancy-related bureaucracy, constructing pregnant identities, and even embodying the pregnancy vicariously.

I draw on in-depth ethnographic fieldwork conducted among gestational surrogates and intended parents in Israel over a period of eight years. The choice of Israel as the location for this study is not incidental. Israel is one of the few countries in the world where surrogacy is legal and where contracts are valid in a court of law. The small geographical size of the country enables research into the hitherto little-explored area of the surrogate–intended mother relationship, as these dyads are able to interact more intensely than surrogacy participants elsewhere, who often live at great distances from one another, for example, in different states in the United States or even different countries. This geographic proximity also affords the anthropologist access to and observation of the often hidden inner workings of the arrangement; even if the same type of emotionally intense relationships do exist elsewhere, it would be impossible for the anthropologist to study them. In the few ethnographic studies to date of surrogacy arrangements, all carried out in the United States, it is no surprise that access to informants was limited to phone and e-mail contacts or that the studies concentrated on only individual surrogate-couple triads.[18]

Israel is also an eminently suitable context for studying the cultural elements shaping women's personal experiences of surrogacy because the very concepts being negotiated in these arrangements are amplified in both Jewish religion and in Israeli national discourse. Motherhood, family, and the importance of bearing children have historically been valorized as having crucial significance for the survival of the Jewish people. Within the context of the Israeli-Palestinian conflict, pronatalist national ideologies and demographic policies have imbued motherhood with major national significance for both sides and have made living childfree by choice an uncommon and socially unacceptable option.[19] Jewish women's bodies, within this context, become a symbolic site in which national and religious boundaries are constituted, particularly because most Orthodox rabbis view birth from a Jewish woman's womb—whether or not the sperm and egg have come from Jewish genitors—as making the newborn a Jew, and, thus, an Israeli citizen.[20]

Examining how surrogates and intended mothers negotiate maternity, kin relations, bodies, and boundaries in a context where these stakes are so high amplifies what we might find among surrogacy participants in other cultural contexts. This local version of a global set of surrogacy practices has important implications for the human experience of surrogacy in general. Comparative notes woven throughout the text highlight how the subjectivities that emerge from this local, national, and religious context might emerge differently in other local arenas of the global subculture of surrogacy.

Birthing a Mother will be of interest to cultural anthropologists and to scholars and students specializing in medical anthropology, medical sociology, and the anthropology/sociology of reproduction. It also intervenes in wider debates of interest to an interdisciplinary academic audience concerned with issues of gender and sexuality, kinship and family, and science and technology. More broadly, the book provides a comprehensive ethnographic account of surrogacy for policy makers, mental health practitioners, and medical professionals that will enable them to have more informed discussions about surrogacy. It can also be used as a resource for couples and surrogates interested in what makes surrogacy relationships work, as well as for those simply curious to read what really amounts to an insider's account of surrogacy. Even for those not directly affected by surrogacy, thinking about reproduction in these terms is life altering, as it challenges the way we think about the basic structures of society. The magnitude of change involved in a practice like surrogacy alters our horizon of possibilities and invites contemplation.

SURROGACY AS A CULTURAL ANOMALY

In light of the broad and varied opposition to surrogacy and the controversy it generates, it is no surprise that surveys investigating attitudes toward the practice in several countries have indicated that the majority of the public disapprove of the practice and perceive surrogacy as the least acceptable of the reproductive technologies.[21] This public uneasiness with surrogacy and the stereotypes and misinformation that pervade surrogacy's public representation are more illustrative of the cultural anxieties that surrogacy encapsulates than of problems with the actual majority of cases. At the base of these anxieties is the subversive nature of surrogacy, which represents a fundamental "cultural anomaly" or incongruity.[22] Anomalies are deviations from the natural order or usual method; cultural anomalies emerge when a given culture's conventions of order and classification are contradicted by an object, person, experience, or event.[23] Cultures mark off phenomena that defy classification as anomalies to protect the social structure and moral code.[24]

Birth, Davis-Floyd argues, is treated as a cultural anomaly in the United States because its unpredictable nature undermines contemporary American beliefs about the superiority of technology over nature.[25] Contractual surrogacy, which presents classificatory challenges to two of the most fundamental conceptual structures of modern society—family and motherhood—represents an even more blatantly anomalous phenomenon than birth. In an era when the modern, nuclear family structure is increasingly "fragmented" as divorce rates rise and alternative family forms flourish, surrogacy represents the height of destabilization of the family concept.[26] Surrogacy upsets the moral framework in which reproduction is regarded as a "natural fact" grounded in love, marriage, and sexual intercourse.[27] Surrogacy constructs families through the marketplace, making them a matter of choice rather than fate. By threatening the understanding of families as biological facts, surrogacy reveals instead that families are social constructs.[28]

The cultural anxieties provoked by surrogacy in relation to the family are further amplified by the anxieties surrogacy raises over loss of maternal wholeness, as the perceived unity of motherhood is deconstructed in surrogacy and the parts distributed among at least three potential mothers: genetic, gestational, and social. Giving birth to a child for the purpose of relinquishment also defies mainstream assumptions that identify pregnancy with the birth mother's commitment to the project of subsequent lifelong social mothering and threatens dominant ideologies in many cultures that assume an indissoluble mother-child bond. Directly challenging the "ideology of motherhood," surrogacy reveals that the belief in motherhood as the natural, desired, and ultimate goal of women in general is also constructed.

In addition, surrogacy disrupts the stability of the concept of nature and the ability of the discourse of the natural to maintain the classificatory categories of motherhood and family discussed above. Nature, social constructivists argue, is a culturally produced category; we need the concept of nature to put order in our thoughts.[29] Cultures have employed nature as an idiom to describe what they understand to be the essential principles by which the world is ordered.[30] Keeping the concept of nature neatly defined has, therefore, been central to maintaining the power hierarchies of gender and race that are naturalized in many societies[31] and to maintaining the idea that technology is superior to nature, which is a basic tenet of technological societies.[32] Surrogacy, like other reproductive technologies, disrupts nature's ability to serve as the ground on which motherhood and family are constituted as "natural facts."[33] Surrogacy thus reveals the fragility of the conceptual system according to which many Western cultures organize themselves.

How do surrogates and intended mothers react to being thrust into this boundary-blurring, category-challenging practice? How do they make sense of the surrogacy process? What does surrogacy mean to them? How does surrogacy affect their ongoing articulations of identity? How do they relate to one another during this process? How does each of them relate to the baby? Furthermore, when questions about the identity of the mother and about whose family is being gestated in the surrogate's womb are constantly in the background, how do the women sort out these dilemmas? How do surrogates preserve their personal identities as mothers—for, in Israel, all surrogates must already have given birth to their own genetic children—while partaking in this potentially deviant role, and how do intended mothers construct a maternal identity? What broader cultural implications do their experiences have for the way we think about gender, motherhood, and family?

In this book, I examine these questions as well as the way surrogacy affects how we think about the body. Gestational surrogacy, which is the variant I explore in this study, is facilitated through IVF. When an embryo, formed in a test tube with IVF technology from the egg of the intended mother and the sperm of the intended father (or from anonymous donors), is implanted in the surrogate's womb, the previously taken-for-granted distinctions between individual bodies is blurred. This transgression of bodily boundaries challenges the once familiar depiction of the body as a whole, interconnected system, complete unto itself with secure bodily boundaries.[34] What impact does this challenge have on the way the women involved think about their bodies, especially about where the boundary of one's personal body ends and the other woman's body begins? How does this affect a woman's sense of individuality and her sense of ownership of her body? What implications does this have for the way we think about the relationship between the body and the self?

THE CULTURAL POLITICS OF SURROGATE MOTHERHOOD

Because surrogacy does not comfortably fit the cohesive and internally consistent Western system of conceptual categories, many lawmakers have approached it with discomfort. As Rachel Cook, Shelley Day Sclater, and Felicity Kaganas note, "What emerges from any consideration of the ways in which surrogacy is dealt with in different jurisdictions is that a sense of profound anxiety and ambivalence has tended to pervade the thinking of policy makers and legislators where surrogacy is concerned."[35] The most popular strategy has been to treat surrogacy as a deviance that must be censured and as a social problem needing to be strictly regulated or entirely banned. It is prohibited in Islam and in some forms in Catholicism.[36]

As Markens notes of the ban on the practice in New York in 1992, opposition to surrogacy in the United States has created some "strange bedfellows" among policy makers and special interest groups, including alliances between the Catholic Church and feminist activists.[37] In government discussions on surrogacy in many countries and American states, ethical issues have been raised in connection with the commercial nature of the agreement and the potential exploitation of the surrogate. Popular objections to the practice have also been related to Christian ethical concerns over the use of IVF technology and have been tied in with moral debates over fetal rights, cloning, stem cell research, and abortion. Italy's 2003 law banning surrogacy and restricting the use of other reproductive technologies was influenced by a cross-party alliance between Roman Catholic politicians and the prime minister as well as support from the Vatican, which urged approval of the proposed legislation, saying it protected the rights of unborn children.[38] Canada's Royal Commission on New Reproductive Technologies, headed by Catholic activist Dr. Patricia Baird, rejected all forms of surrogacy arrangements on the grounds that surrogacy commodifies children, exploits women, and is generally harmful to society.[39] Even in the United Kingdom, where noncommercial surrogacy was eventually legalized, the British Warnock report concluded that "surrogacy is almost always unethical."[40]

As a result of their ambivalence toward surrogacy, the majority of governments around the world have felt justified in banning the practice entirely,[41] and those countries that do allow it do not explicitly endorse such contracts, yet permit them to varying degrees. Some governments—Australia (Victoria), Brazil, Hong Kong, Hungary, Israel, the Netherlands, South Africa, and the United Kingdom—enforce partial bans, authorizing court-approved contracts under specific rules and conditions. A small number of jurisdictions allow the practice without state interference, either offering voluntary guidelines (Australia [five states], Korea, and some U.S. states) or avoiding any regulation at all (Belgium, Finland, Greece, and India). As Weisberg has observed, those countries and American states that allow surrogacy agreements do so grudgingly;[42] lack of any clear and comprehensive regulatory framework leads to inconsistency and considerable uncertainty in case of disputes.[43]

The U.S. federal government has not enacted any laws on surrogacy, and the most common response to the issue at the state level is lack of legislation.[44] Most surrogacy issues have been determined by state courts and legislations, many responding to specific cases;[45] statutory law in states that have a regulatory scheme and case law in states that do not are both piecemeal rather than comprehensive.[46] California has held the reputation as the most surrogacy-friendly jurisdiction since a gestational surrogacy agreement was upheld there in 1993 in the *Johnson v. Calvert* decision.[47] The national and international surrogacy markets clustered in California as intended parents from restrictive states and countries sought surrogacy arrangements there.[48] Although other states now have similar legal precedents, California still remains the center of the global surrogacy industry today and boasts the highest number of surrogacy agencies and clinics. California surrogacy births—counted in the thousands—far outnumber the mere hundreds of births that take place in the United Kingdom and in Israel; these two countries lead in surrogacy births outside the United States at the present time. Although India has recently become an increasingly popular site for surrogacy-related medical tourism, it is still too early to know whether it will become a major player in the surrogacy market or if legislation will curb the practice.[49]

The specific ways in which surrogacy is regulated in California, the United Kingdom, and Israel are shaped not only by politics but also by each culture's key values. The liberal allowance for surrogacy in California extols the core values of individualism, capitalism, and the superiority of technology over nature, all values that have been identified by Davis-Floyd as central to the American cultural approach to childbirth in general.[50] It also speaks to U.S. hesitancy surrounding the issue of state intervention in private reproductive lives.[51] In California, an unregulated commercial market of private agencies has prospered since the early 1980s; each agency screens, matches, and regulates agreements according to its own criteria and without state interference.[52] Most California agencies extend this option to persons of any age, nationality, marital status, sexual identity, or degree of infertility and also assist with altruistic surrogacy within families. And although traditional surrogacy, whereby the surrogate herself provides the egg, is no longer popular, these agencies continue to offer it as an option. A growing number of American surrogacy agencies now cater specifically to a clientele of same-sex couples and facilitate surrogacy arrangements for intended parents who are single. Most American agencies also work with an international clientele of couples who travel to the United States expressly to pursue surrogacy because it is not legal in their home country, and some agencies specialize in surrogacy tourism from a specific country, such as Japan.[53]

In contrast to this liberal market model, state regulations in the United Kingdom are mainly intent on keeping surrogacy from becoming a commercial venture by ensuring that no private agencies can profit from the agreements. The U.K. Surrogacy Act of 1985 exhibited the opposition of British national values to American capitalist culture and the perceived threat of commercial surrogacy to British national identity during the last quarter of the twentieth century. Franklin asserts that the negative reaction to surrogacy in the British Parliament was "no doubt in part because it was an American initiative, undertaken during a time of resistance to the Americanization of Britain under Thatcher," who was attempting to redefine British citizenship through "enterprise culture" and was encouraging privatization of the market, consumerism, and individualism.[54] As a result, surrogacy is permitted in the United Kingdom, but contracts are not enforceable, and the third-party profiting of private agencies from commercial surrogacy is explicitly prohibited. The surrogate is legally recognized as the baby's mother, and her name is written on the birth certificate until the intended parents obtain a court order to transfer custody. The U.K. regulations specifically prohibit payment to the surrogate and encourage intrafamilial and altruistic surrogacy arrangements.[55] In actuality, however, U.K. surrogates often receive remuneration, labeled "compensation," equivalent to the fees paid to U.S. and Israeli surrogates.[56]

In contrast to California and the United Kingdom, Israel took a markedly different legislative approach to surrogacy. As D. Kelly Weisberg notes in regard to the Israeli surrogacy law, "no other nation or American state goes so far in permitting surrogacy."[57] Passing uncommonly quickly through all legislative channels and accruing support from secular and religious legislators alike, the law, approved on March 7, 1996, regulates compensated surrogacy. A state-appointed approvals committee screens all surrogates and couples according to a centralized set of criteria, and all contracts are signed in the committee's presence. In general, the committee does not encourage surrogacy and tries to ensure that it remains the last resort for persons who have exhausted all other options to achieve genetic parenthood. Even if all applicants meet the strict criteria of the law, most contracts are only approved after a significant waiting period and much bureaucratic hassle. This type of state intervention in intimate natal issues is not foreign to Israeli demographic policy. The intensity of Israeli state involvement in surrogacy, however, may be more explicit than in other natal issues, for the state is essentially made accountable for each and every surrogacy arrangement carried out on Israeli soil.

From a cultural perspective, the influence of Jewish religious ethics made surrogacy a less morally contentious issue in Israel than elsewhere. Instead of being regarded as immoral and tied to abortion politics, as it was in much of the United States and Europe, surrogacy was discussed in Israeli parliamentary debates as a positive solution to infertility, in line with the strong reproductive imperative that has historically characterized the country's approach to legislation on reproductive technologies.[58] In contrast to British policy concerns about commodification, the Israeli surrogacy law does not prevent the surrogate from receiving payment, nor does it preclude the involvement of commercial agencies.

Of main concern to Israeli lawmakers was addressing the symbolic threat surrogacy represented to national and religious boundaries. Media coverage and policy debates in the years surrounding its legalization expressed a recurrent concern with the "chaos" that could result if surrogacy were to be practiced locally in a legal vacuum: non-Jewish foreign workers might give birth to babies for Jewish-Israeli couples, or non-Jews from abroad might pay Jewish-Israeli surrogates to gestate their embryos in the Holy Land.[59] Judaism is conferred by a Jewish mother through birth; hypothetically, if a non-Jewish woman were hired to gestate the genetic embryo of a Jewish couple, the child would not be considered Jewish by many Orthodox rabbis because it would not be born from a Jewish woman's womb.[60] This would pose a religious threat to the halachic status of babies born through surrogacy and, metonymically, a threat to the nation's boundaries.

The surrogacy law therefore brings to the forefront clauses that make surrogacy compatible with Jewish law and with the state's Zionist nationalist ideology. The law strengthens, rather than challenges, national and religious boundaries through regulations ensuring that children born in surrogacy are unequivocally recognized as full-fledged Jews and as Israeli citizens. Surrogacy is permitted only to citizens and permanent residents of Israel, preventing international surrogacy. While the law opens the possibility of surrogacy to all denominations, it requires that parties share the same religion. This precaution was meant to ensure that when Jews entered surrogacy arrangements, their offspring would be considered Jewish. One consequence, however, is that no Muslims and very few Christian Arabs have participated in these arrangements: Islamic prohibitions against surrogacy and strong stigmas surrounding the practice in the Christian-Arab community render it impractical within those groups. To my knowledge, most Israeli surrogacy arrangements to date have been between Jews.[61]

The law also takes precautions to prevent any infractions of Jewish religious law that might prejudice the "kosher" status of the child. For instance, some rabbis view intrafamilial surrogacy as a form of incest, and the impregnation of a married surrogate by the sperm of a man who is not her husband as a form of adultery.[62] Consequently, the law prevents intrafamilial surrogacy and directs that the surrogate cannot be currently married. An additional clause maintains that the intended parents must be man and woman and that the intended father's sperm be used in fertilization. These precautions were formulated to avoid as many rabbinical objections to surrogacy as possible.

These directives also exhibit a conservative approach to the family that stands out against the cultivation of new kinship options and alternative family forms in U.S. surrogacy. Although Israeli policy in general has been liberal toward the use of reproductive technologies by single and lesbian women and has legalized adoption by same-sex couples,[63] the surrogacy law prevents these parties from hiring a surrogate by limiting the option only to married or legally paired heterosexual couples. The only families that the law helps to create are heteronormative, nuclear families, to the exclusion of same-sex couples and single individuals.[64] This conservative approach to the family may be a reaction to the potential confusions raised by surrogacy. The law responds to the challenges surrogacy presents to the concepts of motherhood and family by keeping them neatly defined. The law's terminology deems the couple the "intended parents" and the surrogate the "carrying mother," specifying that the couple is *intended* to parent the child and the surrogate is only meant to *carry,* and thus be an instrument in the nuclear family's creation. Elsewhere, I have discussed the Israeli surrogacy law from this perspective as "the last outpost of the nuclear family."[65]

The Israeli surrogacy law is a fascinating artifact for cultural analysis, and others have provided in-depth accounts of its formulation and its cultural and social context. Weisberg's sociological account of the "birth" of the Israeli surrogacy law tells the story of the events leading up to its enactment and interprets them using feminist and legal-studies frameworks for discussion,[66] while Kahn's cultural account of reproductive technologies in Israel sheds light on the religious debates that helped shape the law's guidelines.[67] I too have analyzed specific clauses of the law in the context of Zionist-nationalist ideologies.[68] Markens's sociological study of the legislative responses to surrogacy in the states of New York and California sheds light on the common ground of concerns that shape surrogacy as a social problem in different legislative contexts, playing out differently even while employing variations of the same basic discourses of gender, family, race, and motherhood.[69]

Birthing a Mother focuses on the experiences of the people who are left to navigate the sometimes hazardous shoals of surrogacy within these public discourses and, in particular, under the specific conditions of the Israeli surrogacy law. Significantly, despite the central role that the law and the surrogacy approvals committee play in regulating participation in the contracted agreements, there is little state intervention in the process after the contract has been approved. Committee members are generally not aware of the outcomes of most surrogacies, and no official national statistics related to surrogacy births have yet been compiled. Couples notify a welfare officer of the estimated delivery date during the surrogate's fifth month of pregnancy, but there is no other contact with state representatives until after the birth. After receiving committee approval, the members of the triad are left on their own to navigate fertility treatments, pregnancy, and their relationships with one another without formal direction or an institutionally provided map.

STRUCTURES OF SURROGACY

Common to most commercial, gestational surrogacy arrangements, wherever they occur, is the general sequence of events involved. Israeli surrogates and intended parents are sometimes introduced to one another through "matching" agencies that also assist with submission of their file to the surrogacy approvals committee, but these agencies do not usually have any subsequent role in the surrogacy arrangement. Like small agencies in the United States, they may offer support groups for surrogates or aid with referrals to clinics, but they do not employ psychologists or social workers to serve as case managers during the entire process, as some large U.S. agencies do. Still, no matter where couples choose to undergo surrogacy and no matter how their arrangement is facilitated, the general stages of their journey are similar.

As their first step, couples search for a surrogate, either through an agency or independently.[70] In the majority of commercial surrogacy arrangements, the surrogate is screened for psychological and physical health, although the extent of screening varies. In Israel, where the state centralizes screening criteria, couples submit a file to the approvals committee that includes documents attesting to their and the surrogate's clean police records, a full medical history, and the results of recent medical tests showing that they are all healthy, disease free, and not substance abusers. An Israeli surrogate also has to be between the ages of twenty-two and thirty-eight, unmarried, and raising at least one child of her own. She will not be approved by the committee if she has had two or more cesarean operations, past miscarriages, or past experiences with toxic pregnancy, low-birth-weight infants (under five pounds) or early deliveries (before the thirty-sixth week). Surrogates can also be rejected if they are obese, if they smoke, or if they have taken antidepressants or undergone gastric bypass or other cosmetic surgeries in the past.

In general, the screening process is much less stringent in other locations where surrogacy is practiced. U.S. agencies usually have their own sets of criteria for screening surrogates, some stricter than others; some agencies report that they screen out 90 percent of applicants. In Britain, by way of comparison, where arrangements are not subjected to the screening criteria of commercial agencies or state committees, van den Akker observed that little screening was actually done in the clinics she studied.[71] This lack of comprehensive screening might explain how a woman who would have been screened out elsewhere became one of

Britain's most prolific surrogates. Interviewed in the press after having had babies for seven different couples, she reportedly had no children of her own, took antidepressants through several of her pregnancies, underwent gastric bypass surgery, and attempted suicide following her seventh surrogacy because of anxiety over her weight. Still, she had recently initiated her eighth surrogacy agreement.[72]

In some U.S. agencies, the intended parents must also meet particular health or social criteria, for instance, relating to infertility or marital status; in Israel, intended parents undergo intensive screening. In addition to being heterosexually paired or legally partnered, they must present convincing medical evidence that the intended mother cannot carry a child to term. The intended mother must provide medical proof that she has tried IVF at least eight to ten times,[73] has repeatedly miscarried, or has a convincing medical reason to contract a surrogate such as prolonged infertility, the absence of a uterus, or severe risk to her health. Initially, committee guidelines directed that the intended mother be aged twenty-two to forty-five if providing the ova and twenty-two to fifty-one if using donor eggs, and specified that couples could not apply if they had more than one genetic child prior to surrogacy. Over time, these criteria were challenged by applicants, and the committee now addresses age and family size on a case-by-case basis. The intended father must be able to supply his own sperm. The couple must be able to provide the money for the procedure up front, including the surrogate's fee of approximately $25,000 and additional costs of approximately $9,000. U.S. surrogates earn roughly $20,000 to $25,000, although second-time surrogates may ask for higher amounts.

After the surrogate and couple meet, they sign a contract. This contract may or may not be legally binding, depending on the jurisdiction. Contracts in Israel and elsewhere usually stipulate how much contact the surrogate and couple want to have with one another during the pregnancy and after the birth. Contracts also verify whether the surrogate is willing to undergo prenatal testing, such as amniocentesis, and her willingness to undergo selective reduction or termination if abnormalities in the fetus are detected. The contract includes the schedule of payments, which are usually made in regular installments only after pregnancy is achieved, with the major monetary sum paid after the birth. The contract also states the number of embryo transfers that the surrogate and couple agree to try; in Israel, this is usually six attempts. In the United States, it is often three attempts.

After the contract is signed, treatment begins. In the majority of cases, this stage involves IVF, in which an embryo is formed in a laboratory from the egg and sperm of the intended parents. If fresh embryos are to be used, then the surrogate and intended mother's menstrual cycles are synchronized: the surrogate receives hormones in pills or injections while the intended mother receives daily injections to hyperstimulate her ovaries so that multiple eggs will mature in one cycle and be ready for extraction when the surrogate's uterine lining achieves optimum thickness. The intended mother's ova are then extracted and fertilized through IVF in a Petri dish with the intended father's sperm, and the resultant embryos are implanted into the surrogate's uterus within forty-eight hours, or after five days in some cases.

In cases in which the intended mother cannot produce viable eggs, donor eggs are used. If frozen embryos are used, only the surrogate's body is monitored. If conception does not occur, this treatment cycle is repeated the next month. If conception does occur, the surrogate continues to receive hormonal medications for approximately the first twelve weeks of the pregnancy until her body takes over and "natural" pregnancy resumes. In Israel, several attempts are usually made with the intended mother's eggs before resorting to donor eggs, even if the intended mother is past the age of forty, when chances of conception are lower. Some U.S. surrogacy agencies and fertility clinics advise couples to revert to donor eggs sooner, after only one or two failed attempts with the intended mother's eggs, because each embryo transfer is more costly in the United States than it is in Israel.

If the surrogate does become pregnant, she usually has regular contact by phone, by e-mail, or in person with the intended parents throughout her pregnancy. Most U.S. agencies urge the intended parents to meet with their surrogate several times before the birth, but in most cases, much of the contact between parties is by e-mail and by phone because the sheer distance between areas makes it impractical for the intended parents to meet often with their surrogate; likewise, in cases involving intended parents from other countries whose surrogate is in the U.S., meeting is often nearly impossible. Depending on their geographical distance from one another, surrogates and intended parents can meet for the first time via conference call, at the time of the embryo transfer or even after the surrogate is pregnant. In the majority of U.S. surrogacy arrangements, the intended parents attend the birth; in some cases, they also travel to the surrogate's location to attend an ultrasound scan in the second trimester. In some transnational Indian surrogacy arrangements, the surrogate and intended parents do not ever meet; sometimes they even remain completely anonymous throughout the process.[74]

In Israel, a geographically much smaller country, the parties are usually separated by no more than two hours' travel. This proximity makes for much more frequent meetings during the pregnancy, and usually, the parents accompany the surrogate to the embryo transfer, most pregnancy-related medical appointments, and delivery. Israeli surrogates and intended parents, much like their counterparts elsewhere, also have the option of participating in Internet message boards offering information, guidance, and support from other persons involved in the surrogacy process.

Surrogacy births, wherever they take place, usually happen in hospitals. In California, the intended parents are given a prebirth order, so that their names are immediately written on the baby's birth certificate. In the United Kingdom, the baby is recorded under the surrogate's name, and if she is married, under her husband's name as well. The intended parents apply for a birth order from the court, and the baby is issued a new birth certificate after the order has been issued. In Israel, the state welfare officer is made official sole guardian of the baby immediately following the birth and for the first weeks of life, until the parents are awarded a birth order in a family court. The intended parents are made temporary custodians of the baby, whom they take home directly from the hospital.

Once the baby goes home from the hospital, the shared journey of the surrogate and intended parents comes to an end. It is a journey that begins with a potentially distant, contracted relationship but develops through body-centered interactions into a type of close camaraderie, and it is formulated retrospectively by many surrogates as a heroic quest. My own journey into this world of surrogacy began when I took an unexpected detour, as I relay below.

DOING FIELDWORK: A PERSONAL NOTE ON METHOD

I became interested in surrogacy in 1998, soon after the birth of the first Israeli surrogate twins in February of that year. At the time, I was a new graduate student in anthropology working as an interpreter for D. Kelly Weisberg, a visiting law professor at Hebrew University who was researching the events that led to the legalization of surrogacy in Israel—research that culminated in her recent book.[75] One day, I accompanied Dr. Weisberg to an interview with the woman I call Yael in this book, who had been central to the passing of the surrogacy law and who was just beginning the surrogacy process as an intended mother. It was the first time I ever heard the personal story of someone who had struggled with infertility; I had not actually given motherhood, or the challenges some women face in pursuit of motherhood, much thought before that time. I was profoundly touched by Yael's story and made sure to keep in touch with her after that day.

Yael and I became good friends, and my interest in the surrogacy process grew as she shared her personal triumphs and setbacks with me. Until that time, I had thought that I would pursue research related to folk art; due to my relationship with Yael, my focus changed. Because surrogacy was only in its "diaper" stage at that time, locating informants was not a simple task. There had been only four births by the time I began my search for interviewees, and those involved in surrogacy agreements were not part of any formal network. Whereas researchers on the topic in the United States and Britain were able to turn to commercial surrogacy agencies and nonprofit umbrella organizations to access participants for their studies, there was no such option when I began my work.[76] This dilemma made collecting anything remotely involved with surrogacy an agenda in itself. I collected every type of legal document connected to the passing of the Israeli surrogacy law available,[77] and I also began to collect newspaper articles about surrogacy from the Israeli press.[78] I continued to gather these materials throughout the study. One by one, as surrogacy births occurred in Israel, I was able to locate surrogates and intended mothers to interview using a word-of-mouth network.

My work reflects how surrogacy arrangements have grown quickly in numbers over the years, growth that facilitated my access to the surrogacy population. To date, I have conducted forty-three formal interviews with twenty-six individual surrogates and forty-five interviews with thirty-five individual intended mothers. Nineteen of the surrogates and twenty-three of the intended mothers were interviewed after the surrogate relinquished the baby. Most of these in-depth, qualitative interviews were done in the interviewees' homes,[79] where I was often able to look at home videos and photo albums, which supplied me with supplementary forms of data. In some of these cases, I interviewed intended mothers and surrogates involved in the same agreement; in the remainder of cases, I interviewed only one of the parties. I was also able to maintain regular contact by phone and in person with a significant number of surrogates and intended mothers throughout most of their surrogacy process and thus learn about their progression through each stage.[80] I also interviewed eight intended fathers and two common-law husbands of surrogates, as well as professionals involved in surrogacy arrangements: four doctors, one lawyer, two psychologists, two agency directors, six social workers, and four approvals committee members.[81] In all cases, names and identifying data of informants have been changed. Comparative data on surrogacy in the United States and Britain were primarily gleaned from media coverage, agency brochures, and interviews with the directors of three U.S. surrogacy agencies and with two reproduction lawyers.

My access to informants grew after a surrogacy community began to form in 2001 out of the online exchanges of messages between surrogates and intended mothers on a public Internet message board. The members of this forum also meet in person several times a year at one of the members' homes. I have participated in both the online and face-to-face gatherings of this forum as a participant observer since its inception.[82] I was also able to access a much larger number of surrogates after the establishment of a surrogacy agency by one of the intended mothers I had interviewed for my study. I volunteered to help her organize a monthly support group for surrogates through her new agency, and as co-organizer of this support group, I attended all of its meetings from its inception in early 2002 through July 2005.[83] Through these venues, I have come to know many surrogates and couples besides those I interviewed for this study.

Over time, my involvement in the Israeli surrogacy community has led couples to seek me out as a source of knowledge and advice about the process. They have asked me for referrals to doctors and other professionals involved in surrogacy arrangements and for advice on how to screen potential surrogates and manage surrogacy relationships. After articles appeared in the Israeli press about my research,[84] I found myself contacted by rabbis and by social workers at hospitals who needed more information about surrogacy to establish hospital guidelines and by couples who thought I could help them find a surrogate. In a reversal of the ethnographer's role, after sharing my findings with members of the surrogacy support group and Internet forum, I have encountered surrogates and intended mothers quoting my research in interviews they have given to the popular press and on television. This has led to my work crossing over in some ways into a type of action research, a tradition within public sociology.[85]

There are no official statistics on surrogacy births in Israel, but my own estimated guess is that approximately 350 children have been born through these arrangements since the first birth in 1998.[86] I would also estimate that, through the various sites of my research, I have met and interacted with, online or in person, two-thirds of the persons involved in Israeli surrogacy arrangements between 1998 and late 2005. In the years following the births of their children, I have maintained contact with many of the persons I interviewed; I have watched some of the children born in these arrangements enter first grade, and I have attended a surrogate's wedding at which the twins she delivered, then age four, were seated with their parents at the table reserved for the bride's immediate family.

One of the biggest challenges of this research came from dealing with the highly emotional stories I heard. I found myself coming to know these women very well and I became emotionally invested in their stories. My relationship with informants involved straddling a careful line between the intense connections that developed between us during fieldwork and the distance that theoretical analysis entails. I attempted to juggle this precarious position while holding on to my feminist intentions, empathy for informants, and commitment to a balanced ethnographic representation. I conducted most of my fieldwork before I had children of my own, a position that often made surrogates explain things to me in a way they might not have had I been an experienced mother. This positioning also seemed to make me less threatening to the intended mothers; as I describe in part 3, learning of new pregnancies among friends and family while they struggled with infertility was excruciating for many intended mothers. It was only nearing the end of the study, in September 2005, that I became a mother myself. Throughout my pregnancy, I continued to attend monthly support group meetings with surrogates, who were eager to see me become a mother. Nevertheless, I completed all of the interviews with intended mothers by the time my pregnancy was showing, and I did not attend in-person surrogacy forum gatherings while heavy with child out of respect for them.

A final word must be paid to terminology. The choice of words with which to write this book was not a simple one. The English term "surrogacy" has been widely discussed as problematic in many ways because it suggests that the surrogate is a substitute or replacement.[87] The recent trend toward referring to gestational surrogates as "gestational carriers" is equally problematic, as it implies an instrumental role for the surrogate and trivializes her contribution. My choice of words is further complicated by the fact that I am writing in English about surrogacy practiced among Hebrew speakers. It has therefore been challenging to construct a terminology that would simultaneously represent the "field" and embody its complexity. In Israel, the popular term to describe the surrogate role is "innkeeper mother" (*em pundekait*).[88] The term *pundekait* evokes as many political connotations as the word surrogate does, and perhaps more.[89] My choice to use the terms "surrogacy," "gestational surrogacy," "surrogate," and "intended parents" was mostly for purposes of clarity, because these terms are the most commonly used in legal and popular texts in English. Moreover, the use of the term "surrogate" instead of "surrogate mother" reflects the women's belief that the surrogate is not the mother of the child.[90] I use the term "intended mother" rather than the term "commissioning mother" to stress that becoming a mother through surrogacy is not just about economics but rather involves many intentional acts.

THE WOMEN OF THIS STUDY

One of the questions I am most frequently asked regarding my research is "Who are the surrogates and why are they doing this?"[91] In comparison to the data available on participants in surrogacy in the United States, the women in my study differed on several variables. The American surrogate population has been described as predominately non-Hispanic, Protestant whites, working class, with an average age of twenty-seven years.[92] In her interviews with surrogates in the late 1980s and early 1990s, Ragoné found that the average American surrogate was married with three children; approximately 30 percent of the surrogates in her study were full-time homemakers.[93] Ragoné's description still seems to accord with the profiles of the "typical surrogate" assembled by many U.S. agencies today; some agencies also claim that up to 50 percent of the surrogates they currently work with are military wives. The Israeli surrogates in this study, by contrast, were significantly older, ranging in age from twenty-three to forty, with an average age of thirty-four.[94] Unlike the American surrogates, none of the surrogates in this study were married, although they were all raising at least one child and had an average of 2.54 children.

All participants in this study shared the same Jewish religion and Israeli nationality and thus shared cultural knowledge, which might not be the case among international and interdenominational surrogacy pairings. The majority of surrogates and intended parents were born in Israel, but they associated themselves with a wide variety of ethnic heritages and degrees of religious observance.[95] Although systematic quantitative data on the proportion of particular ethnic identities were not collected for this study, no one group—Eastern European Jews (*Ashkenazi*) or Jews descended from Muslim-majority countries (*Mizrahi*)— was numerically dominant in the sample. Couples pursuing surrogacy often came themselves from different ethnic backgrounds, and it was not uncommon for the pairings to present a mix of ethnic heritages, a factor that played a part in the surrogates' articulation of identity, as I discuss in part 1. It was thus not uncommon to find a Persian intended mother married to a Yemenite man contracting with an Ashkenazi surrogate, or similar cross-ethnic pairings.

Geographically, the women in this study were dispersed along the entire length of the country. In terms of education, most of the surrogates did not hold advanced educational degrees, while some, although not the majority, of the intended mothers held bachelor's or master's degrees. Intended mothers were between the ages of thirty and fifty-two. Most had steady jobs, whereas many of the surrogates had temporary jobs or did not work. Yet there were exceptions to every rule: I met surrogates who had undergraduate degrees and some who were nurses, teachers, or had higher-paying jobs than their intended mother. Still, most of the surrogates, whether or not they were employed in steady jobs, were struggling as single mothers to support their children.

Unlike U.S. surrogates, who can be rejected from surrogacy programs if they are not financially secure or are receiving government assistance, the surrogates I met were usually pursuing surrogacy specifically to supplement their income. Moreover, while some U.S. surrogacy programs reject candidates if they do not have a sufficient support system at home, such as a supportive husband, Israeli surrogates are necessarily unmarried yet raising their children on their own. Finally, U.S. surrogates are screened out of agency programs if their stated motivations are primarily financial. The Israeli surrogates in my study shared many of the same stated motivations as U.S. and British surrogates, such as love of pregnancy, empathy for childless couples, and the desire to make a unique contribution, but they were also unapologetic, honest, and upfront about money being their primary goal in pursuing surrogacy (see also part 3). They expressed diverse economic goals that ranged from the immediate, such as paying off huge debts and providing for their children's basic needs, to the less immediate, such as saving money for the future.

In general, the surrogates in this study fell into three economic classes. The first group (roughly 30 percent) could be described as Israeli middle class to lower-middle class. Women in this group worked at steady jobs, owned cars, and lived in pleasant homes. They wanted the money to set aside for their children. These women usually lived with boyfriends; they would sometimes tell me that surrogacy was the only way other than winning the lottery that they could earn a substantial amount of money all at once to provide for "extras" for their family.

Women in the second group (roughly 50 percent) could be described as Israeli lower class. They worked at odd jobs such as house cleaning and most of them lived on welfare stipends or government aid of some sort. They wanted the money to give them a financial "push" forward in life, and especially to enable them to move to a better apartment or to pay off debts. This category includes surrogates who lived in government housing and even one who lived in a three-room caravan, but inside their homes they had food, clothed children, and electronic appliances including VCRs, DVD players and computers.

The third group (roughly 20 percent) lived in very run-down apartments in low-income areas and could be described as very poor. These women desperately needed the money they earned as surrogates. They sometimes mentioned that surrogacy was a better option for resolving their situation than other options they had considered, such as selling a kidney. The percentage of this group has declined over the years of my research because the approvals committee is hesitant to approve women who are in such severe financial situations.[96]

Economic and class differences exist between surrogates and couples in Israel, but they are smaller than those between U.S. surrogates and couples. Surrogacy has been an option available primarily to the wealthy in the United States, where agency fees, surrogate fees, private medical insurance, and the costs of each IVF attempt in gestational surrogacy (between $5,000 and $20,000) mean that the total costs range from $50,000 for an independent surrogacy to $120,000 for an agency-arbitrated arrangement that includes private health insurance for the surrogate.[97] This does not mean that all intended parents approaching surrogacy in the United States are wealthy; indeed, in a significant number of American surrogacy agreements, a friend or relative of the intended parents offers to be their surrogate without compensation, and in some cases the intended parents' medical insurance helps to offset some of the costs of the fertility treatments. However, for the majority of cases in which these costs are relevant, surrogacy is scarcely affordable to the middle class.

This is not necessarily the case in Israel, because Israeli national health insurance offsets the costs by financing medical care and fertility treatments, so that Israeli couples pay significantly less out of pocket. Their major expenses are the surrogate's fee (roughly $25,000); the extra costs required by the committee, which are partially refunded if not used (roughly $9,000); the costs of the psychological screening (roughly $1,800); and the agency fee, if one is used (roughly $8,000). As a result, instead of being reserved for the economically privileged, commercial surrogacy is more readily available to Israel's middle class. No more than five couples I met could be characterized as wealthy; most had found creative ways to pay for surrogacy, including receiving loans from wealthy friends, using their parents' life savings, taking out a special "surrogacy mortgage" from a mortgage bank, selling their car, selling their house and renting a smaller apartment, or living with their own parents during surrogacy to save on expenses.

OVERVIEW OF *BIRTHING A MOTHER*

The chapters that follow address the personal experiences of surrogates and intended mothers both individually and through their relationships. Part 1, "Dividing," looks at the ways that surrogates experience the process. In it, I examine the ways surrogates negotiate the meanings of nature, motherhood, and family by inscribing symbolic lines of demarcation on their bodies, thereby producing a body map. Through this body map, they distinguish between parts of the body they wish to personalize and parts they wish to distance, both cognitively and emotionally. On the basis of their body maps, the women conceptually divide their bodies into different parts that they view as varyingly detached or connected to their own body and to their intended mother's body. Surrogates use the body map to form an interlinked, networked connection with their intended mother for the duration of the pregnancy. They also employ the body map as a tool during the pregnancy to conduct distancing "emotion work" from the fetus and to manage interpersonal boundaries between themselves and their couples.

Part 2, "Connecting," concentrates on the intended mother and on the surrogate–intended mother relationship. Intended mothers engage in various "claiming practices" to establish their role, status, and identity as mother and to claim ownership of the fetus that the surrogate gestates. Surrogates and intended mothers also engage in joint practices to symbolically remove the pregnancy from the surrogate's body and append it to the intended mother. This leads me to a discussion of the intended mother's resultant manifestation of a "pregnant identity" and her own body's response to the pregnancy. Conceptualizing this as a shifting body, I look at the ways in which this shifting of pregnant embodiment, experience, and identity is supported and co-constructed by the medical system and the women's significant others. In some cases, women describe the intensity of this bodily connection in terms of inter-changeability, marriage, or merging into unity.

Part 3, "Separating," examines the postbirth period. In this stage, the medical system and the state emerge after the surrogate delivers the baby to ritually separate the women. The intended mother's own postnatal incorporation of her new role, identity, and status as mother is also explored. This public and private promotion of separation between the surrogate and intended mother is counterpoised with the surrogate's differing expectations regarding the aftermath of the surrogacy agreement. The surrogate's desire for acknowledgment beyond the monetary payment is related to her understanding of the relationship in gifting terms.[98] The future of the women's ongoing relationship, or lack thereof, is contingent on the intended mother's adoption of the surrogate's gifting logic or her refusal to acknowledge the obligations that receiving the surrogate's gift entails.

Part 4, "Redefining," looks at the way surrogates formulate their surrogacy journey as a quest or odyssey that leads them to acquire self-definition and self-knowledge. I discuss this heroic framing of the surrogate role against the backdrop of the many constraints and potentially disempowering elements that are part of the structure of the surrogacy process as a whole, particularly in Israel. I propose several explanations for the apparent paradox between the restrictive circumstances of the surrogacy process and the women's experience of empowerment.

In the conclusion, I offer a more in-depth discussion of the links between the women's narrated experiences and Israeli nationalism, Jewish religion, and the type of civic maternalism particular to Jewish-Israeli culture. I then look at the ways the ethnography reflects on some of the main theoretical concerns surrounding surrogacy and on the implications for state control of reproduction more widely. Finally, I suggest ways in which the data that emerge from this study might contribute to more informed public policies on surrogacy around the world.

PART ONE

Dividing

THE DOMINANT IDEOLOGIES SURROUNDING MATERNITY in many countries focus on the "natural" role of women as mothers with special bonds to the children they bear.[1] Through their contractual relationships with childless couples, for whom they carry children to term in exchange for payment, surrogates risk doing something popularly believed to be "against their maternal nature" and a violation of the natural order. With this in mind, psychosocial studies have hypothesized that women who choose to become surrogates may be nontraditional thinkers or somehow different from the majority of the population.[2] However, most studies have found that surrogates subscribe to conventional beliefs about sex roles and motherhood and believe ardently in the conservative values of having children and being good wives and mothers.[3] Reconciling their role in surrogacy with their self-perception as "good mothers" to their own children was also at the forefront of concern for the women in this study, much as Ragoné found in her study of U.S. surrogates.[4]

The great weight that preserving the reputation of their own motherhood carried for the Israeli surrogates I encountered may also be attributable to the amplified cultural veneration of motherhood in the Jewish religion and to the pronatalist ideology of the state. Some writers have suggested that Israeli women participate in what has been described as a "cult of fertility," in which reproduction is, and historically has been, constructed as the Jewish-Israeli woman's "national mission."[5] In this cultural climate, in which being childfree by choice is not socially accepted and reproductive technologies are widely available and nationally subsidized for the infertile, surrogacy becomes an especially explosive terrain to navigate. In relinquishing the babies they bore to others, the surrogates in this study risked being seen as engaging in "unnatural" or deviant behavior and also as violating their gendered national duty and expected cultural role.[6]

In this section, I explore the surrogates' attempts to ensure that their actions do not negatively affect their personal, social, and national identities. I pay particular attention to the rhetorical and embodied strategies that surrogates use both to maintain distinctions between the traditional concepts of motherhood, family, and nature and to preserve interpersonal boundaries. Chapter 1 concentrates on the way surrogates interpret conceptive technologies and their own pregnancy symptoms using an idiom of "nature" to distinguish between that which is personal and that which is foreign to their bodies. Chapter 2 focuses on the lines of demarcation—the body map—that surrogates inscribe on their bodies to define whose kin, motherhood, and nature are being cultivated during surrogacy. Surrogates engage in cognitive and bodily distancing practices that help them maintain these separations. Chapter 3 explores how the body map aids them in their attempts to distance themselves from the fetus and protect themselves from being "suffocated" by the contracting couple. The operationalization of this "mapping" serves as a crucial tool in helping the surrogate manage within the limiting structure of the surrogacy contract. The body map enables surrogates not only to endure what could otherwise be an extremely subjugating experience but also to manifest personal agency in constrained circumstances.

I want to clarify at the outset that my exploration of surrogates' lifeworlds does not address their personality characteristics or motivations for surrogacy. Indeed, I view the attempt to characterize surrogates as somehow different from the general population, measurable by particular personality traits or moral shortcomings, as insinuating that these women are maternally deviant.[7] My point of departure is to take at face value the findings of study after study that surrogates are primarily "intelligent, self-aware, stable adults" who are "down to earth, practical, decent people."[8] Moreover, I do not assume that most surrogates are regretful or remorseful about relinquishment or that they feel exploited by the process. Following Lomsky-Feder's approach to researching the personal narratives of war veterans and Sharp's approach to the study of transplant recipients,[9] I view the underlying assumption that surrogacy is necessarily traumatic for surrogates as eclipsing the meaning of the process for surrogates themselves.

It is only by moving beyond preconceived ideas that we can begin to listen to the way that surrogates articulate their experiences and uncover the personal meaning of surrogacy for them.

CHAPTER 1

Surrogate Selves and Embodied Others

There are a number of metaphors that I observed surrogates using to describe their bodies during the process. These metaphors could easily be considered most feminists' worst nightmare: woman as technovessel, implanted with the seed of the patriarchy and lacking control over her body, which is nothing more than a vehicle serving wider systems. They could also be interpreted as mere reflections of the mind/body separation that goes hand-in-hand with the body-as-machine metaphor that is so central to the mechanical model of pregnancy and birth in postindustrial, capitalist societies.[1] However, paradoxically, these kinds of images were often conjured up by surrogates in the context of rebutting ideas suggested in radical feminists' critiques and as assertions of agency and autonomy. During a conversation with Neta, thirty-three years old and the mother of one when she gave birth to her couple's baby, I was surprised to hear her express anger at "those feminists" who critique surrogacy as reducing women to "mother machines" and then refer to herself through a mechanical metaphor:

> What do they think? That we are robots with no feelings? . . . I am here in order to help. . . . I don't even call it a womb for rent. I call myself an oven. . . . An oven that bakes the bread for hungry people. I just help them. . . . Like if my friend needed a loan, I would save from my own food, and I would give her a loan. Would they then say that I am being used? What idiocy that is.

Why did Neta call herself an oven? The explicit self-objectification of the body that the metaphor expressed was alarming to me, especially when many radical feminist opponents of surrogacy employ similar metaphors to argue that reproductive technologies exploit women. These authors use technological images to describe surrogacy as reducing women to "uterine environments," "living laboratories," "test-tube women," "mother-machines," "fetal containers," and "vessels." In addition, they draw from agricultural images to compare women to "fields" for men's "seed," "breeders," "stables of reproductive whores," and "women-as-cows" on patriarchal "factory farms."[2]

It struck me as contradictory for Neta to reject being called a robot while at the same time asserting that she was another kind of mechanical instrument. Two years later, I spoke alongside Neta at a national conference of IVF doctors. There, in front of a large audience, Neta again responded to a question about surrogates as victims by firmly stating that she was not a victim but "the oven that bakes the bread of hungry people." While I was still puzzling over what Neta was trying to express through this metaphor, I interviewed Shahar, thirty-two, who was already a mother of five when she gave birth to twins for her couple. While narrating her experience, Shahar applied another seemingly dehumanizing metaphor:

> I am only carrying the issue, I don't have any part in the issue. . . . I mean, I gave them life, because without me they would not have life. Because [the intended mother] couldn't carry them. Only someone with a womb, a good womb, could hold the children for her. So I am the one. . . . I just held them in my belly, like an incubator. I was their incubator for nine months! . . . And the second that they were born, I finished the job and that was it.

Like Neta's oven metaphor, the image of the incubator connotes the technological colonization of women's bodies. Some radical feminist opponents of reproductive technology, such as Raymond, have pointed to the example of U.S. surrogates describing themselves as incubators as evidence of how far women using these technologies internalize patriarchal views of their bodies.[3] Overall has interpreted surrogates' use of the incubator image as a sign that surrogacy is an extreme form of alienated labor that negates the surrogate as a person (see figure 1).[4]

If ovens and incubators are both machines, could these women be using such metaphors to express the idea that they are technological instruments—mother machines—during surrogacy? If so, then, why did Batya draw on images from the world of plants, rather than machines,

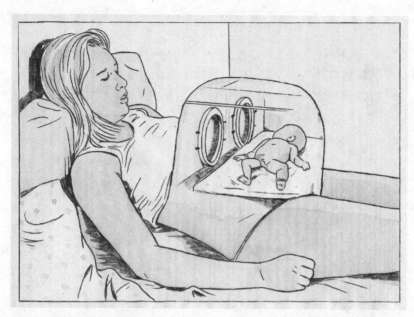

Figure 1. Illustration depicting a surrogate attached to an incubator. Originally appeared in *Haaretz* newspaper. Reproduced with the permission of the artist, Ruth Gwily.

to describe her body during surrogacy? Aged thirty-one and a mother of five, Batya arrived at our interview with her sister-in-law, who actively participated in our meeting. When I asked Batya if she would ever donate an egg, she immediately answered, "Never!" and then went on to explain why she saw egg donation as completely different from gestational surrogacy:

> *Batya:* There's a difference! It [the egg] is mine! It is created from me!!! Here [in surrogacy] it is not created from me! It is his egg and sperm . . .
>
> *Sister-in-law* (interrupting her): She is just storing it [*me'achsenet*] . . .
>
> *Batya:* Yes! . . . I am just like a hothouse [*hamama*]!
>
> *Sister-in-law:* Like a refrigerator. Like a wrapper.

Batya describes her womb as a *hamama*—a hothouse or a greenhouse in which plants are grown in conditions of controlled temperature, irrigation, and sunlight. Like the oven and incubator metaphors, the "seed and the soil" have had their fair share of attention as images linked to

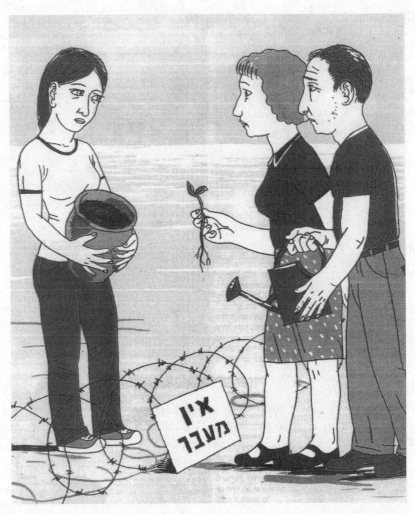

Figure 2. Illustration depicting a surrogate holding a flowerpot for the couple's sapling. Originally appeared in *Yedioth Aharonot* newspaper. Reproduced with the permission of the artist, David Polonsky.

the patriarchal control of women's bodies.[5] Batya's use of this imagery could thus be understood as reflecting the influence of patriarchal kinship ideas on her thinking: perhaps she is implying that she sees herself as the soil in which men's seeds grow, as Rothman's work might suggest (see figure 2).[6] But what can we make of Batya's correction of her sister-in-law, who described her as a wrapper and a refrigerator versus her assertion that she is a hothouse?

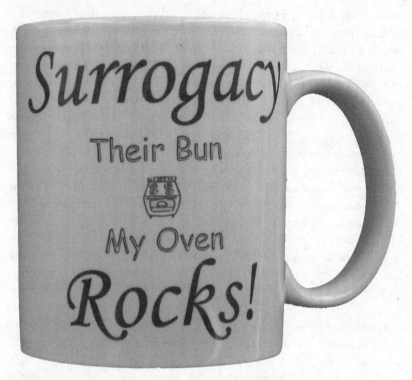

Figure 3. Photo of a mug sold by a three-time surrogate mother on her website, depicting an oven and the popular slogan "Their bun, my oven." Reproduced with the permission of the artist, Meg Kampel (http://www .megscustomcreations.com).

SURROGATE METAPHORS AND MEANINGS

The specific set of metaphors described above share similarities with those prevalent among U.S. surrogates.[7] Indeed, the slogan "their bun, my oven," has become so commonplace among American surrogates that it appears on products sold online, such as T-shirts and license plates (see figure 3). Israeli surrogates I spoke with also used variations of this idea, speaking of "an oven baking a cake" and "a kiln baking a sculpture." Yet U.S. surrogates also used a variety of other metaphors, such as "gardens," "cows," and "baby machines,"[8] that were rarely used among Israeli surrogates.

Following the many studies that have revealed the world of meanings encompassed by metaphors in reproduction narratives,[9] I decided to try to decipher what these metaphors alluded to beyond their patriarchal surface connotations and what the slight differences in imagery might reveal. Kirmayer notes that metaphors are microcosms of meaning that relate to the larger context of a narrative.[10] They also extend the scope of expression of the narrative and open up new paths for exploring it by gesturing toward other stories that may not be overtly taken up by the narrative.[11] I suggest that underlying the dominant surrogate metaphors of baby incubator, hothouse, and oven is a conceptualization of the body during surrogacy as a complex map of nature and culture (technology), depicting parts that can be integrated or detached. Whereas a garden and a cow can be solely ascribed to the natural realm and the "baby machine" to the technological one, the way dominant metaphors are used reveals that the linkages between these two realms are important to how Israeli surrogates envision their bodies and roles.

All of these metaphors designate the surrogate's womb as an artificial, containing environment in which the couple's "nature" is nurtured to viability in a controlled, warm temperature, as in a baby incubator, hothouse, or oven. The metaphors suggest that the couple's nature has been formed even before entering the surrogate's body: the couple's baby, sprouted sapling, and kneaded dough originate in the couple's egg and sperm, but additional processing is needed to produce their final form as infant, plant, and bread. Surrogates therefore are implying that they do not *create* the fetus in any way but develop an already prepared fetus to viability. Eva, who gave birth to twins for her couple, said this explicitly: "I took them [the twins] when they were small, fed them and helped them grow, and then sent them home." The metaphors thus encapsulate the general conceptual scheme that surrogates apply to their bodies in surrogacy: each surrogate sees her body as a complex puzzle, constituted by the coexistence of her *personal nature,* the *artificial womb* she embodies, and the *couple's nature* that she gestates inside it.

In a particularly clever twist on the nature/culture/other nature amalgamation, Batya's hothouse metaphor implies she is an artificial environment that simulates the natural habitat in which precious, valuable, expensive, and cultivated plants grow. Shahar's incubator metaphor draws on a device that is routinely used in hospitals to temporarily replace and simulate the pregnant mother's "natural" womb. Incubators are used in the IVF process to keep the embryo alive before it is implanted in the woman's uterus, and, in the world of premature babies, an incubator's task is to "artificially gestate to maturity" a baby born before thirty-eight weeks' gestation.[12] Consequently, Shahar's incubator metaphor positions her on a continuum of artificial environments used to simulate the "natural" womb without threatening the "natural" mother's claim as the only mother of the child.[13]

In addition, all three metaphors encapsulate a tension between external control and personal agency. Specifically, it is not the surrogate herself who turns on the oven or who places the plant or baby in the artificial environment, which suggests that she is controlled by the baker/gardener/doctor. The idea that the pregnancy is "switched on" and controlled externally enables the surrogate to emphasize its non-naturalness but does not negate her view of herself as the most essential person in the process. In this light, Shahar asserted that she was an incubator because she "gave them life, because without me they would not have life," that is, the twins she bore would not have been born without her warm, embodied, artificial life-support system.[14] Her use of the word "them" leaves the question of to whom she "gave life" open to interpretation: the twins she bore or the couple for whom she bore them.

The metaphors thus encapsulate the complex power structure of surrogacy: the surrogate may be structurally constrained and, as popular portrayals of surrogates in the media have highlighted, she may have become a surrogate to "feed [her] children,"[15] but she sees herself as powerful. Neta's use of the oven metaphor vividly evokes this power, for she is feeding not only her own child and the fetus, but also the "hungry" couple, helping them by baking the bread that they would not otherwise have. Their hunger, as a classic signifier of powerlessness,[16] is positioned in opposition to her power to feed, upturning any connotations that the couple is more powerful than she in the relationship.

Finally, we might understand the metaphors as each affirming that bringing the fetus to viability depends on the surrogate's own nurturing, warming capabilities. An oven, an incubator, and a hothouse are all necessarily warm environments, in contrast to the cold, distant connotations of a "mother machine." Each apparatus maintains a constant, controlled temperature that is needed to warm the couple's nature to viability. Batya's assertion that she was a warm hothouse, as opposed to her sister-in-law's description of her as a cold refrigerator or a neutral wrapper, highlights the centrality of warmth in the women's imagery.

Roberts points out that technology is usually assumed to be cold but that it ironically "warms up" the process of surrogacy by creating connections between the parties involved through the hormonal synchronization of the two women's bodies, the ultrasound, and labor induction.[17] Tempering Roberts's claim, I would suggest that, through the metaphors they use, surrogates assert that it is not technology that is warming up surrogacy but they themselves: they warm up their artificial womb simulators to provide the warmth assumed to be necessary for gestation.

Technology cannot produce the comfort that the surrogate can, as Yana expressed several weeks after birthing her couple's child: "I just gave him [the baby] a warm and comfortable place to be, so that he would be happy to enter this world." This is a human warmth that emanates from the surrogate's heart, rather than something "artificial." As Tamar told me when she was seven months pregnant with her couple's child, "It isn't a womb for rent . . . it isn't quick money and finished." Instead, she asserted, "It is a warm place, both in the belly and in the heart. . . . We surrogates prepare this fetus, feed [it], give him life. We need to develop what is inserted into us until it is ready." To sum up, if "culture" is the cold, instrumental hand of medical technology and "nature" is the warm, nurturing womb, then surrogates are using culture to simulate nature as they artificially incubate other nature in an artificial womb.

PARTITIONING NATURE AND THE ARTIFICIAL BODY

Central to most of the surrogates' narratives was the belief in an all-powerful nature that makes conception occur (through sexual intercourse) and fosters an instinctive emotional attachment between women and their "natural" babies. Idit, thirty-two years old and the mother of two, told me that during surrogacy she "didn't feel an emotional connection" with the fetus as she had during her pregnancies with her *own* children, when she had "felt joy with every development." Explaining this difference in terms of nature, she said, "Nature created it in a woman . . . the woman's attachment [to the fetus] is a part of the process of biological pregnancy. . . . It cannot be explained."

Idit's idea of nature encompasses women universally in biogenetic pregnancy, as she established by referring to my own potential future motherhood and to the commonality of innate emotions that I, too, as a woman in nature, would hypothetically develop in pregnancy. Yet she believed that this force does not uncontrollably spring forth from "deep inside" the "body and soul" of a woman when the pregnancy is "artificial":

Nature and the body make sure that the work is done. From the moment that it is your own egg, then automatically the woman feels that it is her pregnancy. Even if she doesn't want it, and even if she miscarries, she will feel that it is her child, deep inside, in her soul. I hope that you will be a mother one day, and you will feel it, because it is hard not to feel that feeling. Also, when the mother gives birth, how does she receive the baby? Naturally! In a natural way. So that way, in the same natural and biological way, the mother feels toward the fetus. [But here] . . . it is all artificial! Everything is artificial . . . so what is there to become attached to?

Technologically assisted conception, to Idit, is far from natural. She describes it using the Hebrew word *m'lachuti,* meaning artificial, simulated, unnatural, and man-made. By aligning the IVF conception process with artifice, Idit stresses its departure from the nature she has described; to her, the technology is a substitute, copy, or simulation of a natural process:

It [conception] was done in an artificial way. . . . First of all . . . the conception itself. It isn't biological. The fetus in the womb isn't aware of this during the pregnancy, but the initial development of the pregnancy was different from a regular pregnancy. When the pregnancy is regular, you get pregnant by your [male] partner and it unites [the sperm and egg] in a natural way. Here, the pregnancy isn't mine. It's from other genes . . . from him and from her . . . and you use artificial hormones to keep the pregnancy.

Like Idit, all of the surrogates that I spoke to aligned ideas about nature and artifice with a conservative cultural script about the way maternal emotions operate. They all believed that women have an innate love for their *own* children when those children "come . . . from nature," as one surrogate put it. This attachment was considered part of every woman's "biology" and related to the way female "hormones" work. Nearly all of the women contrasted the strong emotional attachment they felt to their own children prenatally to their emotional distance from the surrogate child. The intensity of their comparisons between their *own* gestations and surrogacy hints at "an internal sense of transgression"[18] that surrogates may experience upon realizing that their emotional distance from the fetus might be publicly interpreted as a sign of deviance. Surrogates routinely told me about comments to which they were subjected on a daily basis. For instance, Shiri noted, "People are so ignorant. They look at you like you are doing something bad when you tell them. They ask, how can you give away your children? This [points to belly] is *not* my child!"

Surrogates endowed the technology involved in the conception process with the power to undo the natural tendencies they believed bond them with the children they carry. Idit emphasizes that the technology facilitates her distance from the fetus: "The technology today is so advanced . . . you even see the embryo on the ultrasound the day that they implant you with it and you see that it isn't yours." The technology makes her separation from the fetus certain, logical, visually recognizable, and convincing, enabling her to assert, without hesitation, that as a logical outcome of the conception process she felt no attachment to the fetus throughout the pregnancy: "In a pregnancy, when it is yours, you will feel maternal intuition and feel somehow that it is yours, and here I didn't have that."

The fertility treatment that the surrogate undergoes to prepare her body for the embryo transfer paves the way for the perception that technology overrides nature.[19] First, the surrogate receives injections or pills of synthetic hormones to synchronize her menstrual cycle with the intended mother's cycle and to prepare her uterus. Next, she undergoes blood tests and ultrasound scans to monitor her hormone levels and uterine lining thickness. After the couple's embryo is implanted in her uterus, she receives additional hormonal supplements through injections or suppositories up through the twelfth week of gestation to maintain the pregnancy until her body "takes over."[20] Sima, age thirty-four, who gave birth to surrogate twins between the births of her first two children, explained how this process subdued her body's personal nature but did not erase it entirely:

> You get ten days of injections, every day, in order to suppress your . . .
> biological system. To suppress it and prepare your womb for absorption of
> something else, [something] strange, in an artificial way.

Sima delineates the hierarchical relations she embodies: technology suppresses her "biological system," holding her nature dormant so that culture (technology) can command her body. Like Sima, Orna, who was thirty-six and a mother of three when she became a surrogate, endows the hormone treatment with a powerful, external agency that has the power to draw a virtual line through the body, circumscribing a woman's nature beneath her body's surface and preserving it like a sacred, untouchable substance until after the pregnancy. Orna claimed that the technological takeover of her body was so complete that her brain didn't even register the pregnancy:

It is not mine. It is all artificial. . . . The hormones do it all instead of me. My brain doesn't even know that I am pregnant. My brain is suppressed with the shots that they give me. It turns my brain back to zero. Then all that is needed is given through pills. Through hormones . . . the brain is the injections. Instead of the brain ordering one, two, three, the hormones need to go up, need to go down, and then the injections do everything.

In these comments, Orna clearly outlines set relations among parts of the body, delineating which parts "know" that she is pregnant and which parts—such as her suppressed and zero-calibrated "brain"—are unaware of the hormonal "takeover." In a radio interview, Orna further explained that the treatment she received to prepare her body for surrogacy was intended to "neutralize the body," and "then the doctor starts to give the body hormones, to give order to the body. To neutralize everything and to prepare the body to receive the embryo."[21]

Orna's perception of the conception process reads as that of a woman willingly relinquishing command of her body to a medical professional and to medical technology. From one perspective, her words are an extreme example of the social consequences of reproductive technologies most feared by feminist scholars: total male, medical, institutional control of women's bodies and of "natural" childbirth. Yet as ethnographic studies of women's encounters with reproductive technologies have established, individual women may use these technologies in pragmatic ways and even engage in self-objectification and self-medicalization as a form of agency.[22] Accordingly, Orna embraces the potential of external medical control of her body to maintain clear separation between the categories of nature and artifice.

RECOGNIZING THE ARTIFICIAL BODY

The surrogates I spoke to saw the entire pregnancy as "unnatural." Rinat, a thirty-eight-year-old mother of five when she became a surrogate, promptly became pregnant with her sixth child after birthing a son for her couple. Comparing her body during surrogacy to her body during her own pregnancies, Rinat asserted:

It isn't normal. You have to take their hormones, because the hormones aren't yours. And you start to get bloated. . . . In the beginning, I got a bit round. . . . And I am usually very small in my pregnancies! . . . But here [pointing to a photo of herself pregnant, with her arm around the intended mother] I weighed 70-something kilos [154 pounds] from the injections and the hormones that they gave me. . . . Suddenly I got a bottom, I got a tummy, I got thighs . . . from the hormones. The hormones change your body. And my hair fell out . . . because of the hormones. They aren't yours. The hormones that enter your body are strangers. They give them to you in injections. It is hormones for the baby to develop well. . . . They give them to you for a month and a half and that's it. But afterwards, it affects the pregnancy until after the birth.

Rinat views the hormones as "strangers" entering her body from outside and disrupting the "normal" and routine way it had behaved during her own pregnancies. She believed that the hormones made signs of her body's naturalness fall away: her hair fell out in bunches, and her belly and bottom grew round. Like Orna's description of her brain being selectively taken over by the hormones during treatment, Rinat's idea of her belly, bottom, and hair being overpowered by the hormones shows that the imaginary dividing line that separates nature and artifice in the surrogate's body can be selectively mapped onto different parts.

Just as she suggested that the "unnatural" beginnings of the pregnancy "affect the pregnancy until after the birth," Rinat described the birth of the surrogate child as strange and miraculously different from the birth of her own children:

> Suddenly I go to bed, lay in bed, and I have labor pains. In my own births, I don't have labor pains . . . not in the births of any of my children. . . . Suddenly I felt these pains. . . . If I ever have labor pains, I get them in my back. And these didn't come in my back. Here, I really felt pains in my belly.

Women's descriptions of their bodies during surrogacy almost always included examples of how the body responded differently to artificial pregnancy than it had to "natural" conceptions. Ravit reported that "this pregnancy is making me experience all sorts of strange and unexpected things with my body." Since surrogates had previously experienced, on average, 2.54 pregnancies, they were certain they "knew" how their bodies "normally" reacted to pregnancy. They so often compared three models of the body in their narratives—the natural everyday body, the natural pregnant body, and the artificial surrogate body—that I ended up incorporating the comparisons into my interview questions.

For some of the women, the artificial surrogate body acted oppositely from the natural pregnant body. Sapir claimed that when she was pregnant with her son, she "was always sleepy. I would wake up like a prima donna, feeling faint. My mom would wake me up around 11, and I would go into the living room and continue to sleep until 12." She compared this prenatal lethargy to the insomnia she experienced during surrogacy: "I couldn't sleep at night, so all night I would be awake and during the day I would sleep, and my whole daily schedule was turned upside down."

Some women felt uncharacteristically good physically during surrogacy. Idit, who had birthed two children and had terminated several additional pregnancies, said that during surrogacy she felt "healthier than in any of the other pregnancies. . . . No swelling, not anything. [In my pregnancies] there were more problems than in this pregnancy." Batya found that her surrogate pregnancy, after five pregnancies of her own, was the least symptomatic and the most comfortable. She explained that "in my pregnancies . . . I have fainting spells. Here, I didn't have any! . . . Actually, in this pregnancy, I just bloomed, really!"

For the majority of women, however, the "artificial" body caused unexpected suffering. Tamar pointed out that when she was pregnant with her daughter she "was active, energetic," whereas during surrogacy, "I had no strength, I felt heavy and ugly and fat." Moreover, during her daughter's gestation, she "only gained 12 kilos [26 pounds], and I didn't vomit at all, but in [her intended mother] Miri's pregnancy, I vomited and gained 20 kilos [44 pounds]. In the end, I weighed 86 kilos [189 pounds]! It's also from the hormones, because they aren't natural. So physically, this pregnancy was completely different than the pregnancy with [my daughter]."

Like Tamar, many of the women contrasted their suffering during surrogacy to the relative ease and uncomplicated nature of their previous pregnancies. In fact, in line with their U.S. cohort,[23] one of the reasons they had chosen to become surrogates was their previous experience of easy pregnancies and uncomplicated deliveries, and it was on the basis of their generally good health that they had passed the stringent medical screening of the surrogacy approvals committee. The surrogates referred to details of these previous pregnancies to highlight the unanticipated behavior of the artificial body in surrogacy. Some said they would not have chosen to become surrogates if they had known it would be so physically difficult.

Neta claimed that she was "not a sickly type," so she was surprised to discover that during surrogacy she "was very ill that winter. I was ill around three times. With antibiotics." Belle experienced bleeding, pain, vomiting, tiredness, and dizziness during surrogacy, after having gone through "great" pregnancies with her own three children. She was hospitalized several times, and in the twenty-second week began to experience

swelling in her left hand and then in her right. Soon her feet began to
swell and cause her pain throughout the day, returning to normal only
after she gave birth. When I asked Belle why she thought her illness had
occurred, she asserted that the "hormones" had caused the bleeding and
the pain:

> The pregnancy was different from a bodily perspective, but that is clear. . . .
> Here it was with hormones that change your moods and everything. It is
> because of the hormones that the pregnancy is different. It was also differ-
> ent because the hormones made me hungry, like the hunger that you get
> before you have your period. It's the same. I also had a lot of bleeding. The
> bleeding continued up through the end. . . . And there were also all differ-
> ent unexplainable pains, like contractions of the uterus, things that have no
> explanation. . . . Look, the pregnancy is not natural, so there is always a 50
> percent chance that it will take or that the body will push it out.

Belle understands her bodily reaction to the pregnancy as a direct
result of medical technology. However, such tales of bodily disruption
occurred equally among surrogates who received hormone injections
and those who conceived on "natural" cycles with no hormone preparation at all. Other factors, such as the amount of elapsed time since their
most recent pregnancy, did not seem sufficient to the women to explain
their body's unfamiliar response to surrogate pregnancy. Instead, they
seemed to strategically search for signs of otherness to maintain their
classification of the pregnancy as unnatural.

The surrogates' descriptions of their symptoms as indicators of an
"abnormal" pregnancy may be a narrative strategy they used to stress
their distance from the role and identity of mother. This idea is further
strengthened when these women's pregnancy experiences are compared
to those of their nonsurrogate cohort. A study conducted in the United
States showed that nearly 90 percent of pregnant women surveyed
experienced nausea or vomiting during pregnancy, and for 25 percent
of these women, the symptoms continued through the twentieth week.[24]
These symptoms were so common that the conventionally pregnant
women Murcott interviewed interpreted them as signs that their pregnancies were "normal."[25]

Miller argues that physiological events have no meaning until actors
choose to ascribe meaning to them, and that the same set of physical
symptoms can be ascribed opposite meanings depending on the social
role and identity with which they are associated.[26] Miller found that those
U.S. women who had planned their pregnancies and were ready to adapt
to a "pregnancy identity" and social role interpreted symptoms such as

nausea as a sign that they were pregnant. By contrast, those who had not planned their pregnancies and were not expecting these symptoms interpreted them as illness. In this light, surrogates' interpretation of these symptoms as signaling illness rather than a "normal" pregnancy may be an expression of their desire to distance themselves from the role and identity of mother-to-be indicated by these bodily signs. This may be why the surrogates do not normalize their illness or downplay its significance but embrace its narrative power to stress the otherness of the pregnancy.

These illness narratives can also be interpreted as subversive somatic commentary on the unpleasant effects of conceptive technology, which the surrogate blames for making her vomit, gain or lose weight, and lose her hair. Coker interprets the illness narratives of Sudanese refugees in Egypt as somatic testimonials to their political powerlessness and the loss of their land and community.[27] Since the same pattern of symptoms and interpretations occurred among surrogates who conceived on "natural" cycles without hormones and among those who were medically prepared for conception, I would suggest that the surrogates, like the refugees, are expressing a type of somatic and narrative resistance to their situation. The cause of her bodily disruption is always *other* to the surrogate; it lies with the "artificial technology" or with the foreign couple/embryo that has taken up temporary residence in her body. The illness is never caused by her nature, and it nearly always contrasts with her earlier relatively easy personal childbearing experiences.

The illness narratives may thus be considered symbolic expressions of the surrogate's lack of freedom and structural powerlessness under the restrictive contract and surveillance of the body politic, medical institution, and contracting couple. In general terms, these illness narratives reminded me of spirit possession, which not only occurs predominantly among women but is also frequently interpreted as a reaction to structural powerlessness or being colonized.[28] In an article published over thirty years ago, Graham explicitly compared the characteristic features of regular pregnancy with spirit possession;[29] this comparison seems even more apropos when the body's uncommon reaction during pregnancy is ascribed to synthetic substances and an embryo fertilized outside the body using another woman's eggs. As I show in the following section, surrogates not only express symptoms of illness during surrogacy in common with the possession idiom, but they also experience cravings for particular foods, which is another characteristic of possession. In these ways, the surrogate somatically alludes to being possessed not just by technological artifice but also by her couple's nature.

THE OTHER NATURE SPEAKS UP

To this point, I have outlined the nature/artifice dichotomy as it is inscribed on the surrogate body. Yet as their metaphors demonstrate, women's complex embodiment during surrogacy also includes the couple's nature, which they incubate in the artificial body. Surrogates, thus, not only recognized how the artificial body differed from their own natural body but also identified the foreign presence in their bodies as the couple's nature. This foreign presence in the body was most often seen as deriving from the intended mother alone, rather than from both members of the contracting couple. The presence of this other nature in the body was communicated most vividly in a surrogate's food cravings, which she ascribed to her intended mother's personality. Tamar, for instance, felt that her insatiable hunger during surrogacy could be attributed to her intended mother's appetite:

> I had an appetite and I suppose, I think, that maybe that is because Miri, bless her heart, loves to eat. And her genes are also fat genes. . . . Because in my pregnancy with my daughter I didn't have an appetite, and in my pregnancy with [Miri's daughter] I ate a lot. I wanted to eat all the time.

Tamar attributes her change in appetite to her intended mother's genetic tendency toward fatness, as though by carrying her couple's embryo, the characteristic tendencies of their nature could cause her to engage in unfamiliar binges. In addition to consuming large amounts of food, many surrogates claimed that they developed an affinity for foods they had not known or liked in the past. Most of these cravings were for foods consistent with a couple's ethnic heritage. Sapir, for instance, whose background was Georgian, found that she intuitively craved the foods of her couple's Ashkenazi ethnic cuisine:

> On Wednesday they did the return [embryo transfer], and on Thursday I knew that I was pregnant. . . . Because in my whole life, I never ate soup. I am not the soup type. Suddenly, I feel like having soup. How could you not see that I have an Ashkenazi inside? Suddenly, I want soup. And I would finish a whole pot every two days. And rugelach [an Ashkenazi sweet].

Sapir identified her cravings as specifically linked to a heritage that is foreign to her yet connected to her couple. This aided her in distancing the pregnancy from herself and in reassuring herself that there was no possibility that the child she carried was her own child. In Israel, Jews of European descent (Ashkenazi) have been privileged over other immigrant groups, including Jews who immigrated to Israel from Arab countries (Mizrahi). In this light, one might interpret Sapir's cravings as a critical commentary on the colonization of her Georgian body by an Ashkenazi couple. However, ethnic differences were also commonly operationalized in the cravings described by Ashkenazi surrogates gestating the embryos of Mizrahi couples and by surrogates who associated themselves with various affiliations within the broad Mizrahi category. Thus, I interpret the communication of ethnic cravings in this context as a powerful signifier of differentiation.[30]

The communication of ethnically inspired pregnancy cravings also served to encourage intended mothers to foster a sense of identification with the pregnancy. Yael, an intended mother, told me how her surrogate's cravings had affected her:

> *Yael:* One day, she called and said, "Yael, you know, I have a craving for this kind of soup that Moroccans cook." I said, "I'll tell you the truth. I don't know how to make it, but I will ask my mom."
>
> *Elly:* Is she [the surrogate] Moroccan?
>
> *Yael:* No, she is Iraqi.
>
> *Elly:* You are Moroccan.
>
> *Yael:* Yes. So I came and said to my mom, "Listen mom, it's like this." "What's the problem?" [mimicking her mom's voice]. At that same moment she prepared it, one-two. I took it to her [the surrogate], and she drank it. . . . What my mom says is, "If it was you, wouldn't I do it for you? If you had the craving? So this is the same thing."

Her surrogate's craving for a soup particular to Yael's Moroccan heritage and foreign to her own Iraqi ethnicity gave Yael the opportunity to involve her mother in the pregnancy and to feel more connected to it herself, as if it were occurring in her own body. In a later conversation with Yael, I learned that this soup was particular to the part of Morocco from which her parents had immigrated, very specifically identifying the pregnancy with Yael and distancing it even more clearly from her surrogate.

Other surrogates also emphasized the distinctive nature of their food cravings and interpreted them as strange and particular to surrogacy. Tilly, who was Iraqi, referred to her couple's ethnic background when she claimed to have "a real taste for Ashkenazi food during this pregnancy." Likewise, an Ashkenazi surrogate named Sherry told me that that she had a particular taste for the spicy condiment *harif* during the earlier months of the pregnancy, which she thought might reflect the food tastes of her Mizrahi couple. The surrogates seemed to experience

cravings that accorded with their intended couples' ethnic heritages to
different degrees of specificity, depending on the extent of knowledge
of couples' backgrounds. For instance, Ariella, whose surrogate was
a recent immigrant from Russia, reported that the surrogate craved a
food that was not particular to her own ethnic group but that seemed
to generally symbolize her ethnicity to her surrogate:

> *Ariella:* I asked her if she wanted me to make her something, if she had a
> desire for something. So she said, "I bet that Yosi's [Ariella's hus-
> band's] mother cooks well." So I said to her, "So do I." So she said,
> "I have a taste for couscous."
>
> *Elly:* That is not a food she regularly eats, is it?
>
> *Ariella:* Are you kidding? She's Russian. They don't even cook, the Rus-
> sians. They only buy prepared food. And never couscous—what's
> the connection at all between her and couscous?
>
> *Elly:* But you are Persian. Do you eat couscous? What is Yosi?
>
> *Ariella:* Yosi is Egyptian. But I do make couscous. And anyway, I think
> that she didn't know exactly what we were. She thought that we
> are Mizrahim and that Mizrahim eat couscous.

The cravings described by surrogates are particularly interesting in
light of studies of conventionally pregnant women showing that they typically crave foods they normally eat.[31] The women Murcott interviewed
interpreted whatever food aversions or cravings they had as "normal"
symptoms of pregnancy and as part of their general attempt to frame
pregnancy as an ordinary experience. They refused to indulge in or to
live out any of the bizarre stereotypes of pregnancy behavior popularly
characterized as odd or peculiar.[32] This normalizing behavior stands out
against the surrogates' emphasis on the distinctive nature of their surrogacy appetites. When surrogates crave the salty soups of their couple's
ethnicity, for instance, they stress the naturalness of the pregnancy for
the intended mother and its distance from the surrogate's own ethnicity. Moreover, they illuminate the relationship between self and other
within their bodies. As Lupton observes, when eaten and absorbed, food
becomes part of us.[33] Food crosses our bodily boundaries, becomes part
of us for a temporary period, and then is expelled from the body. After
we ingest it, food enters a liminal phase in the body, which Lupton com-
pares to the liminal presence of a fetus in a pregnant woman's body.

The surrogate's craving for her couple's ethnic foods expresses the
ambiguous situation she embodies: she encourages the couple (their
food and their nature) to cross the boundaries of her body for a temporary period. It is clear to her all the while that her hunger is not her

own but the hunger of the foreign nature she carries. The presence of the couple/fetus in the body thus affects her behavior, but she recognizes it as "other" than herself.

The ability to identify the couple's foreign nature within the artificial body was most vividly portrayed by Ye'ara, who was a surrogate twice, for different couples. The intensity of Ye'ara's portrayal may be linked to the extreme differences in ideology and lifeworld that existed between her and her couples. Both couples were ultra-Orthodox Jews, while Ye'ara was not just secular but antireligious. Indeed, she had not married her common-law husband, Natan, who had been her partner for fourteen years, out of protest against the religious authorities that govern marriage in Israel; she vowed only to marry when civil marriages were permitted. Yet she had deliberately chosen to contract with ultra-Orthodox couples because she was interested in bridging differences between the secular and the religious and felt that the surrogacy experience in each case would be an interesting challenge. Natan, whom I also interviewed, observed how Ye'ara displayed behaviors foreign to herself in each of the pregnancies. In both pregnancies Ye'ara was nauseated, which she had not experienced while gestating her own two children. Moreover, Natan reported that during the first surrogacy Ye'ara craved certain condiments she usually abstained from, became ill at the thought of meat, and was repulsed by food in general:

> She changed all of her tastes. . . . She liked to eat only this and that. It was as if a *dibbuk* [spirit] had possessed Ye'ara and was carrying out the process through her. . . . Things that [she] never ate, like ketchup and mayonnaise . . . there were all different things that you could see that it wasn't the same person that was there before.

The second pregnancy, by contrast, gave her an unusually ravenous appetite, a particular taste for cola, and a craving for barbecued meat. As a participant observer in Ye'ara's surrogacy experiences, Natan identified the foreign presence in his wife's body during surrogacy by reference to a *dibbuk*—a Jewish idiom referring to possession by an often-troublesome spirit. His spontaneous comparison between the surrogate pregnancies and spirit possession recalls Graham's observation that, in both pregnancy and possession, the individual's body is "invaded" by an alien being whose presence explains her behavior and exempts her from responsibility for her actions.[34]

Yet the presence in Ye'ara's body was not an abstract entity but directly linked during each pregnancy to the intended mother's personal characteristics. Thus, Natan observed changes in Ye'ara's behavior as manifestations of the intended mother's personality. Describing the intended mother in Ye'ara's second surrogacy as a lethargic, sickly, terrified, and hysterical woman, Natan observed that Ye'ara's usual good health, optimism, courage, and rational thinking temporarily vanished, leaving her uncharacteristically unsure of herself, needy, physically weak, and plagued by irrational fears. He even ascribed Ye'ara's temporary aversion to her usual compulsive tidying up of the house to her intended mother's characteristic untidiness.

Ye'ara, on her part, saw these changes in her personality and tastes as the logical outcome of surrogacy, explaining that it "sounds so logical to me. It really makes sense. Because it is another person's baby, a different [person's] personality and different hormones." Throughout the second pregnancy, she knew, she said, that what she was experiencing was the intended mother's nature making itself known: "All of the heavy feelings and the difficulty and feeling unwell, I'm not like that. . . . But I had days here that I couldn't even move a glass from one place to another. It wasn't me. That's why I was so eager to give birth already, because I wanted to get my life back." Indeed, during the birth, Ye'ara experienced a marked transition back to her former self: "The fact is that during the birth, I returned to be who I am."

The idea evoked in the women's tales of the foreign nature in their bodies is similar in many ways to a phenomenon found among organ transplant recipients. Fox and Swazey note that both givers and receivers of organs engage in an animistic, magic-infused thinking.[35] Donor families often feel the need to meet the persons who received the cadaver organs of their loved one and to have contact with the part of their deceased relative that "lives on" inside the recipient's body, and recipients sometimes describe changes to their personalities after receiving a donor organ that they liken to the donor's characteristics.

Sharp found that this occurred even when the recipients did not know who their donors were (organ donation is usually anonymous).[36] Recipients still imagined that they had acquired some of a donor's characteristics, especially when the transplanted organ carried strong metaphoric and symbolic meanings, as in the case of the heart. Sharp interprets this behavior as the recipient's attempt to restructure his or her self after the transplant, a feat that can be achieved either by the incorporation of the organ into the recipient's "transformed" self or by neutralizing the organ's origins and mechanistically considering it a "spare part" that has no effect on the recipient's self.[37]

Surrogates combine both strategies of restructuring the self while temporarily "carrying" the foreign organ/embryo. They selectively distance some bodily phenomena by ascribing them to "artificial" technology and other bodily occurrences by referring to them as manifestations of the couple's nature. Together, both strategies not only aid them in signifying what parts and behaviors are "other" to themselves but also help them recognize the boundaries of their personal selves within their "occupied" bodies.

THE NATURE OF NATURE

Why do surrogates hold so steadfastly to this scheme during surrogacy? What other meanings does the nature idiom carry, and what is at stake if it is not carefully preserved? One explanation may be that, by emphasizing the naturalness of their maternal attachment to their own children, surrogates are able to confirm their normativity as women and as mothers. Their articulations are consistent with those discussed in other studies of assisted conception that often employ nature as an idiom for reconciling technological paths to parenthood with normativity.[38] Indeed, Thompson has shown the power of this idiom across different technologically assisted contexts in which consumers "strategically naturalize" genetic, gestational, or social elements, depending on the procedure they use.[39]

Yet surrogates' distinctions between nature and artifice are not entirely consistent with studies of women's attitudes toward fertility treatment more generally. Studies in the United States and Britain have shown that IVF patients tend to discuss the technology itself as "natural," as a "bridge" to nature, as giving nature a "helping hand," or as keeping it on course before the body picks up and itself continues a pregnancy "naturally."[40] The emphasis that the surrogates in my study put on the *unnaturalness* of the technology speaks to the importance they ascribe to keeping their personal "nature" untouched by the surrogacy process. It is the unnaturalness of the process that enables the surrogate to explain her distanced emotional response to the baby and to confirm to herself and to others that she is not deviant, even as she engages in the nonnormative act of agreeing to relinquish a child that she births.

Surrogates' attempts to denaturalize technology are also revealing about their stance vis-à-vis the technology itself. Whereas persons influenced by dogmatic Christian beliefs may view human intervention in "nature" as an affront to G-d's will, many Jewish scholars agree that such technology is not necessarily morally contentious.[41] Indeed, Israeli policy makers have expressed fewer serious ethical and moral reservations regarding reproductive technologies than have been raised in other Western countries.[42] In Judaism, the divine commandment to "be fruitful and multiply" is regarded as binding, especially in the realm of human reproduction; it is telling that this commandment is combined with a second divine command to "subdue the earth." In the realm of reproduction, humans are thus not only entitled but also mandated to "interfere" with G-d's creation—it is morally permissible and mandated to alter "nature."[43] Thus, surrogates' emphasis on the unnaturalness of technology may be influenced by a decidedly Jewish approach to technological intervention in "nature."

Surrogates' approach to "nature" also has repercussions for gender. As feminist anthropologists have long argued, following Ortner's influential essay on the essentialist conflation of biological functions and social characteristics,[44] in many societies women have historically been hierarchically affiliated with nature, whereas men have been associated with culture. Strength, firmness, and aggression are represented as the natural characteristics of the male body, and liquidity, animality, and leakiness are represented as the natural condition of women.[45] Surrogates seem to be upholding these "naturalistic views" of the body that legitimize gender inequalities.[46] Their idea of nature is that of an uncontrollable, emotional, instinctual, and dangerous substance that must be controlled, subdued, and contained by medical technology, an arena considered in the radical feminist literature to be dominated by men. The surrogate's idea of nature is also used to maintain a sense of normativity that equates womanhood with motherhood—an equation that feminists have made great efforts to break apart.[47] This idea thus seems to express subjugation and surrogates' willingness to submit to male control of their bodies to override the supposed hysterical qualities of their allegedly inferior female "nature."

At the same time, surrogates' narratives reveal an important subversive commentary that simultaneously upends and reifies the patriarchal idea of biology as women's destiny. Surrogates may be submitting their bodies to a doctor's control, but only to use that external harness to control the outcome of their own actions. In particular, they may believe in an essentialist idea of nature, but they also exemplify the empowering idea that a woman can become independent of the influence of her so-called nature. Engaging in actions similar to those Thompson has described as "agency through objectification,"[48] they invoke the same technological representations (IVF, mechanistic metaphors), which critics see as alienating women, in order to exercise personal agency.

These women believe that by embracing the power of technology to control their bodies and through their own complex cognitive classifications (nature, artifice, other nature) and self-objectification (mechanistic womb metaphors), they have the power to overcome any innate emotions and "natural" uncontrollability that may stem from their bodies. They may therefore believe that women are destined to become mothers, and they may submit themselves to patriarchal control, but they also subversively use the tools of patriarchy—medicalization, objectification, and technology[49]—to make sure that "maternal nature" manifests itself only where and when they want it to.

CHAPTER 2

The Body Map

To this point, I have explored how surrogates conceptualize their bodies as composed of a personalized nature that carries their emotional bonds to their own children but remains dormant during surrogacy; an artificial presence that subdues their personal nature and makes sure that their wombs remain separate, neutral spaces; and the intended parents' nature, which they temporarily warm inside their wombs. Although surrogates viewed technology as a necessary tool for creating these separations, they did not see it as sufficient to maintain them throughout the pregnancy. Surrogates imagined the unwanted effects that might result if the personalized nature and the intended parents' nature were allowed to mix: it would no longer be clear who the mother of the child was or to whose family the child belonged, and the surrogate might emotionally connect with the fetus. To maintain these separations, surrogates made constant efforts to clearly distinguish divisions in their bodies, creating what I call a body map delineating areas for their personal nature, kin line, and maternal identity that are separate from those designated for the contracting couple to inhabit (see figure 4). The surrogate's body map complicates any simple equation between body and self.[1] Viewing their bodies as segmented, the surrogates believed that specific organs could retain personal identity even when detached from the body, while others could be depersonalized within the body. In the following discussion, I decipher the topography of the body map.

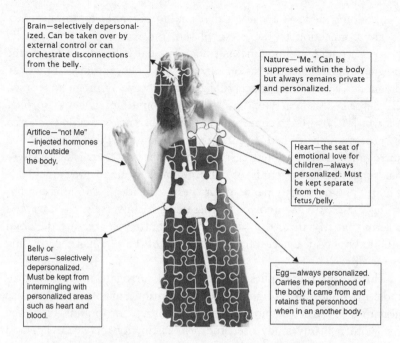

Brain—selectively depersonalized. Can be taken over by external control or can orchestrate disconnections from the belly.

Nature—"Me." Can be suppresed within the body but always remains private and personalized.

Artifice—"not Me" —injected hormones from outside the body.

Heart—the seat of emotional love for children—always personalized. Must be kept separate from the fetus/belly.

Belly or uterus—selectively depersonalized. Must be kept from intermingling with personalized areas such as heart and blood.

Egg—always personalized. Carries the personhood of the body it came from and retains that personhood when in an another body.

Figure 4. Illustration depicting the surrogate's body map, which she uses to differentiate between personalized and distanced parts of her body. Photo reproduced with the permission of Elana Leventhal.

INNKEEPERS, BABYSITTERS, AND RENTED HOUSES

In the body maps devised by my interviewees, the womb was consistently denuded of personal traits, whereas the egg was consistently identified with the woman and the family at its genetic source. Surrogates believed that the eggs implanted in them were extracorporeally associated with their intended mothers' personhood and kin line. For example, Sapir's description of her initial phone call to a surrogacy agency conveys that the womb and the egg held divergent meanings for her from the start:

> I was very interested [in learning] if it is something that I [would be personally] involved with. If it was something that I was involved in then I would have immediately rejected the option . . . I mean, like if it was my egg, if this child had part of me. In the beginning, I thought it was like a woman needs to deliver a child and put him up for adoption. . . . So they told me no, that it is a couple that cannot have children because the woman has a problem with her womb. But she has eggs and it is just, you just have to carry it. So the process looked really good in my eyes.

In Sapir's view, as an organ that has no potential for connectivity or any connection to the personal self, the womb can unaffectedly "carry" a child without making her personally "involved with" the pregnancy. Sapir's emphasis on *carrying* links conceptually to the way pregnancy is popularly conceptualized in Hebrew; all pregnant women are described as "carrying" or "lugging around" pregnancy [*sochvot herayon*]. It also links conceptually to the current terminology chosen by professionals in the U.S. surrogacy industry, in which they describe surrogates as "gestational carriers" or simply as "carriers."[2] As Ivry has suggested in her study of cultural conceptions of pregnancy, one can be "pregnant with meaning" or "gestate an idea"—notions emphasizing the creativity involved in these acts.[3] Conversely, to "carry" is a term that trivializes the woman's contribution to creating the child and downplays the necessary contribution of the surrogate to creating the family.

This perspective implies that gestational surrogates might not promote the importance of genetics over gestation but instead emphasize gestation to garner acknowledgment for their contribution. However, the women in my study used the firm distinction between eggs and wombs to maintain cognitive separation. As "carriers" rather than genetic originators, surrogates clearly designate themselves as "carrying" motherhood and kin ties for someone else. Sapir used this logic to explain her role as a surrogate to her young son:

> In the beginning I said that Shoshana [the intended mother] wants a child. So he said, "But you aren't going to give me away to her!" I said, "Never, no way, not a chance in the world. But we have a chance to help her. She has a baby in her belly, but she can't continue to have the baby grow in her belly, so she wants someone to take care of and protect him [*lishmor alav*] for her. She wants to give me the baby so that it will be watched over in my belly. And in exchange for that, she will buy you lots and lots of gifts."

The babysitting analogy helps Sapir clarify for her son the definitive kinship boundaries between the two families and her different responsibilities toward him and toward the surrogate child. Sapir was adamant that these boundaries remain clearly drawn terminologically and that she not be socially labeled the *mother* of the surrogacy-born child. When I referred to the intended mother during our interview as "the second mother," Sapir's immediate reaction clearly indicated that, from her perspective, I misspoke. The ensuing dialogue clarified how delicate a matter my reference to her as a "mother" was:

Sapir: Look, I don't know if I am called the second mother, because I am not a second mother.

Elly: No, she's the only mother, right.

Sapir: I am second to her.

Elly: You are the second mother.

Sapir: But I don't see myself as a second mother. Because . . . nothing in the child belongs to me. It is as if I would go now, and I would tell you, "Elly, look after my child for me." It is just like that. It is from the beginning [literally, from the belly and birth], the *original child* of Shoshana and Itamar. So I didn't feel any [connection].

Sapir insists that the surrogate child is unaffected in any way by its development in her womb, just as Sapir's own child would be unaffected if she asked me to babysit him. The babysitter idiom is also a popular vehicle for surrogates to express their embodied relationships in the United States,[4] where contemporary surrogates often describe themselves on online message boards as "prenatal nannies" or as "the baby's house for a while." Lihi takes this analogy one step further, describing herself as gestating a *couple,* rather than merely a *baby,* in her womb. Appearing on Israel Channel 10's *Behind the News* program, she explained this concept:

In surrogacy you need to insert a couple into your belly, your home, your family. There is nothing biological of mine. They are in me but they are not biologically mine. I didn't feel like a vessel [*kli*]. There are people who use their brain as their vessel. My womb is my vessel.[5]

Making it very clear that being a surrogate does not affect her self-conception ("I didn't feel like a vessel"), Lihi maintains that her personal self, nature, and kin remain in her own "biological" substance (her egg), while her womb is mechanically divided off as a "vessel." She can then host her couple in her neutral womb, her home, alongside her own family, without letting the two families mix. During my interviews with Lihi, she repeatedly used similar descriptions to illuminate the clear divisions between the families in her body. She suggested that being a surrogate was like looking after her neighbor's children when they came over to play with her own two daughters: "You watch over them even more carefully than your own, because they are not yours." This analogy also helped Lihi to clarify the kinship boundaries between her own family and the family she was helping to create, and to distinguish between her different responsibilities toward each of them. Lihi also compared her womb-home to a house that the couple/embryo rents without owning it or thinking that it is a permanent home: "It is not yours. Nothing. Not the egg, not the sperm. . . . It is just like I am living in a rented house."

The imagery evoked in Lihi's statement demonstrates a conceptual analogy between wombs, houses,. and homes—a linkage that recalls Carsten's observation that "kinship is made in houses."[6] The imagery also connotes the popular idiom used for discussing gestational surrogacy in the United Kingdom—"host surrogacy"—and the popular term for surrogacy in spoken Hebrew—"innkeeping," or "*pundekaut*" (see figure 5). This term has even been used in Israeli courts to define the practice.[7] Nearly all of the surrogates I spoke to described their role using this terminology, and some even extended it into a metaphor for describing their role in the agreement. For instance, Orna explained to me, "I have no connection to this child. It is just like it's called, a literal inn [*pundak*]. I am a guesthouse [*achsania*] for nine months." She later declared in a radio interview: "I am altogether just the birthing mother, the inn [*pundak*] mother, the innkeeper [*pundekait*] only. It is not my egg, and I have no connection to this child."[8]

The widespread use of this idiom, which downplays the surrogate's influence on fetal outcome and reduces her role to "host" or "carrier," reveals that the tendency to privilege genetics over gestation is a widely accepted folk model for understanding pregnancy in the Israeli public. In contrast to cultures such as Greece, where gestation is privileged,[9] popular perceptions of pregnancy among Israeli biomedical professionals and laypersons alike tend to trivialize gestation and follow a strongly geneticized model of pregnancy.[10] Ivry found that the pregnant Jewish-Israeli women she studied and their obstetricians tended to embrace prenatal diagnostic testing of the embryo while downplaying the importance of environmental factors such as nutrition, weight gain, rest, and overall care for personal well-being during pregnancy.[11]

In fact, adherence to this geneticized model of pregnancy might even help explain why surrogacy has met with acceptance and little ethical debate in the Israeli media and public in general, and by doctors and infertile couples in particular; gestational surrogacy basically accords with Israeli cultural understandings of reproduction.[12] In contrast, although gestational surrogacy is permitted in Greece, it is rarely practiced because local beliefs hold that the "blood" conferred through gestation and childbirth establishes maternity.[13] Gestational surrogacy is culturally incomprehensible and thus outlawed in countries such as Japan, because the womb environment is understood to be crucial in

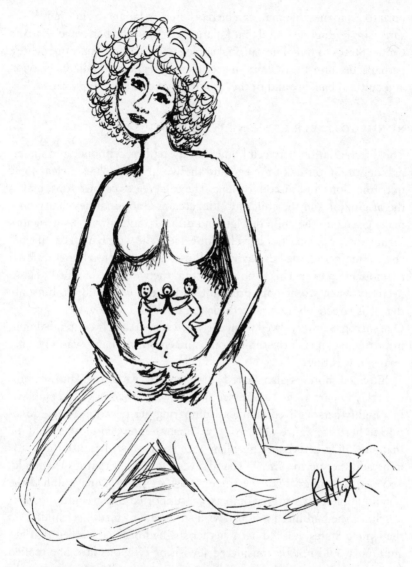

Figure 5. Illustration depicting a surrogate as an "innkeeper" hosting a family in her womb. Reproduced with the permission of the artist, Rhisa Teman.

determining fetal outcome.[14] It is not surprising, then, that in March 2007 the Supreme Court of Japan handed down a judgment denying the parenthood of a Japanese couple whose twins, although genetically related to them, were birthed by a surrogate in the United States; the denial was justified on the basis that only children who are physically born to a Japanese woman can be registered as Japanese children.[15] Not surprisingly, Ragoné found that Japanese couples who had traveled to the United States to find a gestational surrogate preferred Asian surrogates, perhaps because the womb environment, pregnancy-related behavior, and cultural background of the "carrier" were of such importance.[16]

NONNEGOTIABLE EGGS, NEUTRAL WOMBS

The differentiation between home, family, nature, selfhood, and maternal identity in terms of the egg and the womb formulates a clear logic of connections and disconnections. The egg creates connections, makes the originator and the child into kin, creates emotional ties that would make giving up the child deviant and difficult, and entails a surrogate's separation from a part of herself. Conversely, the womb is an "artificial" environment, regarded as having no kin-creating potential or emotional tie-inducing power. This is not to say that the womb is denuded of connectivity when women are pregnant with their *own* children, but only that it is selectively neutralized for the term of a surrogate pregnancy. One surrogate interviewed in an early newspaper article contended that, in surrogacy, "it isn't the same womb and emotions that it was when my own son was there."[17]

Intended mothers also shared surrogates' views of eggs and wombs: as I relay in part 3, they addressed the subject of their eggs and embryos in a highly personalized manner. Comparing her rejection of egg donation to her acceptance of surrogacy, Dina, an intended mother, told me that she "didn't have any problem with [surrogacy] because the egg is mine and the sperm is my husband's. . . . Here, I felt that it is my child, 100 percent mine." Like the surrogates I spoke to, Dina nullified the potential influence of the womb as she supported the strength of genetics. Since she had hired a non-Jewish surrogate to birth her children in the United States, I asked her whether she had been concerned that her children would not be considered Jewish by religious law. She replied that, in her eyes, her daughter is "a completely pure Jew," even describing her as "100 percent kosher." The womb was so insignificant vis-à-vis the egg, she explained, that she did not care about the surrogate's looks or skin color:

> It is my egg, so she has no influence on how the child looks. . . . I knew that the child would look like me. And I don't have any problem with it [the surrogate not being Jewish or] even if she was black.

For Dina, gestation in the womb of a non-Jewish woman would have no effect on her daughter's Jewishness, just as the womb of a dark-skinned woman would have no effect on her daughter's whiteness. Her words stand in contrast to the scholarship on donor preference, which has illuminated the central place of racial considerations when genes are concerned; these studies have pointed to an overwhelming preference for "whiteness" among Israeli ova recipients, as well as among Israeli recipients of donor sperm.[18] Consistent in surrogates' and intended mothers' views alike was the idea that genes were central to kinship and fetal outcome, while the womb was denuded of any such influence. This consistent logic diverges from the flexible approach to eggs and wombs that other anthropologists have encountered in U.S. surrogacy. Ragoné reports cases of women in the United States entering surrogacy agreements as gestational surrogates and later becoming traditional surrogates.[19] These women shift between contradictory kinship models, first privileging genetic kinship over gestation and later privileging social motherhood over genetics and gestation.

This cultural tendency to trivialize gestation and to privilege genetic determinism perhaps eliminated certain conflicts between the Israeli surrogates and intended mothers I studied; by way of comparison, when gestational influence is believed to be highly consequential to fetal outcome, conflict may erupt, for example, over the surrogate's nutrition during pregnancy. American gestational surrogates have reported their couples' requests that they stay away from fast food, increase their intake of fruits and vegetables, and eat only organic foods. Others have reported their intended parents' requests that they only use plant-based cleaning supplies or refrain from pumping gas.[20] The Americans in Griswold's collection of intended mothers' personal stories describe their worries over their surrogate's exposure to secondhand smoke, stress, and toxic chemicals. As one reflected, "Even though I try not to worry about every little thing, it is difficult sometimes. They [the surrogate's family] have a cat, for example, and for a long time I worried about Laura changing the litter. . . . They also have a Jacuzzi, and she dyes her hair occasionally, and sometimes she goes to a tanning spa. She did the same things when she was pregnant with her own children."[21]

Israeli surrogates and intended mothers, by contrast, did not usually come into conflict over these issues: intended mothers were generally more preoccupied with the outcome of prenatal genetic diagnostic tests than they were with their surrogates' nutrition. There were, of course, exceptions to this rule, and some intended mothers bought their surrogates healthy foods or hired cleaning help for them to prevent them from physically exerting themselves during pregnancy, but the downplaying of gestational influence was the norm. In contrast, the personalized status of the egg was crucially nonnegotiable among surrogates, as affirmed in the following interaction excerpted from my field notes:

> In an impromptu conversation with three surrogates—Tamar, Reli, and Ravit—as we made our way to visit a fourth surrogate who had just given birth, I told them that in the U.S., surrogates were not as adamantly opposed as Israelis to using their own eggs. I explained that a U.S. surrogate sometimes does two in vitro attempts with her couple's embryos, and then goes on to do inseminations with her own eggs for the couple when the IVF attempts fail. The three women stared at me with expressions of shock. "With their own egg?" Reli pressed. "Yes," I answered. "Would any of you be surrogates with your own egg?" I was surprised at the emotionally charged answer, as they all shouted in unison, "No!" I asked, "Even after you knew your couple and wanted more than anything to give them a child?" Again, a unanimous no from all three. Interested in the extent of their conviction, I pressed on: "For $100,000?" "No." "For a million dollars?" "No!" "Not under any circumstances, then?" Each answered in turn "No" or "Never."

Why is the egg personalized so strongly by these surrogates? Beyond the "geneticized" cultural model of pregnancy discussed above, the intensity of the surrogates' nonnegotiable stance toward their eggs may be explained by other factors. First, the egg/womb dichotomy may help these Jewish-Israeli women to establish clear kinship boundaries in the context of two divergent "cultures" that influence their thinking: the culture of biotechnology and Jewish culture. Whereas all surrogacy arrangements carry the underlying question of whether the surrogate or the intended mother has priority claims to kin ties with the child, this question is amplified in the Jewish context. The biotechnological view posits that kinship is ruled by genes, blood, law, and "nature." This is the predominant kinship model that Schneider identified as basic to American kinship[22] and that others have identified as central to Euro-American understandings of the kinship outcomes of reproductive technologies.[23] Biomedical understandings of kinship inform the prevailing folk model among the non-Orthodox population of Israel as well.[24]

Conversely, Jewish law has historically privileged the womb over genetics in matters of kinship: in the view of a majority of rabbis, a Jew can only be born from a "Jewish womb" and not from a "Jewish egg" that is gestated in a non-Jewish woman's womb.[25] Most interpreters of Jewish law also agree that the woman who births a baby should be viewed as the mother, so a majority of rabbis would consider a gestational surrogate to be the mother. As Kahn discusses fully in her ethnography of assisted conception in Israel, the influence of Jewish law penetrates many aspects of the practice of infertility medicine in Israel, and religious parties are often vocal in governmental debates over reproductive issues.[26]

Since these divergent cosmologies coexist in Israel's fertility context, the fixation on the genetic kinship model must be assessed against the backdrop of Jewish law and its privileging of the womb as an organ of connectedness. The surrogacy law actually embodies both views, since it mandates that Jewish couples hire Jewish surrogates, thus privileging the Jewish womb. Simultaneously, however, the law insists that the sperm be provided by the man who will raise the child, thus privileging a patriarchal genetic kinship model that departs from rabbinic thinking. Consequently, participants in surrogacy agreements may be downplaying the contribution of the womb and centralizing the importance of the egg in creating kinship to override the possible connotations that the rabbinical approach generates: that the surrogate is the "real mother" because she provides the womb.

In addition, the egg may be consistently personalized because of its relative significance in comparison with other body parts to the woman's gender identity. Elson analyzed women's experiences with hysterectomy, revealing how gender identity was symbolically ascribed to the egg and the uterus differently.[27] Following her analysis, I would suggest that the uterus, a symbol of childbearing potential, can be neutrally shared by the surrogate with the intended mother or "borrowed" by the intended mother from the surrogate. In contrast, the egg, as a symbol of the core of feminine identity, cannot be shared because it is iconic of the woman's whole self as a feminine subject. In the next section, I continue to outline how the surrogates mapped their kin lines and personhood onto other parts of their body and self, including the blood, heart, and soul.

KINSHIP IN THE BLOOD

The blood system was consistently personalized by surrogates, and, just like the genes, it was understood as a potent symbol of connectivity. Blood has many strong connotations, according to Euro-American kinship ideology. As Schneider famously argued, blood relationships are believed to be the strongest.[28] Beyond the realm of kinship, blood also

serves as a potent symbol of the self, the soul, love, unity, and the relations between people who are not related but are very close friends.[29]
In Jewish-Israeli culture, blood is also linked to popular idioms such as
"blood brothers" and "love sanctified by blood" that describe close relationships among friends and comrades-in-arms.[30] Surrogates maneuver
carefully around the vital substance because they believe that inadver-
tent mixing of surrogate and fetal blood lines could connect them to the
baby. Batya referred to the separation of blood systems to refute others'
allegations that she had any kin ties to the baby she carried or that surrogacy could lead to such transgressive acts as incest:

> Some woman says to me . . . "Let's say, when she grows up, the girl, your
> son meets her. You know, the world is a wheel. . . . So if he goes with her,
> it is incest." I said to her, "What nonsense, what a line of thinking. . . . She
> was not born from me, she was not created from me. She [visited] me, yes.
> But she was not created from me. She was not created from my husband's
> sperm. She is a stranger! She doesn't even have my same blood type!"
> . . . [mimicking the woman's voice] "But she grew by you [in your house/
> womb]." . . . Correct, she grew by me . . . but she is not mine!

Batya shares her own blood system with her kin and not with the surrogate child. From a blood-gene-biotechnological viewpoint, families
share the same blood, and since she and the child have separate blood
systems, future incest between one of her own children and her surrogate child is not a possibility. Batya's insistence on blood and genetic
separations is especially important since she is religiously observant and
is aware of the rabbinic view that the birth of her genetic and surrogate
offspring from the same womb might render them siblings. Like Batya,
Rinat also referred to blood to securely counter any notion of surrogacy
leading to transgression:

> Some [neighbors] said, "Oy vey, she is giving away her children." They
> just couldn't digest that it wasn't mine. Nothing of mine is there. Nothing,
> nothing is mine here. It is only theirs [the couple's] . . . nothing of him, not
> my blood. No. It is all theirs . . . what was put into me is a whole baby. It
> is ready. A baby that is formed from the sperm and egg together and was
> created as a baby and only then inserted into my belly. And then what is
> attached to me is just in the placenta and the umbilical cord. But nothing
> else is mine. Nothing, nothing is mine. . . . And that is why I am telling you,
> that you don't have feelings [for the fetus] like you would expect.

Rinat conceptualizes her body and the fetal body in mutually exclusive systems, existing side by side but never mixing. The "whole baby"
carried in her womb has its own parents' blood and is connected to her

only via two physical structures—the placenta and the umbilical cord. Rinat maintains that she shares nothing—as she repeats six times—of her personal bodily system with the baby she gestates other than through these two limited links. This clear map of connections and dis-connections enables her to logically explain why she is not in violation of the cultural imperative to fall in love with the child she carries. She uses the same kinship logic to explain to her children that the surrogate child is not their brother, because he does not share their blood. Rinat's preteen daughter asserted that the surrogate child "is not related to us. His blood isn't our blood. Nothing is ours. It is the blood of the biologi-cal mother, of the parents. I would like to have him as a brother, but he isn't ours." Rinat's daughter's explanation reveals just how consistently and clearly the symbols of surrogates' body map were drawn.

Orna's narrative offers an even more powerful illustration of the connective and separating powers of blood. Orna locates her strong determination to become a surrogate and to give her couple a child as existing within her blood, her heart, and her soul: "It [surrogacy] entered my blood. . . . Without it, I would not be able to live. It is like air to breathe for me. . . . It had entered my heart, really my soul."[31] Blood carries her personal emotions, hopes, and dreams with such intensity that failing in her goal would kill her. It is no wonder that such an emotion-transmitting personalized substance must be kept so strictly separate from the fetus, which Orna sees as connected to a completely autonomous blood system:

> The egg and the sperm aren't mine, right? There are cells, I just develop those cells. I mean, the cells divide with his genes. For instance, when you get a blood transfusion, you don't change all of your blood. . . . The blood that they give you, it helps you make more of your own blood. It has to be the same type of blood, because you can't mix two different types of blood, but it just helps your own body recover by itself. It is the same thing here. You have a cell, an embryo, and it just needs a little help from outside in order to develop into a fetus. The genes of the child aren't mine. . . . I feed him, develop his genes. But not mine. My genes are something else. His looks, his personality, he takes nothing from me. It is all there in four little cells, eight cells, the first cells, everything is already there. Even the shape of his nose is in those two cells. . . . I have nothing to do with this embryo. I have no genetic connection to him. . . . I have no connection to him.

By comparing her relationship with the fetus and couple to a blood transfusion, Orna also positions herself as personally saving the life of the couple by aiding them in replenishing, or continuing, their bloodline.

As Waldby and colleagues note in their study of blood donors, blood is a renewable substance that is replenished by the body a few weeks after donation.[32] Donated blood is depersonalized, anonymously pooled, and banked before transfusion. Thus, just as a blood donor can depersonalize the donation act and donate repeatedly without necessarily believing that he or she has given part of his or her personal self, so Orna can depersonalize gestation while simultaneously equating it with a blood transfusion's capacity to save lives. This image joins with the metaphor of the "warm womb" explored earlier to show that surrogates view their distanced, depersonalized, yet warm, nurturing womb work as "giving life" to their couple and saving them from childlessness.

Orna's deliberations on blood also symbolically express her perception of boundaries between different types of persons. She sees blood not only as unifying families by replicating their distinctive genetic characteristics but also as creating disconnections and difference between persons whose blood types cannot be mixed. These distinctions illuminate the symbolic link between the personal body and the body politic, for, as Douglas has famously argued, ritual attention to women's bodies is particularly symbolic of collective concerns.[33] Accordingly, Orna also warned me of the dangers she perceived in mixing different *national* types of blood. Comparing surrogacy to international adoption, she claimed that an adopted child from abroad "is not yours. The genes are not yours. He won't look like you, he won't have your personality, you will always have the feeling that you didn't give birth to him. You don't know the feeling, the fun of being pregnant when you give life from within your belly." When I reminded Orna that the intended mother will never experience being pregnant either, she replied,

> But it is her genes, it is much more than adoption. Adoption you go to Brazil, you go to places where you don't know the parents at all, you don't know anything about them, one day you will suddenly find out that it is an Arab, that you are raising an Arab. He has Arab blood. One day he will come and throw a stone at you and he won't know why at all. Because it's . . . it's in the blood, you can't do anything about it [in] the genes, and genes are very, very strong. So when you have surrogacy, with this law, you know that it is yours, the personality will be yours. The looks. He'll look like you. Do you understand?

Orna's suggestion that recognizing separate blood systems can keep Arab and Jewish families from mistakenly crossing national boundaries hints at levels of meaning embedded in one's personal nature that go beyond the individual and the kin network. Her words echo the aversion expressed by Jewish-Israeli ova recipients interviewed by Nahman toward Palestinian women's eggs, which led Nahman to suggest that practices surrounding ova donation can be viewed as another way of symbolically constituting the boundaries of the nation.[34] The divisions that separated blood systems can maintain, however, are particularly vivid when they are counterpoised against the connections that blood can forge. Orna employed the same blood metaphor to divide herself from the fetus and to express her close, emotional connection to the intended mother:

> They took blood tests from the two of us, and our blood was matched, her blood type to mine. Then they gave us hormone shots to synchronize our menstrual cycles. That way my womb is ready to receive the embryos as soon as her eggs are ripe. It is a parallel process for both of us. My body couldn't do it without her. It has to be together.

Like Orna, other surrogates told me of the strict blood and genetic divisions between themselves and the fetus and, in the same breath, described being "one bloodstream" with or having a "blood connection" to the intended mother. Just as they saw separate blood systems as distancing any suggestion of a kin connection with the fetus, they viewed the blood they symbolically shared with their intended mother as establishing simulated kin relations between them, a topic explored in part 3.

The significance of Israeli surrogates' adherence to the body map scheme is brought into sharper focus when viewed in the context of the Indian surrogates studied by Pande and by Vora.[35] The gestational surrogates in these studies, who were mostly rural Gujarati women, were not versed in the biomedical kinship script when they were hired by a clinic in Anand, India. Indeed, both observed that the clinic director "educated" the women about biogenetic kinship connections to shape their conceptualization of their role as the "house" for the intended parents' embryo.[36] Yet as Pande's ethnographic observations reveal, the blood-gene-womb script was not always convincing to or accepted without question by the women. During interviews, some made claims to the children they birthed through surrogacy, asserting that their "blood, sweat and tears" shaped the child and that "it was their [the couple's] genes, but my blood."[37] Some of the surrogates who had not yet given birth imagined the pain they would feel at being parted from the baby, and one even fantasized in her interview with Pande about keeping one of the triplets she would bear for her couple. This comparative case illuminates the centrality of the biogenetic kinship scheme to the Israeli surrogate's distancing regime as well as the power of the body map trope as a preparatory tool for relinquishment.

WHERE THE HEART IS

Along with the blood, the heart emerged from the surrogates' narratives as a highly connective organ. Yet unlike the blood, the heart was not directly symbolic of kinship or relatedness.[38] Rather, the heart was used to symbolically express emotions and identity, much as anthropologists have discovered in other cultural contexts. For instance, Good found in his study of illness in Iran that the phrase "heart pain" expressed loss of identity, community, and culture.[39] Coker found a similar expression among Sudanese refugees in Egypt, who, in addition, related the heart to qualities such as strength, stability, and devotion to family.[40] Anthropological studies of organ transplant recipients in North America have revealed that heart transplant recipients are more concerned than other organ recipients about the gender, ethnicity, and moral character of their anonymous donors.[41] Western cultures privilege the heart as the organ most closely associated with personal identity, and therefore the belief that it retains the donor's qualities in a mystical, animistic manner after transplant is more pronounced than is the case for other organs.[42]

The powerful association of the heart with personal identity and emotions explains why surrogates believed that the heart had to be kept separate from the neutral belly where the fetus was held. Rinat, for instance, described how embodied messages from her midsection were separated from her heart during surrogacy:

> You have to understand that the feelings were [in surrogacy] completely different. For instance, now [in her subsequent pregnancy] I feel that it is my heart and that it is all mine. And I am eager for it to come into the world. Look, also for her [the intended mother], I looked forward to it coming already, that she will see it and it will be fun, but I didn't have the feelings of a mother.

Rinat positions her own pregnancy as something that she "feels" because "it is my heart," in contrast to the surrogate pregnancy in which her heart was not involved. Her idea that maternal feelings come from the heart corresponds with Ragoné's finding that traditional surrogates in the United States, who were both genitor and gestator of the surrogate child, credited the intended mother with being the one to conceive the baby "in her heart."[43] The idea that the heart can measure just how much the surrogate feels toward the baby was central to Masha's explication of the body map:

> Look, 80 percent of it is business but there is still some emotion. We still do have a heart. . . . Whoever comes and tells you that that she is closed [*atuma*] and that she seals off her heart [*otemet et halev*], she is a liar. I won't accept that there is someone who is cold-hearted, because she couldn't do this [if she was].

Masha views having an "open" and "warm" heart as an important part of being a surrogate and believes feeling a measure of emotion toward the fetus is necessary and natural. Yet she too maintains clear demarcations in her body map, which are evident in her comments below:

> *Masha:* This is a mission with a lot of emotions. It is a mission of giving life. . . . It is not an object.
> *Elly:* Do you put your soul into this fetus?
> *Masha:* My soul?! No! No way, no! If I give my soul, then it means that I am giving away my . . . my soul is my own daughter's. This [the surrogate baby] is not mine. There is emotion but not . . . there is affection, there is physical contact . . . but not . . .

Nearly all of the surrogates with whom I spoke explicitly personalized their hearts and their souls. The centrality of the heart connects back to the metaphors of the oven, incubator, and greenhouse as descriptors of a warm womb. Consequently, it seems that although she kept her heart and soul symbolically separate from the fetus, the surrogate radiated a warmth from her heart toward her couple that provided the necessary climate for the development of their child in the oven/incubator/hothouse womb. Hence, Neta, who had described her role as the "oven that bakes the bread of hungry people," expressed how surrogacy was about giving from the heart, saying, "If I can give someone this happiness on the other side, for me it is everything. That feeling of your heart filling up. The heart fills and expands when you are giving to someone." Likewise, Belle, who had used the hothouse metaphor elsewhere, explained,

> If you don't do this deep from inside your heart and your soul, then no money in the world can help. It has to come from inside you, the desire to give, with love, to give with all your heart and soul. This is where emotional fortification enters [*po nichneset hasinut nafshit*]. If a person does it from his heart, from his soul, then it really is a feeling of perfection. There's no doubt he won't feel pain or emptiness afterwards, because he knew his aim from the start of the process.[44]

Like the others, Orna emphasized that the heart was the locus of her determination and that it was the organ on which her ability to give depended. In a radio interview, she used the heart metaphor to describe her decision to be a surrogate as "just something that comes from inside the heart." Later in the broadcast, she described her feeling of personal failure when she did not conceive after the first attempted embryo transfer, saying that "the hard part is after you have begun the treatments . . . and after a month of injections and hopes, in the end they tell you that you aren't pregnant. Tears burst forth from your heart, and you feel pain, despair, and disappointment."[45] In a similar manner, she told me of the "heart cleansing ritual" that she enacted each time she experienced a failed embryo transfer, saying, "I need to let it out of my heart, to let out the tears. When the heart is clean, I can go out and start to burden it again."

Not only was Orna's heart the place where her ability to give and her determination to be a surrogate existed, but it was also the locus of her emotional relationship with the intended mother, whom she described in radio broadcast as "my friend in heart and in soul." Because the heart was such an important, personal locus of emotions and love, it had to be kept completely separate from the fetus so that no emotional connections would inadvertently develop between the two. Orna's determination to uphold her bodily map and to keep the heart and the womb separately situated led her to physically show me the lines of demarcation on her body:

> So I was like this. Me [points to her chest and upward], not me [indicates area from chest to mid-thigh]. Completely disconnected. I totally disconnected myself from my belly. I mean, whatever I felt in my belly, I didn't feel. I mean, I was always saying that I am divided in three. From here to here is me, from here to here isn't me, from here to here is me. And everything to do with my belly, I ignored. Very simple. I got fat, so I got fat. I didn't pay any attention to my belly at all. No touching. It was fun to . . . feel him move . . . because he was alive. But not to feel him move with my heart.

For Orna, the heart remains personalized as an organ of feelings, and during surrogacy the midsection of her body—the belly—is disconnected so that no feelings related to that part of her body reach her heart. Orna's clear positioning of the heart as the seat of her private emotions, empathy, and desire to "succeed" in surrogacy at the same time that she describes her disconnection suggests that she wants to be sure to maintain her self-image as a feeling person and a loving mother—but not to direct those emotions toward her disengaged body parts.

Surrogates may also assign importance to distancing the heart from the belly because it is symbolically substituting for the organ that, in Jewish-Israeli culture, is usually believed to contain the emotions. In modern Hebrew, the idea that emotions are housed "in the belly" [*babeten*] is widespread and part of what might be seen as a "folk model" of the body.[46] The word *beten* refers to the entire midsection, which houses both the digestive system and the reproductive organs and which is where babies are "carried." Thus, if emotions are generally carried in the belly, then the belly must be cleared of potential hazards during surrogacy by deferring the surrogate's emotions to the heart and increasing that organ's figurative weight.

Shirley best summarized this idea. Seven months into her pregnancy, Shirley told the women present at a meeting of the surrogacy support group that surrogacy had taught her to channel emotions through her heart: "I learned to express words from the heart and not to keep them in the belly." Ravit, then in her fifth month of pregnancy, rejoined, "That is because your belly is occupied." The joking interaction, which I entered into my field notes without realizing its potency, embodies the flow of emotions in the body map: emotions may be channeled through the heart but must carefully avoid the contents of the belly.

BODY MAPS AND OCCUPIED TERRITORIES

I chose the metaphor of the body map to describe the surrogate's ordering of the body despite the fact that none of the women I met actually referred to their body in cartographic terms. On the basis of simple comparison, I found the map metaphor appropriate because maps have routes, borders, and boundaries that change over time in response to historical processes. The surrogate's body map expresses her spatial world and the relationships that she embodies[47] in terms of territories, routes, and mobility. First, the surrogate re-creates the body in a graphic way that demarcates spaces of ownership and identity. Next, she strategically opens up certain spaces and cordons off others, creating a hierarchy. Finally, she traces routes of possible mobility for herself and for her intended mother. These include a route of social mobility for the other woman that will result in making her into a mother and a route of financial mobility that she herself can pursue without harming her own social status as a mother. This process allows her body to serve as a conduit for the other woman's transformation to motherhood without being permanently marked.

Another reason I found the map metaphor appropriate is because maps are "good to think with"[48] about how power relations play out on women's bodies. Nash posits that in contemporary visual art and literature, maps appear in artistic projects metaphorically or visually projected onto women's bodies. These maps are used to theoretically critique "uneven geographies of power and pleasure, of space and the body," within the larger project of feminist geographers to deconstruct cartographies of colonial territories "as powerful tools of domination and authoritative and power-laden forms of representation."[49] As Nash argues, maps—or creative representations modeled on maps—can reveal "geographies of conflict, solidarity, power and resistance over the course of women's lives."[50] Maps can thus evoke the differentials of power and the themes of occupation and possession that emerge from the surrogates' narratives.

Who is in control of the territories on the body map? On the one hand, if to map is to claim the right to territory and to control it, then it is significant that it is the surrogate herself who is doing the mapping and allocating of spaces. On the other hand, at the same time that she may be the one marking the dividing lines, she must also remain within the lines she has marked, confining her embodied self to a restricted space. The body map thus exhibits two perspectives on her situation: that of a colonized body and that of an effort to prevent colonization. This is also evident in the surrogate's relationship with her couple, as the body map becomes a tool for negotiating their mutual boundaries. As I discuss in the next section, the surrogate uses the body map to protect her personal space in the body, to limit the couple's movement, to temper the couple's efforts at policing her boundaries, and to refute their attempts at colonizing her entire body.

Finally, the map metaphor hints at the presence of the body politic within these embodied relations. It is in this context that the constellation of women's bodies and maps is linked to another aspect of colonization. Specifically, as Das discusses in the case of the India-Pakistan war, the bodies of women have historically served as "surfaces on which texts were to be written and read—icons of new nations."[51] Das interprets the abduction and rape of thousands of women during that war as a sign that "the men of the other community would never be able to forget that the women as territory had already been claimed and occupied by other men." Although comparable only in terms of the symbolic conquest and possession of territory, one observer has noted that the

Israeli military usually designates land targets by the names of women's body parts.[52]

Drawing on the idea that nations claim control by possessing women's bodies, we might read the surrogate's demarcation lines as an imprint of state interests. Israel is a country in which the government intervenes in the natal lives of its citizens, and, as studies of pronatalist and antinatalist policies have long established, these policies are carried out on the bodies of women through abortion policy, family planning policy and contraception, and incentives or punishments for curbing or increasing birth.[53] In Israel's pronatalist society, the surrogate's mapping of her body might be seen as an act of making the womb provide for the nation—an act of self-domination, in which surrogates, as "docile bodies"[54] or "disciplined bodies"[55] offer up a disembodied womb to others in an agreement sanctioned by the state. One might even go so far as to propose that a surrogate is ultimately allocating space in her body to produce a child for the nation, since the state is directly involved in commissioning the child. The fact that a state representative becomes guardian of the child immediately after the birth for a short period of time, as described in part 3, reinforces this idea.

From a semiotic perspective, the body map can also be interpreted as an inscription of the values of the body politic on the surrogate's bodily scheme. It stabilizes national priorities by reflecting social boundaries within the lines of the map: Jew versus Arab, ethnic divisions, and the gender divide. The surrogate demarcates her body and confines her personal space, living within the lines of this map, just as she lives within the maps that society prescribes as appropriate for a woman, mother, and gendered citizen. Her body map also serves the interests of the body politic because it maintains the traditional classifications that the state aims to preserve and protect—motherhood, nature, and family—and because her mapping efforts trace a route for the creation of a heteronormative, nuclear, "natural family" through her marginal, single-parent body.

Still, without falling into the trap that Abu-Lughod calls "romanticizing resistance,"[56] I suggest that the body map is also a creative expression of personal agency. Das suggests that the women raped during the India-Pakistan war converted the passivity of being written on into agency by actively allocating space within the depths of their bodies to hide and gestate the pain, refusing to allow it to be born. One woman, consequently, told Das that she was "designing a body that is appropriate for the time, for in those days . . . women had to grow two stomachs—one was the normal one and the second was for them to be able to bear the fruits of violence within themselves."[57] The surrogate's allocation of separate and isolated spaces within the body for her couple to pass through thus enables her to feel that her own self has privacy and remains liberated even while her body is "occupied" by "guests." The body map preserves her sense of a personal space in which she can breathe rather than feel choked or bounded.

CHAPTER 3

Operationalizing the Body Map

In this chapter, I suggest two ways in which the body map is activated by surrogates as a boundary-policing tool to deal with the tangible challenges of surrogacy: it is used, first, to maintain an emotionally distant relationship with the fetus, and second, to maintain interpersonal boundaries with their couples. Surrogates employed several means for emotionally distancing themselves from the fetus. One was to react to any movement emanating from the belly area nonemotionally. The need to engage in such "emotion work"[1] stemmed from a surrogate's perception that the fetal movements she sensed had the potential to create emotional ties or bonds between herself and the child she gestated. The body map helped women distinguish between bodily sensations that could create emotional connections and those they could defer. Idit explained that surrogacy involved deep classification work: "You have to really classify your emotions . . . classify, sift apart. [My] children are [my] children, my family life is my family life, surrogacy is surrogacy, and their fetus is their fetus."

This strategy of emotion management drew on the idea that the mind could command the body to selectively interpret a sensation as a personalized emotion or to neutralize it. Belle, for instance, described how she deliberately "decided" to neutralize any potential emotions stemming from fetal movements:

During the pregnancy, I neutralized myself from the baby. If he moved, that's great—moved, kicked, turned around. And I always encouraged the mother, so that she'd get used to [the idea] that she is going to be a mother soon. But my feelings I totally neutralized. I didn't develop any feelings. I simply decided that I wouldn't have feelings. I decided that I am going forward. I just didn't look to the left or to the right. I had it in my head all the time that I am capable of neutralizing my feelings, and I succeeded.

Tilly described the ability to "decide" what to feel and to command the body to abide by that decision as "pressing a button." Likewise, Nina described it as "a switch in the mind," and Lihi compared it to "translation." Explaining why she "didn't become attached" to the twins she carried for her couple, Lihi reported, "I felt them in my belly, but I didn't interpret everything I felt, and I didn't translate it into who they are. . . . Okay, they are moving. . . . I felt nothing. I just disconnected myself from all of the expectations and the feelings."

Neutralizing any potential feelings toward the fetus was often undertaken with the help and support of the surrogate's family. Batya's sister-in-law, who joined us during our first interview, told me how the entire family had encouraged Batya's distancing practices: "We also put it into her head a lot. . . . We said, 'Don't think about it, don't look at it, I mean, the pregnancy. Try to act as though it is a stranger.'" The idea that the mind can control the development of potential emotions underlies the women's sense of "self-mastery of the emotions":[2] they choose when they want to feel and when they want to insulate themselves. This mastery was evident when surrogates described "neutralizing" their emotions and feeling "nothing" toward the fetus at the same time that they described moments of strong fear, concern, or excitement. For instance, it was not uncommon for the women to report feeling nothing toward the fetus and then to describe their fear of miscarriage or surgery or how they wept with emotion when they realized what an important gift they had bestowed on the couple.

Extending this neutralizing practice, surrogates did not merely nullify their own potential emotions toward the fetus but also transposed emotionality into feelings toward their couple. A bodily sensation that made them feel "nothing" toward the fetus could trigger excitement and happiness for their couple's impending parenthood. Neta reported that when she started to feel the fetus in her belly, "It made me happy that he is all right, that everything is okay." She added, "I didn't feel anything towards him [the fetus] . . . not at all. I was happy for them." Masha attested to having the same reaction, saying,

I knew that she [the baby] wasn't mine and would not remain with me, and I didn't let myself develop feelings and expectations toward her. . . . When I felt her moving in my belly, I got excited for them. I didn't think about myself, but about how they are feeling with the pregnancy.

Another distancing practice that surrogates used was to imagine the belly as disembodied and detached from the rest of the body. This technique usually occurred as the result of very strong distancing and channeling work, to the point that the surrogate no longer identified her belly as spatially connected to the rest of her body. Idit, who explicitly divided her emotions, family, and identity from the belly and its contents, explained that, during surrogacy, she began to feel that her belly "wasn't even part of my body. . . . It isn't connected to me. . . . Psychologically, it isn't mine, it doesn't connect." The distancing of the belly was so intense in her case, she reported, that "sometimes I would even forget that I was pregnant during the process! I just ignored it. I didn't pay attention to the pregnancy."

Like Idit, other surrogates experienced the pregnancy, and the body part that housed it, as spatially separated from the rest of the body. Shahar described how she became increasingly debilitated during the pregnancy, while the twins in her belly grew and developed. The sharp contrast between the healthy babies and her ill health led Shahar to view her body as divided into two, a phenomenon that she encapsulated by saying, "It was as if the pregnancy moved alongside me." Ravit reported the extent of her disconnection from the pregnancy was such that she repeatedly found herself standing in front of her closet and picking out pre-pregnancy clothes to wear, even when she was seven and eight months pregnant: "Only when I put my legs in the jeans and couldn't pull them up, then I remembered that I was pregnant. It was something!"

The ultrasound scans that surrogates frequently undergo during pregnancy also aided in distancing the belly. As several feminist commentators have noted with respect to ultrasound, the procedure creates a disembodied image of the fetus floating in "space" on a monitor, as though it is detached from the woman's body.[3] These authors have critiqued this disembodiment at length for displacing the pregnant woman as the central "knower" of the fetus, enabling the doctor and the father to gaze at the monitor's screen and take possession of "authoritative knowledge" of the fetus that is often privileged above the woman's knowledge.[4] For surrogates, however, the ultrasound worked well as an accomplice in their distancing practices, for it enabled them not only to imagine the belly as a disembodied organ but also to picture it as such through this technological means. Batya, for instance, described how she was able to look away from the ultrasound screen as a further act of distancing herself from the belly and its contents:

> In my subconscious, I said that it isn't mine, and I didn't become attached to him [the fetus]. I didn't have any connection to him, and that's it! I don't bond with the fetus! Even in the ultrasound, I wouldn't look. He [the doctor] would say to me, he is in such and such week . . . she has a girl. . . . I didn't connect at all. Not at all. . . . I would look to the side. . . . It didn't interest me . . . because I said that it is just a fetus that I won't have in the end. . . . I knew that it wouldn't stay with me in the end. And that it wouldn't be part of me. So why become connected to it?

As Batya notes, the spectacle of her womb's contents on the screen was an opportunity for her to meet the "stranger" that she "didn't know"—an opportunity she avoided by looking to the side instead of gazing directly at the projection of the belly and its contents. Most of the surrogates I spoke with reported looking away from the monitor or watching their couple during ultrasounds rather than directly engaging with the image of the fetus, as they had during their own pregnancies.

The final distancing practice that surrogates employed was to manage the contact of their hands and those of others with the belly. Surrogates seemed to understand touching the belly as an act that encouraged bonding with the fetus. For this reason, some of them avoided touching the belly at all during the pregnancy. Ronit, a thirty-nine-year-old surrogate who was interviewed by a local newspaper after giving birth to a singleton for her couple, spoke of struggling to keep her hands away from her belly so as not to connect the rest of her body with it and its contents, leading her to uncomfortable physical manipulations:

> Physically, it was an excellent pregnancy. Emotionally, it was weird for me when I began to feel the fetus. It's a shock, [even] with all of the preparation. Your body is talking, and it doesn't sound right to you [lo nishma lach]. Pregnant women speak to their baby and stroke their belly, and I found myself sitting for the first weeks with my hands at my sides, on my knees, behind my back, just so that I wouldn't bond with him.[5]

Ronit's tactics for separating the belly were relatively extreme in comparison with other surrogates' strategies for managing touch. Most of the women I spoke to simply tried to limit touching the belly to necessity. Nina, in her seventh month when I recorded the following exchange, exemplified this approach.

    Nina: I just put it in my head that I won't bond. . . . I just disconnect com-
          pletely from that part of my body [points to her belly]. . . . I only
          touch it if I feel like she [the fetus] isn't moving and I want to wake
          her up, to make sure that she is okay. But I don't let my children
          touch the belly. . . . I just try to keep them from touching my belly as
          much as possible, or if they touch it, not to touch it as though there
          is a baby there.
    Elly: Did you touch your belly when you were pregnant with your
          own kids?
    Nina: Of course. I bonded with my children. I touched them, caressed them
          all the time.

Most of the surrogates I spoke to did touch their bellies during pregnancy, but only for "practical" reasons, such as making sure that the
fetus was alive. Very few of the women told me that they had touched
their bellies with any emotion. Those who did were careful to temper
their statements, assuring me that the emotion was no different from
what they would have felt for their sister's child, or their friend's child,
unlike the way they felt when they touched their bellies while pregnant
with their own children. Still, most of them believed that a fetus needed
to be touched during pregnancy, and therefore they encouraged their
intended mothers to engage with the belly: to touch it, lay their head
against it, kiss it, and put their ears to it to "hear" the fetus. Together,
these distancing practices activate the demarcation lines of the surrogate's body map, enabling the surrogate to symbolically and experien-
tially detach the belly from the rest of her body at will. In her distancing
of the fetus, the surrogate disembodies the belly, relegating it to a space
that is linked to her body but separate from it. Her efforts at maintaining order among her mapped parts culminate in the birth event.

ORCHESTRATING BIRTH

While surrogates perceive the pregnancy itself as manageable through
their cognitive and embodied efforts at self-control, childbirth is seen as
an uncontrollable event in which anything can happen. Consequently,
the women almost always spoke about the birth in a way that expressed
a fear that the demarcation lines of their body map might become confused in all of the commotion and that this confusion might lead to
threatening emotional consequences.

    Not trusting the doctors and birth attendants to keep their boundar-
ies intact for them, the women chose one of two ways of dealing with

the birth event. One popular strategy was to harness technology to take personal control of the event. This strategy involved requesting an elective cesarean section during the thirty-eighth week of pregnancy. Three weeks after she gave birth to a surrogate child, Neta explained that her decision to opt for a cesarean was motivated by a desire to circumvent the birth entirely: "I said, I don't want an epidural. I want [general] anesthesia. To go to sleep and wake up without it."

Like Neta, who preferred to completely eliminate consciousness of her own presence from the event, other women were wary of the possible consequences of actively birthing the child. Batya, for instance, had already given birth to five children vaginally before becoming a surrogate. Still, she feared that the uncontrollability of a regular delivery might jumble her hard-achieved classifications: "From the beginning I said it would be cesarean. I didn't want a regular birth. . . . I didn't want this birth. . . . I was afraid to bond with the baby." Shahar, who had also given birth to five children prior to surrogacy, similarly thought that there might be something in the childbirth event itself that would bond her to the twins she carried as a surrogate. She explained, "I think a woman that undergoes a regular birth finds it easier to bond with the baby. That's why I didn't want to have a regular birth. . . . I guess that there is something in the birth itself that bonds the mother to the baby."

Shahar was not alone in thinking that women bond with their babies during childbirth even if they have not done so during pregnancy. I did not fully understand the implications of this idea until I met a surrogate named Oranit at a surrogacy support group meeting. She was then in her twelfth week. She told me that the reason she was considering a cesarean was because she had only bonded with her own children when she first saw them after they exited her womb. Oranit's and Shahar's statements echo Ivry's findings that pregnant Israeli women deferred bonding until they had birthed a thriving, healthy baby.[6] Consequently, the local cultural script of post-birth bonding seems to inform the surrogates' wariness of the delivery.

Among the women I interviewed, elective cesareans were requested by more than half. Some were carrying twins and came to the decision together with their couple and doctor, concluding that cesarean delivery would be "safer" and less complicated than vaginal delivery.[7] For others, an elective cesarean represented the ability to end the pregnancy earlier, usually in the thirty-eighth week of gestation, rather than waiting for the onset of spontaneous labor up to a month later. Surrogates cited other reasons as well, such as the ability to feel in control of the progress of the birth and avoid prolonged labor, much as has been described in studies of some laboring women's pragmatic choices to ask for technological intervention in their hospital births.[8] Some degree of influence might also be ascribed to the extra compensation a cesarean promises according to the surrogacy contract, although I would suggest that this had little actual influence over the women's choices. Indeed, several of the women I interviewed confided that their couples had tried to convince them to have a cesarean in the thirty-eighth week and that they had refused, even when tempted with additional payment.

The factor that had the most impact on the women's birthing choices, trumping all of the alternative explanations just considered, was their aim of preserving the integrity of their body map during delivery. In this respect, the elective cesarean procedure served as a strategy for keeping all of the surrogate's mapped parts in place. It prevented the accidental integration of the belly into the surrogate's personalized parts during delivery, since it made her into a passive observer as the doctor, behind a curtain, cut the belly and extracted the newborn.

The same rationale, however, led some surrogates to demand "regular" deliveries so that they would not be left with the scar that a cesarean delivery would produce. A scar would mark the body permanently with the memory of the baby and not allow the woman to finalize the distancing, or, in a manner of speaking, "clean" the belly before reintegrating it into the body-self afterward. Orna expressed satisfaction that she was not left with any stitches after the birth because it helped her "forget" the pregnancy more quickly: "I, from my point of view, have already forgotten giving birth. It was lucky that I didn't need any stitches and didn't have to think any thoughts about the baby in that regard."

Other behaviors surrounding the delivery read similarly as strategies for maintaining the order of the body map. If the surrogate felt the need to refrain from touching the belly and to encourage the intended mother's bodily contact, we see this idea coming to the fore at the time of the birth. Two routine hospital birth practices are of central concern to the surrogate: the resting of the newborn on the childbearing woman's belly while the umbilical cord is cut and the handing of the newborn to the new mother to hold. Masha felt that the act of laying the baby on the birthing woman's belly was an extraordinarily moving experience that transformed a woman into a mother. Therefore, she was relieved to find that the hospital had made plans to ensure that the baby she carried would not be laid on her belly and would be delivered directly into the intended mother's arms instead.

Masha: There are all of these little things that are very special, and afterwards during the birth, the way that the baby comes out and they
rest him on your belly and it is a feeling that is just out of this
world. You forget all of your worries and everything you've been
through. . . . As much as you suffer from contractions, and as hard
as it is, the minute that you hold the baby, nothing can compare to
what you have in your hand at that moment . . .

Elly: But this time . . .

Masha: Tova will hold [it]; that very moment they will give it to her. We
were just at the hospital and they explained how it will be. That I
will give birth and they will immediately let her hold the baby in
her arms.

When this promised choreography was not carried out as planned
and the baby was laid on Masha's belly rather than given directly to
Tova, Masha became very angry. Like Masha, Rinat also became agitated when the doctor laid the baby on her belly after delivery. Telling
the doctor to remove the baby, saying, "The baby has a mother and
father," she communicated the role assignment that she understood as
having been confused in this act. To avoid such confusion, almost all
of the surrogates made sure that the intended mother would be present during delivery. Even during cesarean operations, intended mothers
were often allowed to stand next to the surrogate's head. During her
vaginal delivery, Idit carefully choreographed the medical staff's movements to avoid what she perceived as the danger of the baby bonding
with her through smell.

Idit: Also the smell. The baby also bonds with the smell of the mother the
first time. Who does he smell? The mother! So this way he learns to
identify, by the smell, because he can't see, he doesn't know the surroundings. He is not aware of the environment. He only knows the
first smell of the mother . . .

Elly: But maybe the baby, if he was in your environment, if he smelled you,
then maybe . . .

Idit (interrupting): That is why I made sure that the minute that she [the
baby] comes into the world, they take her right away. And the one to
take her into her arms, is the mother. Not me.

While none of the other surrogates to whom I spoke explicitly
referred to the danger of smell, most of the women giving birth vaginally
described the explicit need to choreograph the birth so that they could
remain in control. Suggesting that the cognitive and emotion work that
she engaged in during the pregnancy had ultimately succeeded in final-

izing her emotional distance from the child, Idit described her feelings during delivery: "I gave birth and I saw her coming out of me. . . . I was very happy for them and very happy that the deal is over. I didn't feel any emotion. It's strange how nature does its thing. How things work out naturally. . . . And the psychological work that I did succeeded. . . . Especially how I penetrated into myself that it is nothing. It was like watching a movie."

Idit may credit nature with some of the responsibility for her neutrality during the delivery, but she ultimately acknowledges her own detachment strategies for her "success" in managing any potential emotions during the birth. Engaging in multiple levels of emotion work,[9] she feels "nothing" toward the fetus but happiness for her couple and for herself. Her self-reliance in keeping order through the birth demonstrates her understanding that she is the one who is ultimately in control. From the beginning of the surrogacy process, the doctor and the technology may have the power to medically command her body, but only Idit herself, with her clever management of the body during the pregnancy and her clever choreography of the delivery, can make sure that everything turns out the way she wants it to.

BACK TO THE BODY

The body map aided the surrogates in reintegrating all of their parts and sections after the birth. Postpartum women are commonly concerned with "getting the body back."[10] Yet for surrogates, returning to the body involves more than physically retracting to a prior figure. The strategic detachment techniques that surrogates employed during the pregnancy enabled many of them to "erase" the pregnancy and birth from their bodily memory. For instance, after her surrogacy birth, Neta said that "it was as if it hadn't happened. . . . I've gone on with my life, like normal." Likewise, after her delivery, Lihi said, "I felt like I had been through surgery, not that I had given birth to children. . . . I mean, the only thing I felt was that I had completed the mission."

None of the surrogates I spoke to reported any postpartum connection to the baby, a matter they attributed to the success of the detachment techniques they employed during pregnancy. Rinat spoke about how she felt the first time she saw the baby: "[I felt] nothing! I also thought that when I saw him I would remember, but nothing. . . . I took him and kissed him and played with him. And it was fun. But not a thing. It was just like my nephew coming in here, or my neighbor's son."

She felt that her body had hastened her final detachment from the child by delivering him much quicker than her own six children (in three hours instead of her regular daylong labors) and by not producing milk: "The doctor said to me, 'You have no milk?' I said to him, 'No.' He said to me, 'That doesn't make sense.' And he checked! And nothing." When I suggested to Rinat in a later conversation that she may have been given pills to prevent lactation, she answered, "They didn't need to. I just didn't have milk because it wasn't mine." Rinat also gave evidence of her body's quick reintegration when she showed me a photo album with a picture of her just a few hours after she had delivered her couple's child. Pointing out her non-pregnant-looking silhouette, she said, "That was not long after. . . . I got out of bed right away. After an hour I was back on my feet." And her belly, she added, disappeared "right away."

Like Rinat, other surrogates interpreted their body's nonproduction of milk after the birth as symbolic proof of the success of their emotional detachment from the baby. It was also common for surrogates to show me their slimmed-down figures soon after the birth as testimony of their body "forgetting" surrogacy and moving on. This was a standard occurrence at meetings of the surrogacy support group, where participants would compliment those who had recently delivered on how quickly they had returned to their "skinny jeans." Surrogates regularly reported losing their pregnancy weight faster than they had after their own children's deliveries. Eva, for instance, told me it had taken her two weeks to lose all that she had gained after delivering twins for her couple, whereas she struggled for two years to lose the extra weight she retained after her own son's birth. Even for those who did not "get the body back" right away, the final detachment from the pregnancy was liberating. Idit, who asked to be released from the hospital the day after birthing a surrogate child, reported, "I was glad that it was over. . . . The mountain had disappeared from me. . . . I didn't return to the same proportions because I was still weak. . . . But I began to function that day. I began to cook, to move."

The postpartum period was also marked by what surrogates described as a "return" to their pre-surrogacy lives and identities. The bodily changes they had experienced during surrogacy did not alter their identities; like the first-time British mothers studied by Bailey,[11] surrogates had a sense of a "continued self" after surrogacy. They frequently spoke of "returning to their selves." Masha noted, after completing her second stint as a surrogate, "I want to return to my life, to go back to my daily routine [*shigra*], to go back to my kids." The notion of "returning to myself" [*lachzor l'atzmi*] implies that the surrogate had been "away" from her everyday life. Surrogacy may not have physically removed her from the home other than during hospitalization, but it did figuratively remove her from her regular functions at home. Neta described a role reversal that occurred between her and her young son while she was a surrogate, noting that he had "suffered a little, because mommy wasn't his so much . . . mom was something else. . . . And he would make his own dinner, close up the house, turn off the lights, take the dog downstairs, tell me goodnight, turn off my light, and go to sleep. And that was hard for an eight-year-old boy. But I kept telling him, 'Look, it will be better afterwards.'"

When the surrogate had a live-in boyfriend or common-law husband, she also temporarily vacated the role of wife during surrogacy. One week after she gave birth to her couple's twins, Shahar reported, "My [common-law] husband can't wait for me to return to myself. . . . He says to me, 'I want you back. I can't stand it anymore. For nine months I had no wife at home.'" Familial roles and daily routines were not all that surrogates returned to after being "away." As Shahar noted, returning to her life after surrogacy also included reassuming aspects of her personality that she had left aside. Still recovering from a cesarean operation and a difficult pregnancy, Shahar added, "I am tired, hurting. I just want to get back to myself. . . . Before the pregnancy I was a very lively type. . . . I am usually full of life, laughing and satisfied."

Returning to their selves also denoted the end of the limitations that being a surrogate involved. Referring to the multiple constraints on their behavior imposed by the surrogacy contract and by their couple's and their doctor's surveillance, surrogates described returning to the freedom to act as they like. Tamar described how she had given up many of the things she enjoyed to be a surrogate, including smoking, drinking beer, going out to pubs, dancing, and having sex; returning to herself meant resuming these activities:

Look, what does it mean to return to myself? All during surrogacy I was constrained. To return to myself is to go out at night, to dance, to smoke. . . . Because when you take a project like this on yourself, then you also give up a lot of things. . . . Part of returning to yourself is that you want to have sex, and in general to do things that you didn't allow yourself to do while pregnant. You were limited the whole pregnancy. . . . I like to drink beer, wine, to have fun, to go out. To return to yourself is also to wash the floor on all fours and to climb up on a chair without being afraid to fall and hurt the pregnancy. I am very hyperactive. . . . But in . . . pregnancy I couldn't be a risk-taker. When you return to yourself, you return to routine daily life.

When the body had been reclaimed and they had "returned" to themselves, the women tended to once again personalize emotions and bodily phenomena and to attribute them to their own bodies rather than to artifice or to the couple's nature. In this way, the reintegration of the body also signified the end of their tendency to explain physical phenomena by reference to external sources. Hence, when Daniella became ill with Crohn's disease soon after delivering her couple's child, and Belle suffered from a stomach infection several weeks postpartum, they both interpreted their illnesses as their own body's reaction to the strain that they had endured in surrogacy.

Emotionality was similarly personalized. For example, tearfulness was ascribed to the surrogate's own "natural hormones" resurfacing from their dormant status. As Tsila remarked, "I cried the day after because I thought I was losing her [the intended mother] as a friend, but my sister told me that it was just my hormones, like in a regular birth, and then it passed." As in all mentions of post-surrogacy blues, Tsila is careful to describe her tears as relating not only to her nature resurfacing but also to her friendship with her intended mother. None of the women ever interpreted their emotionality as a sign of attachment to the baby: postpartum emotionality, viewed as potentially overwhelming, reinforced the importance of the divisions they had established and the importance of keeping their own "nature" dormant during the pregnancy.

Several surrogates also reported being surprised by a painful engorgement of the breasts several days after the birth. Yet despite the medical explanation that a childbearing woman's milk does not usually come in until three to four days after she gives birth, the surrogates were often surprised to experience any signs at all of lactation. Surrogates interpreted the body's refusal to lactate immediately postpartum as proof of their detachment during the pregnancy, and it convinced them of the success of their mapping techniques, for they were able to stave off expressions of the "natural body" until their surrogacy "labor" was done. At the same time, however, the sudden, uncontrollable tears and the milk secretions represented a danger to the idea that the surrogates wanted to convey about relinquishment being a non-traumatic event: indeed, in rare cases when surrogates have refused to relinquish, some have explained their change of heart by saying, "My hormones changed."[12]

The surrogates' strategic management of detachments and selective connections thus encompasses rhetorical and embodied strategies to manage emotions that they must constantly keep in check so as not to disrupt their carefully molded conceptual models. Their constant strategizing, neutralizing, categorizing, and selective personalization require careful cognitive, emotional, and physical effort. Their orchestration of the body map belies the idea that surrogacy is a simple task; it makes the references to rented wombs, outsourced wombs, and gestational "carriers" that are so popular in surrogacy discourse seem not only derogatory but also severely misrepresentational of women's actual undertakings. More than the womb is involved in their fulfillment of surrogacy; so also is a full repertoire of painstaking skills.

CONTRACTED CONSTRAINTS

In addition to managing the imagined internal boundary within their body that separates them from the fetus, surrogates used a variety of strategies to maintain a clear boundary between themselves and the couple. With their boundaries in place and using the skills discussed above, the women were able to manage a situation that could otherwise be interpreted as one of total invasion and colonization of their bodies and lives.

Specifically, standard contracts create circumstances in which surrogates are confined in their behavior, medicalized to a notable degree, and constructed as commodities to be bought and sold.[13] Indeed, in many ways, surrogacy arrangements have the potential to fulfill the prophecies that radical feminist commentators made regarding the process in the 1980s.[14] Gestational surrogacy, whereby conception depends on IVF technology and the intervention of fertility specialists, is a strictly medicalized process from beginning to end. After completing the medical treatments entailed in the conceptive process, surrogates must comply with the structure of prenatal care. Since Israeli prenatal care is notably centered on the detection of fetal anomalies,[15] Israeli gynecologists often recommend that surrogates undergo prenatal tests ranging from ultrasounds and blood tests to invasive procedures such as amniocentesis. Most contemporary contracts include the surrogate's agreement to undergo amniocentesis or chorionic villus sampling (CVS) if requested by the couple or recommended by the doctor.[16]

In addition, in certain cases, doctors recommend surgical procedures such as embryo reduction (if conception results in more than two fetuses), termination (if certain fetal anomalies are detected), and cesarean operation. In standard contracts in Israel, surrogates are contractually obliged to agree to any and all of these procedures; even though surrogates are protected by the patients' rights law and cannot be forced to agree to such an intervention, refusal is considered a breach of the surrogacy contract. Surrogates are therefore implicitly forced to comply because they would otherwise have to reimburse a couple for all payments made until that point and to pay them an additional fine amounting to thousands of shekels.

The surrogate is also contractually obligated to take any medicines prescribed by the doctor exactly as instructed. Not taking a prescribed medication as indicated can constitute a breach of contract. On her part, if she wants to take any drug at all, even an aspirin, she must first ask the doctor's permission. If the fetus is in danger, the surrogate can be ordered hospitalized or confined to bed rest for any portion of the pregnancy. I have met several surrogates who were hospitalized for up to six weeks or put on bed rest for long periods of time—factors that affected their own families and children. One surrogate was confined to a hospital two hours from her home for the last two months of the pregnancy after complications developed; she had to make constant provisions to ensure that her two young children were cared for by her ex-husband, her sister, and various friends.

In many contracts, surrogates also agree to engage in or forgo certain "freedoms" of the body, including smoking, eating certain foods, and having sexual intercourse. All Israeli surrogacy contracts include the surrogate's agreement not to smoke for the duration of the contract, from the first treatment through delivery, and the surrogacy committee will not approve a contract if a surrogate is known to smoke. Standard contracts even include the surrogate's agreement to undergo a blood test after the child is born to discover whether she has violated this provision. A lawyer who arbitrates these contracts explained to me that if a child is born underweight or with a suspected smoking-related problem, and the blood test shows that the surrogate smoked during the pregnancy, then she is in breach of contract and must return the money she was paid and even pay a fine. In practice, I have never heard of this provision being enforced, and I have met several surrogates who did smoke while they were pregnant. However, the provision created pressures on surrogates, and in one case I followed, a surrogate agreed to her couple's request that she submit to surprise urine tests after she admitted to them that she had been tempted to resume her smoking habit.

Moreover, standard surrogacy contracts include the surrogate's agreement not to engage in sexual intercourse during the twenty days surrounding each IVF attempt. While some earlier contracts I encountered included the woman's agreement not to have sexual intercourse throughout the pregnancy, current contracts specify that she should not have intercourse during the pregnancy without using a condom. A significant number of surrogacy contracts involving Orthodox Jewish couples include the surrogate's agreement to maintain certain religious standards during the process. The lawyer cited above estimated that at least seven contracts he had drawn up required the surrogate to agree to eat only kosher food, fast on Yom Kippur (unless medically prohibited), and to go to the ritual bath [*mikvah*] before each embryo transfer.

Surrogates also encounter constraints that arise from their relationship with the intended parents. Even in the most amicable surrogate-couple relationships, tensions often arise over issues concerning the surrogate's body. Sometimes a couple uses the contract to pressure the surrogate to comply with their wishes, but at other times the issues in contention are not mentioned in the contract at all. One central issue is whether or not the surrogate should give birth by elective cesarean. I have seen cases in which a surrogate prefers a cesarean but the intended parents want her to have a vaginal birth because they believe it will benefit the baby. In other cases, couples try to persuade the surrogate to have a cesarean in the thirty-eighth week so that they do not have to wait out a full-term pregnancy.

In most surrogacy contracts, only one physician is appointed to accompany both the surrogate and the couple through the process and to represent both parties' interests, so the potential for conflicts of interest is great. In the cases I followed, this arrangement also made the doctor the central mediator of conflicts. For instance, doctors often became involved in mediating conflicts over whether the surrogate should travel during pregnancy. Couples routinely became upset if their surrogate wanted to travel by car or bus to a distant location while pregnant with their child. In numerous cases, this issue was debated so heatedly by surrogate and couple that it was only resolved by their doctor's intervention. In two cases, the doctor acceded to the intended mother's pleas to recommend that the surrogate forfeit her plans, and in two other cases, doctors acceded to the surrogate's wishes and reassured the intended mother that the surrogate would not endanger the pregnancy by traveling.

Surrogates also reported arguments with their couples over their conduct while pregnant, such as going out to pubs, taking their medicines at the appropriate times, and not answering their cell phones every time the intended mother called. Some couples reportedly even tried to control who surrogates dated. When an IVF cycle failed, couples would sometimes become suspicious that the surrogate was at fault for not taking her medications on time or for missing a dose. Surrogates were offended by such accusations. Sometimes intended mothers were so concerned about their surrogates working too much, being overtired, or taking unnecessary chances that they asked the doctor to prescribe bed rest. Eva's couple was so worried about her riding on her motor scooter while pregnant with their twins that they gave her their car for the latter half of the pregnancy. With these constant intrusions into their personal space and these constraints on their freedom, surrogates had to keep vigilant guard over their personal boundaries.

MAPPING INTERPERSONAL BOUNDARIES

Surrogates employed many of the same skills explored in the preceding discussion to map out a sense of personal space in the body and ward off the potential feeling of being invaded, exposed, or controlled by the couple, the contract, and the medical routine. Each woman erected a symbolic "stop sign" on her body that demarcated the boundary that others were not to cross. Masha described this boundary as a "red line":

> I think everyone learns where the red line is. There are some private things that a woman wants to keep private. About her body, physical things. For instance, intimate [physical] examinations and that sort of stuff. I think that the couple might want to accompany the surrogate in all of the process, but you have to say *stop* [here she used the English term]. . . . There are things that must be kept separate for the surrogate's privacy. . . . That is why it is important to define those types of things, because when those lines are crossed, it is really frustrating and angering.

The "red line" that Masha refers to was not only invisible, abstract, and different for each surrogate, but it could also shift in what might appear to an observer to be contradictory ways. That is, a surrogate might willingly submit to objectively invasive requests from her couple but object to less obviously intrusive behavior. Tamar, for instance, had no problem undergoing any prenatal screening requested of her, including amniocentesis, but she felt it was crucial that her couple not impinge on her sense of freedom: "I'll tell you something that made it easier for me with this couple. . . . I could tell from the first time that I saw her that she wouldn't be stuck to me twenty-four hours a day. Because . . . I've always liked my freedom. It's very important to me. And she likes her freedom too. I never pestered her, and she never pestered me."

All of the surrogates I spoke to had different definitions of what they considered to be boundary-crossing behavior. Some wanted their intended mother to phone them several times a day, while others preferred they speak together only once a week. One surrogate had no problem divulging intimate details about her personal history, which included several elective abortions, two failed marriages, and spousal abuse, but she refused to let her couple see photos of her own children, let alone meet them in person. Another surrogate did not mind eating the organic vegetables that her intended mother bought for her and asked her to consume, but she refused to stop drinking regular cola, even when indications of gestational diabetes surfaced and her doctor and couple requested that she limit her consumption of the drink. Still another surrogate had no problem obliging her Orthodox couple's wishes that she immerse herself in the ritual bath [*mikvah*], eat kosher foods, and not travel on the Sabbath, but she drew the "red line" when they asked her to abstain from sexual relations (even with protection) throughout the entire pregnancy.

Maintaining the boundary, wherever it was positioned, involved three strategies: detaching, activating the boundary, and discursively eliminating it. The first strategy involved considering any potentially invasive procedures enacted on the body to be noninvasive because they involved body parts the women did not consider to be under their own jurisdiction during surrogacy. When I asked Sapir, for instance, why she had agreed to undergo certain invasive genetic tests, she explained that she couldn't refuse because the tests concerned a part of the body that belonged to the couple—the embryo—and the belly that she had detached:

Sapir: It isn't my business. . . . It is her child; what right do I have to keep her from doing what she decides?

Elly: But it is your body.

Sapir: Now that is why you need to decide beforehand if you want to get into it or not. . . . For instance, if G-d forbid something went wrong for me during the pregnancy and the child was breech and I needed a cesarean, and I was against surgery or something. Do you think I would refuse? . . . Look, you enter into the process when all of the ingredients are theirs, not yours. I mean, it is they who decide, not you. I was really scared, for instance, [about] the comprehensive ultrasound and the nuchal translucency test. And what if the results were bad and I would have to abort? . . . So, of course, that would have affected me, but it isn't my decision.

Sapir's idea that decisions regarding certain areas of her body belong to the couple alone overrides any hesitation she may have stemming from her own discomfort or from the possible consequences of a particular test. As she is very well aware, the prenatal tests could reveal a fetal anomaly and result in the termination of the pregnancy; then Sapir would not receive the majority of the payment that she was promised for a live birth.

Other surrogates also answered my questions about refusing invasive procedures by stating that "the decision isn't mine" because the procedure involves "something that is theirs [the couple's]." Responsibility for such decisions, thus, was completely identified with the couple rather than with the surrogate. Shinkman reports a case in which a couple decided to terminate their surrogate's pregnancy at twenty-seven weeks because of a major fetal abnormality and only informed the surrogate of their their decision after it had been finalized. In that case, the surrogate so fully thought of the pregnancy and of any decisions relating to it as belonging to the couple and not to her that she did not even express alarm that she had not been consulted.[17]

The second strategy that surrogates used to maintain the "red lines" involved activating signposts around their personalized spaces that said "this is my body" and "do not cross." This frequently occurred during vaginal ultrasounds. Surrogates often felt torn between the desire for privacy and the knowledge that their couple wanted to see the image of their child. Neta decided to allow both members of her couple to attend the ultrasound: "I also allowed him, the husband, to go into all of the checkups. Even in the beginning, the vaginal checkups. . . . But I still agreed that he come in, because it was important to me that they both feel that it is their child. . . . If that [the ultrasound] is the little bit that they have, then how can I refuse?"

In negotiating such situations, the surrogate activated the body map in a way that simultaneously allowed the couple (or intended mother) to connect to the fetus and protected the boundaries of the parts of her body that she equated with her private self. For Neta, this was accomplished by covering the areas of the body she didn't want to expose: "So they would leave him [the father] outside for a moment, put a blanket on me, set me up, and call him to enter, so he can see. Even though I didn't always feel comfortable with it. But it is theirs! And I will do everything so that they can feel like they belong to it."

The boundary between public and private parts of the body was drawn differently by each woman, but all of the women agreed that the lines they had secured must be respected. Idit, who also encouraged both members of her couple to observe ultrasounds, described where she drew the line:

> Of course, everything [was] in modesty and privacy. . . . If they would do a gynecological exam, then I would prevent her from entering, not to look, because it is . . . I am a modest woman from that perspective. . . . It is my body and my soul. There is a boundary. So she respected that very well. . . . She participated in the delivery with me. But she didn't stand . . . opposite. Where it is supposed to come out."

Maintaining the boundary around the private body and self—whether by covering the body or diverting the gaze of others—enabled Neta and Idit to feel respected and protected in situations in which they might otherwise have felt that their privacy had been invaded. For others, the problematic nature of such situations was obviated by a third strategy, which involved the surrogate discursively making herself into an invisible link between the intended mother and the baby, so that, temporarily, no boundaries existed between them and, therefore, no potential for trespass existed. Lihi, for instance, reframed her nakedness in her intended mother's presence as a nonissue because she was not the focus of attention:

> To do the embryo transfer next to her, or to take off my clothes in front of her, or to undergo something else next to her. Or the vaginal ultrasound. Okay, so it is something that has to be done, and it is her child. I am the instrument here. I am the mediator. I am not the *issue* [in English] here. I mean, there is something else. I am not the center. That's all.

Although nakedness could be divorced from sexuality and intrusiveness while the surrogate was pregnant, it was clear to all that this situation was a temporary one. Accordingly, when Daniella gave birth to her couple's child, she felt no inhibitions at encouraging her intended father to witness the delivery from "that end." However, as soon as the baby emerged, she immediately returned to her former, everyday boundaries: "The midwife made a motion to lift my gown and check my breast and I immediately pushed her hand out of the way. It kind of took everyone by surprise. It was just an instinct. It was like suddenly I didn't want him [the intended father] to see. My body had returned."

Daniella's account reveals the discursive nature of the erasure of boundaries; the modesty, intimacy, and privacy that Daniella formerly associated with parts of her body resurfaced immediately after the birth and closed access to those parts. Other cases in which intimate body parts are first emptied and then recoded with sexual and social meanings may help to illuminate the bodily negotiations occurring during surrogacy. Henslin and Biggs analyzed the ways in which routine vaginal examinations by male doctors are conducted in ways that denude the encounter of sexual connotations. They note that women routinely allow male gynecologists—often strangers—to insert a speculum or their fingers into the vagina. They explain this momentary boundary crossing by suggesting that social roles and scripts of patient, doctor, and nurse, together with the props and methods deployed (such as the use of drapes, various spatial and temporal arrangements, etc.) all work to support the identification of the interaction as nonsexual.[18] Accordingly, the operationalization of the body map erases the regular cultural conventions surrounding a particular type of interaction and enables temporary boundary crossings that are only socially permitted to occur in the medical clinic or hospital during the out-of-the-ordinary process of surrogacy.

None of the above-mentioned boundary-maintenance techniques could be upheld without the cooperation of the couple. Yet even when couples respected the surrogate's boundaries, they sometimes misconstrued one type of interaction as invasive and nullified the intrusiveness of another seen by the surrogate as objectionable. For instance, Idan and Maya told me that they had demanded that their surrogate stop smoking, that she undergo all of the prenatal tests that they wanted her to have, and that she have the procedures performed by a particular doctor. Idan explained, "With the amnio and all, we can't force her to do it, it is her right to her body, but it was clear to all sides that it was part of the agreement."

However, alongside these demands on her body, both of them felt that it was very important to respect their surrogate's integrity. Idan added, "When we went to the [the doctor] I wouldn't go in. They threw me out, and Maya would be in back of the curtain. The fetus belonged to us but she [the surrogate] doesn't belong to us." When I asked Maya if she touched their surrogate's belly, she reiterated her husband's perspective, saying, "We don't have the right to touch. She would ask us if we wanted to. It was very important to me to protect her privacy. It is her body. . . . I don't think I have the right to do that."

Riki, an intended mother, spoke of her own perception of the boundaries of her surrogate's body. Both Riki and her husband attended all medical checkups with their surrogate, including the vaginal ultrasound: "In the beginning, she didn't know if she wanted him to come in, but it happened in such a natural way. You know, she lays down and removes her clothes. He stands next to her, and it is okay." However, while Riki naturalized her surrogate's nakedness, she felt uncomfortable touching her:

> Yes, I put out my hand and softly touch [her belly] when I see her. I say shalom to this one and shalom to that one [twin fetuses]. Look, my desire is to . . . but it is her body and I don't allow myself to. I mean, if I touch her, then, you know, I ask. I don't just do it all the time! Because it is an intimate thing. I mean, it is a body, and a body has its own rules. You cannot invade it. . . . It [the body] has boundaries. And even though there is an intimate relationship between us, because we share the same blood in the end really, but she isn't my husband. I don't feel comfortable touching her. So what I do is I hug her sometimes, give her a kiss.

Maya's, Idan's, and Riki's comments reveal slight differences in their perceptions of the surrogate's body from surrogates' own perceptions. The surrogates were usually sure of the demarcation lines that divided their bodies and were thus uninhibited for the most part in allowing one or both members of their couple to gaze at or touch their disengaged belly. Couples, however, and intended mothers, in particular, saw touching the surrogate's belly as a type of invasion. Unaware of the surrogate's carefully mapped bodily order, they did not have a clear perception of whether or not they were overstepping their welcome, colonizing or overtaking the surrogate's body.

As a result, intended mothers who were not in sync with their surrogate's boundary logic would sometimes inadvertently cross the surrogate's boundaries, unaware that their behavior went beyond the limits that the surrogate had allocated. It was these conflicts in perception that underscored the majority of tensions between couples and surrogates; an extreme scenario in which this occurred is detailed in the next section and illustrates the possible consequences of such conflicting boundary logics.

THE BODY AS ENEMY: SIMA'S STORY

I have argued that, by employing cognitive "maps" of classifications, by doing careful emotion work directed at detaching themselves from the fetus, and by erecting "red lines," surrogates are able to deal with the many intrusions, submissions, and challenges that they are faced with. The intrusions are structurally unavoidable because gestational surrogacy in Israel is a necessarily commodified, medicalized, and technologically controlled process in which surrogates are bound by a strict and harnessing contract. Consequently, I suggest that, if a surrogate does not have an explicit map of classifications and boundaries in place, she runs the risk of "losing her self" in the body.

By looking at an atypical, extreme case that departs from those described thus far, we can consider the extent to which surrogacy can be a harsh and scarring experience when surrogates are unable to operationalize the skills discussed in the preceding sections. Sima, age thirty-four, was the first woman to become a surrogate in Israel, and her personal story was recorded in every national newspaper. Her couple garnered additional attention by marketing the story to both a national newspaper and a documentary filmmaker halfway through the pregnancy. The film was broadcast on Israel's Channel 2, and the intended mother's personal surrogacy journal was published in a national newspaper soon after the birth. Sima's retrospective portrayal of her surrogacy experience must be understood in light of this latter development: she had believed that the intended mother genuinely cared for her despite her overprotective behavior, but she discovered otherwise after reading the journal. When I first attempted to interview Sima not long after she gave birth to surrogate twins, I turned off the tape recorder and changed the subject only fifteen minutes into the conversation because it was too difficult for Sima to speak about it. In the years that followed, Sima and I remained in contact, speaking by phone and visiting about twice a year. Six years after the birth, I was finally able to interview her, but only when I brought along a friend to help me.

At the time she became a surrogate, Sima had a son, a toddler, and she had been involved with her then-future husband since age seventeen. She and her husband now have two more children. My account of Sima's story derives mainly from an interview that was published in a local paper, but also draws from my own conversations with her. From the outset of her surrogacy, Sima felt she was slowly losing control of her body as her couple took over. Both members of the couple administered the hormone treatment preparatory injections to her buttocks, causing her pain: "The husband at least was a combat medic and knew how to do it. Esti [the wife] would shake, get confused, more than once she caused internal hemorrhages in my buttocks."[19]

Unable or unaware of the need to erect boundary signposts early on, Sima felt herself slowly being colonized by her intended mother. At first she enjoyed the intended mother's attempts to merge with her, interpreting it as a sign of nurturing. During the embryo implantation, she said, "Esti leaned on me, and for a moment it seemed as though she was asking for my pain to stop or to be transferred onto her. I felt like she empathized with me and it did my heart good, but it didn't stop the pain, which was unbearable."[20] However, as the pregnancy progressed, Sima increasingly felt as though her body was being taken over. Subjected to her couple's repeated attempts to control her and dictate her conduct, Sima experienced her body as being "occupied" to the point that no private areas remained.

Whereas some surrogates told me they welcomed one or both members of their couple to the vaginal ultrasound after signaling where they had drawn their "red lines," Sima felt she had no choice in the matter. When her intended father accompanied her to this checkup, she felt embarrassed and powerless to refuse his presence: "It embarrassed me that he was present when they did the vaginal ultrasound. I couldn't refuse his presence in the room, but I felt that from the moment that I became a surrogate I was no longer standing alone, on my own. I was part of them, and I couldn't prevent him from participating in this experience just because he is a man." Sima's boyfriend, Ofer, saw her belly as coming between them: "From the minute he found out that I was pregnant, he stopped having sex with me. He felt disgusted by me, by my belly, by my actions."[21]

In the fourth month of the pregnancy, Sima moved with her small son, but without Ofer, into an apartment attached to her couple's house, after telling friends and family that they were going abroad. Sima began to feel like a prisoner in their home as well as a prisoner in her own body. The boundaries between private and public were disrupted in the home as well as in her body, and rather than being bounded off in relation to her other organs, her belly instead took over her entire being, making her a "walking belly":

> I didn't go outside, and when I did, I acted like an escaped prisoner. I wore sunglasses and walked quickly. Most of the time I sat at home, rotting and wilting. I disconnected from all of my friends. . . . I felt choked, lonely, horrible frustration because my independence was taken from me. I had no privacy. Whenever they wanted they would enter my house. The phone line was shared and more than once I felt like they were listening to my conversations. They didn't allow me to move, to clean, to cook. They expected me to sit all day with my legs crossed reading magazines. They didn't want to believe that this was not a normal situation for a pregnant woman. That there is a person in back of this belly.[22]

Sima's portrayal of being trapped within the couple's home like a prisoner contrasts sharply with other surrogates' enforcement of their "red lines." The distance and space that the body map afforded other surrogates makes Sima's depiction of forced stagnation and surveillance all the more jarring. As the couple's occupation of her body and her life expanded, and as her self was increasingly subdued and "suffocated" in the body, Sima began to long for any route of escape:

> Several times I had the thought that I wish I was dead now, I wish a car would run me over. But it remained a thought. One Friday I felt especially suffocated. A friend called and invited me over for Shabbat. . . . Ten minutes later he [the intended father] called me angrily and said he didn't want me to go, that if I went he wouldn't give me the 1,200 shekels, which was the monthly salary they gave me for doing nothing. I was so angry that I forgot to ask how he even knew that I was going to go. He lost control and threatened me that if I go I won't return. From my point of view, that was the sack that broke the camel's back. I was in a state of nervous breakdown. I screamed, I tore out my hair, I hit my belly, I threw chairs. What had I asked? For my freedom? The neighbors heard the screams. I know that someone called here and said they should stop torturing me, and where is their soul?[23]

She moved to an apartment in another city but still felt trapped. Her presence in her body almost completely diminished, Sima began to see the body itself as enemy territory and expressed her rebellion against its colonizers by taking destructive actions against it. In her eighth month, Sima reached a point of crisis; she demanded to be taken to the hospital, where she took a knife and threatened to cut her belly to extract her couple from her body: "I couldn't do it anymore. I wanted to die. I took a razor and played with it. I thought I would cut the veins, cut the belly. The social worker saw this game and notified the doctor, who decided it was time to deliver me."[24]

Sima's threat resounded in newspaper headlines, one of which read, "I wanted to cut my belly and my veins." When I asked her whether she had really wanted to commit suicide, she explained, "I just wanted to warn them. I wanted to be free from them already. To get the fetuses out of my belly and the couple out of my soul." The couple, she told me, "crawled into my skin. My blood, not just my skin. Him too. Him more than her." Sima's body-centered language reveals how strongly her sense of invasion contrasted with the sense of security conferred by the demarcation lines other surrogates inscribed on their body maps: she describes the couple as infesting her soul and her blood, both areas of the body map that other surrogates vehemently personalized and protected from surrogacy. Sima reflected on why she had been unable to protect herself:

I tried not to think about them, but you can't detach your soul from your body. I guess it is an art. . . . I don't know how you can do it. I really wanted to do it. I thought I had succeeded, but I didn't succeed enough, I guess. Alone at least. I guess by trying not to think about it I hurt myself without even noticing. Because it all hit me with a boom. Only after. Not during.

Unlike the other surrogates I met, Sima felt a connection to the children she had carried: she "remembered" the twins she had borne through the inscriptive memory of her body's surface. She told me, "I saw them on television, and suddenly I understood that they were in my belly. It was the first time that I saw them. And I felt an emptiness in my belly, in my hands." When I asked her if she thought about them, she said, "Sometimes. I dream about them." "In your subconscious," I said. "Yes," she confirmed, "I dream about them a lot at night. They come to me in my dreams. I think about them. What they are doing now, how old they are. But more than that I live with the humiliation I went through, with the way they treated me. That is what really left a mark on me."

The mark of the couple's disrespect for her "gift"—more than the babies themselves—left a scar on her conscience that she struggled to efface: "In my subconscious, it is all there. The problem is that I didn't see them, but I heard them. I heard them taking babies out of my belly. . . . I heard them crying. And that was it. It [the crying] disappeared. You understand? Maybe it is better not. Who knows how I would have reacted? I don't know." A year after the surrogacy birth, I asked Sima how she felt about surrogacy in retrospect: "When I see a baby in the street, I get the shivers. I kind of envy them [her couple], now they have two babies and their lives are full. Mine is now empty."

Six years later, Sima still received disability payments from the National Insurance Institute (Israel's Social Security) for emotional damage she incurred as a result of the experience. Unlike the majority of other surrogates, who have seen the babies they bore, Sima has had no face-to-face contact with the twins and does not maintain any relation with the couple. She remembers the surrogacy experience with bitterness and feels that its emotional repercussions made it difficult for her to conceive her second child, forcing her to rely on fertility treatments. I will never forget, when I called her cell phone a few days after the birth of her second child, how her husband answered and whispered to me: "Elly, I am so worried. She isn't bonding with the child. She is apathetic, she has no feelings. I knew that the surrogacy would do this."

I asked Sima to explain how her pregnancies with her own three children had differed from the surrogate pregnancy. Her answer reflects what is at stake in being in control versus being controlled—and the benefits of the body map:

> [When it is your own pregnancy] it is yours. You feel that it is yours. There is no threat, no one is waiting around the corner to take it. No one is controlling your life. It was totally different. You feel it at the moment of birth. It's another world. I thought that it would be almost the same thing but it isn't. And then everything fell down, boom, in my face. No one prepared me for it. Everything floated up and surfaced. Like shit. Like a block in the sewage. It can't be fully blocked.

Sima's story presents a stark picture of the potential consequences of surrogacy on the surrogate's well-being. I stress that Sima's experience is atypical of the majority of cases I studied and that I heard no other accounts comparable in their extremity to hers. What made Sima's case end up as it did? Sima did not have less access to psychological support than the other surrogates I interviewed; most surrogates do not exercise their right to psychological counseling during surrogacy, even though all expenses would be covered by their couple. Moreover, even though some surrogates attend monthly support groups or participate in online message boards, no one "taught" them the cognitive and emotional skills they employed during surrogacy. One explanation for the extreme nature of Sima's case might be that the couple had more controlling personalities than other couples did and that the intended father took on a more dominant role than in other cases I followed. Sima herself claims that she was not properly screened as a surrogacy candidate because her contract was approved before the surrogacy committee had fully developed its screening criteria. Indeed, she later sued the state, believing that she should not have been allowed to become a surrogate and was not psychologically prepared for the experience. The inexperience of the approvals committee and of the medical staff attending to her particular triad may also have contributed to some of the events that took place. The committee instated several amendments to their guidelines after Sima's story garnered wide media attention.[25]

Most of the surrogates I interviewed described their surrogacy experience positively. Yet Sima's story sheds important light on the potential for acute situations to develop in all surrogacy cases. It underscores the importance of acknowledging the measures surrogates take to protect themselves and recognizing the high stakes they face.

FROM FRAGMENTATION TO DETACHABILITY

The surrogate's individuation of body parts could easily be seen as an extension of the argument that medicalization and reproductive technologies fragment women's bodies and alienate women from their selves. Emily Martin proposes that fragmented images of the body are the product of capitalist perceptions of the body as machine.[26] The mechanical model does not position the body as a unitary entity or as an integral part of the self and the emotions, but as an amalgamation of replaceable pieces that can be moved from person to person and purchased or sold.[27]

Martin argues that, for a woman to become sexually female, her body must become an object to her, entailing an inner fragmentation of the self. Suggesting that "women are not only fragmented into body parts by the practices of scientific medicine, as men are; they are also profoundly alienated from science itself,"[28] Martin adds that women may also suffer the alienation of parts of their self more acutely than men. She exemplifies this idea by making reference to medicalized childbirth, suggesting that the hospital-birthing women she interviewed perceived themselves as submitting passively to having procedures "done to" them, revealing a separation of the self from the body and from physical sensations.[29] They expressed a sense of anxiety over their separation from both the event of childbirth and the child, which generated fragmentation and alienation in their conceptions of body and self. On the basis of her data, Martin argues that women feel alienated from medicalized childbirth in a way that is analogous to and worse than the alienation of a laborer from his or her work.

Balsamo looks at several "technologies of the gendered body," including bodybuilding, reproductive technologies, and cosmetic surgery.[30] She interprets the way that these technologies affect women through media representations, critiquing the technologies for fragmenting the female body into isolated parts and rendering the body itself a visual medium. Extending this discourse into surrogacy, Rothman critiques surrogacy for the implied mind-body dualism and the individualization of body parts that thinking about the practice entails.[31] She regards the capitalist logic that wombs can be "rented" as ludicrous, writing that discourses on surrogacy suggest that it is "as if body parts were rented without renting the woman. But pregnancy is not a condition of an isolated organ. Women experience pregnancy with their whole bodies."[32]

The critiques outlined above are applicable to the situation of the surrogates I interviewed. These women are definitely subject to control of their bodies by state, legal, and medical institutions. Moreover, in a certain sense, they passively have things "done to" them by doctors (IVF, medicalized childbirth), by the state (which selects them to serve as instrumental womb replacements for infertile, married women), and by their couples, with whom they sign legal contracts that constrain their actions and may even harm their basic human right to govern their own bodies.

However, the data I have presented also suggest that fragmentation can be a tool for preventing the surrogate from feeling alienated from her body and from the technological process she participates in. Surrogates do fragment their bodies, objectify certain parts, and conceptualize the body as a visual text (body map) and as a machine (incubator, oven). Yet they do not necessarily feel that this is "done to" them or that it has negative consequences. Instead, enacting the script that Rothman sees as oppressing women—distancing the pregnancy to a specific body part and separating it from the rest of the body[33]—is exactly what enables the surrogate to feel in control of the situation and to maintain a sense of being an integrated whole. This is what Thompson is describing in her discussion of "objectification as agency" in the context of women's practices during medical treatment for infertility.[34] Thompson's concept can be extended here to apply to the contractual constraints of surrogacy and the distancing techniques that surrogate embodiment entails.

In this sense, one might conclude that surrogates pragmatically embrace the self-objectification that technological reproduction is conducive of and that they extend it to participate in a type of "ontological choreography"[35] that goes beyond the clinic. In every aspect of their lives as surrogates, these women choreograph serial moves of *embodiment* (of their personal nature, kin, and parts), *disembodiment* (of the intended mother's nature, kin, and parts), *personalization* (of the desire, intent, and will to conceive, provide for their own kin, and make another woman into a mother), *depersonalization* (of any connection to the fetus), and *reconciliation* (of all of this movement into a coherent identity and for a defined purpose). It would thus be devaluing the surrogate's creative choreography of connections and disconnections to say that she is passively fragmented by technology and by the state. Instead, it is through the divisions she recognizes and her mapping of her body that the surrogate is able to realign the innovative form of maternity that she has created with nature and culture, with her personal goals, and with the pronatalist national ideology of maternal service to the nation.

In a paradoxical way, surrogates may actually have more positive pregnancy experiences than conventionally pregnant women because of the classificatory schemes and emotion work techniques that they apply. Their boundary negotiation tools can be viewed as giving surrogates a sense of control that better prepares them to make pregnancy an empowering experience. Social researchers who study Western women's pregnancy experiences have repeatedly discovered that women feel a lack of control over their bodies during pregnancy as they are "invaded" by strangers and friends prodding and poking their belly with little consideration of their private body boundaries and "occupied" or even "possessed" by the baby/stranger/alien inside them.[36]

In contrast to the experiences of conventionally pregnant women, the majority of the women I studied who underwent surrogate pregnancies came to feel a sense of transcendence through the control they were able to exert over their bodies. They were not "out of control" even for a moment, because their mapped bodies and movements were so carefully choreographed. They were not "fragmented" by pregnancy or "divided" by hospital birth, but they intentionally fragmented their own bodies for strategic purposes, and they strategically encouraged the invisibility of their belly instead of feeling that the belly made them invisible. They were aware from the start that their pregnancy was public rather than private and were thus better prepared to negotiate their limits; they expected, controlled, and even encouraged the "invasion" of their bodies and marked the limits of boundary crossings with their "red lines." They did not feel as though they were being passively "delivered" by doctors[37] but that they were actually *giving birth*. Finally, they did not feel a "loss of self" because their nature, family, and self were carefully protected within the sections of the body map that they partitioned off. The surrogates described "returning to themselves" after surrogacy in relation to getting their pre-pregnancy body back and resuming their ordinary activities, but they preserved their pre-pregnancy identities throughout.

As the data presented here demonstrate, one cannot theorize what surrogacy is about without documenting the experiences of surrogates themselves. The majority of feminist critiques of surrogacy, which are theory driven, can provide insights into surrogates' situations but cannot account for the complexity of their experiences. It is only through empirical data that we are able to comprehend how surrogates subversively undermine medicalization, objectification, and technological fragmentation and transform them from tools of oppression into methods for preserving their sense of integrity, their sense of control over the situation, and their sense of personal space and "freedom" in their occupied bodies.

It is only on the basis of data-driven theorizing that one can discuss agency, as ethnographic studies of reproduction have established.[38] The surrogates display agency along three dimensions that coincide with classic themes:[39] cognition, exhibited in their nature/artifice metaphors and cognitive mapping of the body; emotion, revealed in their intense distancing emotion work vis-à-vis the fetus and in the tone and the active voice they employ in their descriptions of being in control ("I chose," "I did," "I took upon myself"); and practice, displayed in the actions and actual behaviors they undertake, such as creating the metaphors and maps, engaging in distancing techniques, and erecting "red lines" in their body boundary negotiations with their couple.

PART TWO

Connecting

CONTRARY TO ONE POPULAR ASSUMPTION that women hire surrogates as a luxury, to avoid pregnancy and birth, the intended mothers in my study arrived at the decision to pursue surrogacy only after they had explored every other option possible to become pregnant and give birth themselves. This was usually after they had made motherhood the central goal of their adult lives. Similarly to Paxson's observations among infertile women in Athens, Greece,[1] the intended mothers in this study were as focused or more focused on becoming mothers as they were on having children in their lives. The majority of intended mothers in this study were childless; a few had given birth to a child before encountering complications in subsequent pregnancies, and three were raising their husbands' children from prior marriages.

Each intended mother had arrived at the surrogacy option knowing that it was her body, rather than her husband's body, that had prevented the couple from becoming parents. All of the husbands could produce viable sperm, and the majority of the intended mothers could produce viable eggs. It was their inability to conceive or to carry a pregnancy to term that brought the women to surrogacy. Some had been born without a womb or with a misshapen womb, and some had had their womb removed after medical complications. Others had suffered multiple miscarriages or had undergone years of failed fertility treatments, and some chose surrogacy because of severe health problems endangered by pregnancy.[2] Common to all of them was the feeling that they were the ones responsible for the failure of their marriages to produce children and that it was their duty to fix this "problem."

Their lives were consistent with depictions that have emerged from other anthropological studies of women who have encountered involuntary childlessness in terms of their experiences with the emotional hurdles, false hopes, and marital strains that often accompany infertility.[3] Nearly all of the women felt the assault of this "reproductive disruption" on their feminine identity, especially those who had been born without a uterus or had a hysterectomy.[4] Those who underwent fertility treatment before turning to surrogacy had significantly longer "infertility careers"[5] than women generally explored in the ethnographic literature. This was because state subsidization of reproductive technologies in Israel enabled them to afford more fertility treatments than women in other countries, where use of these technologies is either not covered or severely limited by insurance providers. All of the previous infertility patients in my sample underwent a minimum of seven failed IVF cycles before turning to surrogacy.[6] Some who had unexplained infertility underwent as many as thirty IVF attempts over periods spanning up to twenty years before finally turning to surrogacy.

The women's experiences of the stigma of childlessness was compounded by Israel's pronatalist, family-centered culture. Israel has been described as "the land of imperative motherhood,"[7] where motherhood has historically been viewed as a woman's "national mission."[8] The women's childlessness was continuously present in their lives in a way that it might not have been in cultures where being "childfree by choice" is a socially legitimate option. Most people do not hesitate to ask women of childbearing age in Israel if they have children or when they are going to have their next child, in a blunt, direct style known as "dugri speech"; this is not interpreted as rudeness but as an accepted cultural form of relating to others.[9] Most intended mothers described the forced smiles they wore while attending the birth celebrations of family and friends, being subjected to questions from unknowing aunts and uncles at family gatherings, and the unasked-for advice that constantly came their way.

As a result of their struggles to overcome childlessness, many intended mothers were exhausted and emotionally drained by the time they came to the decision to pursue surrogacy; they were not necessarily prepared to find that surrogacy, too, would be a "bumpy road" from the start. The first hurdle they faced usually involved finding a surrogate. Many couples began this search on their own, even if they later turned to a matching agency. When I began my research, couples would advertise for a surrogate in the classified columns of newspapers or even tack up notices in neighborhoods near their homes. Some told me of long periods during which no one answered their ads or the only women who answered were married or otherwise incompatible with the criteria of the Israeli surrogacy law. Intended mothers often found themselves traveling alone or with their husbands to the ends of the country to meet potential surrogates. Most told of many awkward phone calls and meetings or of being stood up after having traveled to an agreed-upon meeting. Some spoke of finding the "perfect match" and of cultivating a relationship with a woman for a significant period only to have that woman decide she didn't want to be a surrogate after all or to have her fail the psychological or medical screening. In a few cases, the surrogate was disqualified by the approvals committee after she and the couple had spent as long as six months becoming invested in one another.

Receiving the surrogacy committee's approval to proceed with the arrangement was no simple task. It took tremendous effort for some intended mothers to establish their eligibility for surrogacy, especially in cases of "unexplained infertility." For example, one intended mother had to argue before the approvals committee that she needed a surrogate even after she had experienced seventeen failed IVF cycles, and another intended mother was told to try one more IVF cycle—her eleventh—before considering surrogacy. Her surrogacy contract was only approved after she miscarried following that last cycle. When the intended mother had a life-threatening disease, such as cancer, the committee was also hesitant to approve a surrogacy contract unless her prognosis was favorable or she had been in remission for a significant period. In cases that departed from the committee's guidelines—for example, when the intended mother was older than the permitted age limit for surrogacy—it was sometimes necessary to challenge the guidelines in court to secure the committee's approval.[10] In general, it took a tremendous amount of effort and determination for couples to reach the stage at which they, and their surrogate, could actually begin fertility treatments; it is telling that a huge gap exists between the number of inquiries into surrogacy and the actual number of files that are submitted in full and approved by the surrogacy committee.[11]

When the embryo transfer attempts finally began, the road was usually no less rocky, marked by failed embryo transfers, ectopic pregnancies, early miscarriages, and other challenges. This section looks at the experiences of intended mothers once a pregnancy is underway. It is during this period that intended mothers begin to take steps toward preparing themselves for motherhood, albeit with apprehension, the disappointments that have paved their way always in the backs of their minds. Chapter 4 explores the intended mother's efforts to connect with her expected child and to formulate a maternal identity. Chapter 5 examines the way body-centered interactions between the surrogate and intended mother lead the latter to experience a vicarious pregnancy.

CHAPTER 4

Intended Mothers and Maternal Intentions

In this chapter, I look at the experiences of intended mothers during the surrogacy process, with a particular focus on their "parental claiming practices." Sandelowski, Harris, and Holditch-Davis employ this concept to refer to the strategies used by those preparing themselves to adopt as they wait for that fateful phone call notifying them that they have become parents.[1] Unlike adoptive mothers, intended mothers through surrogacy have access to the time frame of conventional pregnancy and know their child's history from the moment of conception. I examine two claiming practices that intended mothers in this study employed while awaiting the birth of their child. The first, *kin claiming,* focused on rendering the expected child their own kin. Kin claiming was conducted toward an abstract fetal entity, presenting intended mothers with the dual challenges of cultivating a belief in the "realness"[2] of the "object of expectation"[3] and of trying to form emotional attachments to it. The second practice, *maternal claiming,* involved techniques aimed at claiming entitlement to the social label of mother of the expected baby. Maternal claiming centered on identity building and transformation of one's status into that of mother. Even when an intended mother already *was* a mother before turning to surrogacy, she still exhibited ritual behaviors aimed at privately and publicly designating herself *the* mother of the surrogate child.

The intended mother's entitlement to each of these claims was contested by the unavoidable fact that it was not she but the surrogate who gestated and delivered the child. The surrogates did not see themselves as the child's mother or as competing either for the maternal title or for the baby, and in fact, they spent much of their time trying to relieve themselves of any entitlement through their body-centered delineation practices. Intended mothers, however, were not fully convinced that surrogates did not want to be mothers to the children they gestated; even if the surrogate repeatedly reassured her of this, the intended mother still usually viewed the surrogate's gestation of *her* child as generating potential competing claims.

IDENTIFYING WITH EMBRYOS

Intended mothers shared many general perceptions of motherhood, kinship, and the body with their surrogates. Just as surrogates used the idioms of nature and of genetics to preserve their identities as normative mothers to their own children, intended mothers used these idioms to articulate their own burgeoning maternal identities. Like their surrogates, intended mothers viewed motherhood as a woman's "natural" destiny and genetics as constitutive of "natural" and unquestionable kin ties. Theirs was a "nature" realized through extracorporeal fertilization and pregnancy, but it was still the outcome of what most saw as a "natural" need. Sharon, whose son was carried by a surrogate, justified her choice of surrogacy over adoption in these terms:

> It was very important to me that we have a biological child. That's why I went to surrogacy and not adoption . . . it just seems so natural to you. First of all, a natural need. A natural need like any person has. . . . If it is possible, there are eggs, there is sperm, [and] there are beautiful embryos. Technically I can't carry them, but my child is from my genes; it is just a need of the human race that it be yours.

Much like other persons in treatment for infertility, intended mothers applied genetic idioms to formulate narratives of continuity in their identities when their life course met with reproductive "disruption."[4] Like Sharon, other intended mothers spoke about having "natural" motivations for using technology to reproduce and upheld the idea that they were pursuing "natural" and normative goals and creating a "natural family."[5] In addition, just as surrogates viewed ova as highly personalized, inalienable body parts, intended mothers spoke of their eggs as markers of their ownership of the children that would result from surrogacy.

Their personalization of genetics, in general, and their identification with their ova were often expressed in praise for their eggs, their
husbands' sperm, and the quality of their resultant embryos. Miri, for
instance, asserted that "adoption was never an option" for her, especially since "we have excellent embryos. A lot! Great fertilization rates.
Excellent sperm, excellent eggs." Other women quoted the assessments
of medical personnel. Katya reported that "the lab technician told me
that . . . [mine] were the most perfectly round, great-looking eggs she
had ever seen. It made me feel good that at least my eggs were exceptional." Descriptions of "beautiful," "perfect," or "excellent" genetic
material are also common among women undergoing IVF treatments
in the United States and the United Kingdom and are ways of easing
women's feelings of failure or of being at fault for their childlessness.[6]

This genetics-centered model linked the ways Israeli participants made
sense of kinship and identity in surrogacy. Just as surrogates conceptualized their eggs as consistently personalized parts of their "body maps,"
intended mothers saw their eggs and embryos as reflections of their personal selves and as representations of their expected kin. When either
party spoke about her eggs in our interviews, she was simultaneously
talking about an extension and reflection of her personhood—"a part of
me"—and about the abstract image she held of a future child. This use of
genes as multivocal symbols is compatible with observations that the egg
and sperm have become major cultural icons representing kinship and
identity,[7] masculinity and femininity,[8] and even "life itself."[9]

Use of donor ova was always viewed by intended mothers as an
option of last resort. Several intended mothers that I interviewed only
acquiesced to their doctor's suggestion to use donor ova after they used
up the last batches of their frozen embryos or after their surrogates
had repeatedly failed to become pregnant with their eggs. They also
masked the use of donor ova from those outside the marital dyad. On
the surrogacy Internet forum, for instance, few participants knew that
May's surrogate was carrying an embryo created from a donor egg,
even though May openly shared nearly all other details of her surrogacy
experience. Likewise, when some intended mothers told me during
interviews that frozen embryos had been used in their surrogacies, I had
the distinct feeling that they might be concealing the use of donor ova.
This hesitancy to divulge the use of donor ova is consistent with the
masking of egg donation in the Western popular media, which depict
the miraculous births of twins to postmenopausal celebrities without
ever mentioning of the use of donor ova.[10] This trend has also been

documented in anthropological studies of secrecy among families using donor ova and sperm.[11]

Among the five women in my sample who openly discussed their use of donor ova, accessing a genetic link by proxy was cited as crucial to their kin-claiming process. Roni explained that she wanted to pursue surrogacy with egg donation because "at least if it is from my husband's sperm it will be 50 percent mine." Likewise, when Jenny's sister offered to be her traditional surrogate—an undertaking that they were able to carry out using their English citizenship, thus bypassing the Israeli surrogacy law—she remarked, "Daniella and I look so much alike that it is as if it is my child anyway." This fixation on genetics and resemblance as means of asserting kin ties is similar to that observed by Hayden in the case of lesbian kinship.[12] She notes that, because lesbian partners who start a family together cannot both be genitors of their child, they often find ways to simulate genetic kin ties with the co-mother who is not carrying the baby. They either ask a blood relative of the co-mother to donate sperm or choose a sperm donor with the same skin tone and hair and eye color as the co-mother.

For intended mothers who used donor ova, donor choice also served as a medium for facilitating their kin-claiming process. For instance, although most of the intended mothers who used donor eggs had anonymous donors, they were interested in obtaining information about their donors that could help them begin to imagine their future child. Even if they could not garner any specific details about the donor, knowing the general profile of the donor population made it easier to identify with the donor and with the baby. Usually, all they knew about the anonymous donor was her phenotype and where she was from in Eastern Europe, where the eggs were purchased at offshore, Israeli-run clinics.[13] Nili chose to buy ova online from a U.S. agency, even though it was much more expensive than the Eastern European option, because the U.S. donors were not anonymous. She chose a donor whose coloring resembled hers and whose online profile seemed to communicate a "cute personality." Her choice illuminates the importance of being able to identify a reflection of one's self in the egg and of cultivating a tentative kin connection to the awaited child on the basis of resemblance. Nili's identification with her donor began immediately; she told me, "I am already falling in love with her. I dream about her at night."

Whether the egg came from her own body or from a donor, the intended mother in each case attempted to create a symbolic link to the embryo gestated in the surrogate's body. When the intended mother is genetically linked to her future child and the egg is harvested from her body, then the embryo becomes an extracorporeal part, or site, of her body and self. Yet even when she does not have such a link, the partial genetic link through the husband and imaginings about potential donors work to create identification with the embryo as a symbolic representation of the expected child. As in the case of the infertility patients studied by Becker,[14] this "elusive embryo" becomes the intended mother's focus, the one figure she can grasp in her mind during this liminal time. The icon of the embryo, rather than an image of the baby and of herself as a mother, marks the limit of her horizon.

SONOGRAPHIC PROJECTIONS

The iconic embryo remains abstract and ambiguous throughout the first stages of fetal development. This notion is reflected in how easily women veered between personifying the embryo and reluctantly engaging with the fetus. For example, one intended mother told me that while transferring her frozen embryos between hospitals, she handled the nitrogen tank delicately, "as if they were my children already." However, the same intended mother described her hesitancy, once her surrogate was pregnant, to bond with the *fetus* and to fully trust that it would eventually develop into a *baby*. What remained constant in the claiming process was that the intended mother focused on images, projections, ideas, and icons rather than on the material presence of a living, growing fetus in her surrogate's womb. Her maternal claiming practices were more about expanding her potential for transition to motherhood than about actual identity change, and her kin claiming was more about identification than about forming emotional attachments to an expected child.

Ultrasound played a significant role in the women's attempts to grasp the "realness" of their expected child. Once regular ultrasound scans had commenced, the intended mother was able to access material objects (photos) representing her future child. She also had the opportunity during scans to position herself as an actor within the narrative of the child's development. Surrogates were complicit in facilitating these objectives, for just as they used ultrasound to visualize their own separation and detachment from the fetal image, they also viewed the sonogram as providing an important opportunity for the couple to "meet" their fetus. Lying in the supine position while the sonographer decoded the images on screen, the surrogate would symbolically "step aside" to create a space for the couple to take center stage, becoming an audience witnessing their excited response to the sonogram, much like the pregnant women in Sandelowski's study did vis-à-vis their husbands.[15]

This act of "stepping aside" made room for the intended mother to "perform" in the cultural drama of the ultrasound: to enact the role of a soon-to-be mother viewing her soon-to-be child. While the ultrasound may, arguably, demote the body of the pregnant woman to a secondary order of significance,[16] the technology also enables the surrogate to promote the intended mother's experience to a privileged position. Indeed, if visualization technologies such as the fetal ultrasound have been critiqued for exposing the interior of the pregnant woman's body to visual inspection, leaving her bodily boundaries thoroughly transparent,[17] in surrogacy, it is this transparency that enables the intended mother to conceptualize the fetus apart from the surrogate and to access the role she covets.

In her discussion of the enhanced experience of the fetus that the technology affords expectant fathers, Sandelowki suggests that ultrasonography is "an enabling mechanism that permits them access to a female world from which they have been excluded because of their limited biological role in reproduction."[18] In fact, the ritual behavior of intended mothers in relation to the photos produced during ultrasound exhibited just such linking qualities. Specifically, intended mothers considered the ultrasound photos representations of the fetus and of the pregnancy that they could carry with them, keep in their homes, and symbolically retain close to their bodies and selves. As artifacts depicting the fetus as an independent entity floating in free space,[19] these photos served as technovisual "proof" of the fetus's existence and enabled the intended mother to create a fiction of "holding" her child, at least in terms of this one symbolic representation.

Natali, for instance, kept the photos in a file on a shelf in her living room: "I would keep them right here and I would look at them all the time." Other intended mothers displayed the photos in places where they could be regularly viewed, representing the "presence" of the fetus within the home. During my first interview with Riki, she asked me if I wanted to "meet her twins." Puzzled, I followed her to the kitchen, where a recent ultrasound photograph had been posted on the refrigerator door. Stroking the photograph lovingly, she explained: "This way I can wish them good morning and put them to sleep at night." Similarly, an intended mother interviewed in a national newspaper after her surrogate's pregnancy was terminated revealed that she had marked the end of her own symbolic gestation by immediately removing all of the ultrasound photos from her refrigerator and "burying" them in a drawer.[20]

In another variation on this theme, Yael carried her ultrasound photos everywhere she went, holding them close to her body. She told me that she would look at them only infrequently, fearing that, if she looked too much, the images would not manifest as a baby. Agreeing to show them to me, she carefully removed an envelope from her purse, delicately handling the photos as though they contained some intrinsic part of the child. This pregnancy ended in miscarriage, and during her surrogate's next pregnancy, Yael told me that she did not look at the ultrasound photos too often for fear of the "evil eye."

Yael's behavior surrounding the ultrasound photos reveals the abstract and ambiguous nature of her parental claiming practices. On the one hand, the photos enable her to vicariously carry and protect the fetus close to her body and in her own home, serving as prosthetic artifacts of her experience of the pregnancy. On the other hand, this "authoritative proof" of fetal existence does not ease her fears that the pregnancy might not result in a live birth. Her reaction reflects what Taylor identifies as the essential paradox of ultrasound technology: it encourages maternal claiming at the same time that it makes pregnancy more tentative, since it can detect fetal anomalies that might lead to the termination of the pregnancy.[21] This paradox is compounded by the "evil eye" beliefs common among Jewish-Israeli childbearing women.[22]

MATERNAL CLAIMING RITUALS

The intended mother's position can be further understood through a comparison with other nonnormative transitions to motherhood. In her study of mothers of preterm infants, for instance, Landzelius suggests that her U.S. informants were similarly challenged to make sense of their maternal identity and to make kin claims on their babies in the presence of incubators that physically divided them from the infants and replaced their gestational role.[23] Landzelius metaphorically conceptualizes the incubator as an "artificial umbilicus," a "cyborg womb," and a "prosthesis with child," arguing that the mothers were able to formulate emotional attachments to their babies by appropriating the incubator as a virtual appendage to their own bodies.

Landzelius suggests that this connection is constituted through ritual behaviors in which the mothers personalize and "domesticate" the incubator by decorating it with stuffed toys, ribbons, and family photos. Layne identifies the cultivation of similar goals by U.S. women who experienced pregnancy loss.[24] Even if they had lost the pregnancy early on, women engaged in symbolic rites aimed at bonding with and memorializing the *baby* and moving themselves socially into the role of *mother* despite the absence of a child. These ritual behaviors included cuddling, dressing, naming, photographing, and holding a funeral for the stillborn "baby" to transform the dead infant's body into a socially present "daughter" or "son."

The vivid differences between the women in these case studies and the intended mothers in my study reflect the cultural construction of pregnancy in each culture. The U.S. women are trying to bond with a preterm or dead infant that they regard as a *baby* and with whom they actively try to engage despite its liminality. The intended mothers, conversely, were hesitantly trying to connect with a liminal, abstract entity they inconsistently regarded as an egg, embryo, or fetus but not usually as a baby. Their tentative stance is distinctive both of pregnancy in Israel, in particular, and of the escalating technological intervention into pregnancy, in general.[25] It was also directly affected by their prior struggles with infertility, which made it difficult for them to trust the possibility of a positive outcome. Still, intended mothers shared with the mothers of preterm and dead babies described above the goal of transitioning into the status, identity, and role of mother through ritual practices.

Their practices focused primarily on contemporary rituals they believed expectant mothers normally engage in as part of their transition to motherhood. One of these activities was reading about and conducting "research" on pregnancy and fetal development. An activity that is generally popular among pregnant women in many countries, reading information pamphlets, magazine articles, and guidebooks about childbirth was understood as a way of "mentally and intellectually preparing them for motherhood."[26]

While we drove together to a surrogacy-related gathering, I participated in a conversation with two intended mothers, Batsheva and Aliza, on this subject. Batsheva noted that one of her relatives had bought her the quintessential Israeli pregnancy guidebook when she began surrogacy. *The Israeli Guidebook to Pregnancy and Childbirth* is a thick, hardback volume with a movable-wheel diagram on its cover that women can use to estimate their due date. "It is still in the back of the car," Batsheva told Aliza and me. "I decided that I won't take it up to the house until there is a pregnancy." To this, Aliza responded, "I also bought it when I first began IVF. It is on the bookshelf, but I turned it around, so the dial doesn't show. My fantasy is to turn it around and display it on the shelf when she [the surrogate] becomes pregnant."

Surrogates, on their part, refrained from researching the pregnancy, although, during their own pregnancies, they had engaged at least to some extent in this practice. Instead, surrogates noted that their intended mothers would read about pregnancy and follow its stages "by the book." This sometimes created tensions when the intended mother worried about the pregnancy because of something she had read, rather than listening to what the surrogate told her. This recalls Georges and Mitchell's critique of such guidebooks,[27] which demote the status of the embodied, intuitive knowledge of pregnant women and promote disembodied, authoritative messages in its place. However, most surrogates acknowledged that their intended mother's reliance on the guidebooks was more sad than annoying because, as one surrogate noted, reading about pregnancy was one of the only ways the intended mother could experience it. Indeed, although pregnancy guides have been critiqued for conveying the message that a woman can only acquire the culturally appropriate self of a rational and informed mother through educational guidebooks,[28] the ability to consume this message, "just like any other pregnant woman," becomes a way for intended mothers to access the role they long to play.

Alongside pregnancy reading, some intended mothers engaged in journaling as a means of recording their child's way into the world. Although most of the intended mothers who began a surrogacy journal forsook it early on, some persisted. One intended mother recorded every meeting with her surrogate in a handwritten notebook, while two others whom I met through the surrogacy forum created online blogs about their surrogacy journey. As the surrogacy Internet message board became increasingly popular, sharing messages about significant developments became a ritual of authenticating the transition to motherhood. Intended mothers would generally announce major events in messages to the online forum, including their first meeting with their surrogate, signing the contract before the approvals committee, the first embryo transfer, the "beta count" after a positive pregnancy test, and the major diagnostic ultrasound scan. Surrogates less commonly shared these events with the group; for intended mothers, they represented a confirmation of linear progress, significant stepping stones on their path to motherhood. Many intended mothers whom I met through the forum told me how eager they were to be able to share that first long-awaited message—the pregnancy announcement—with the group and how fervently they hoped for the day they could announce the birth and post a picture of their newborn. A message posted by Ilena on the day she returned home from the hospital with her newborn daughter conveyed the importance of this ritual for her. Her message was titled, "Finally, now it's my turn."

Intended mothers also engaged in other claiming practices, such as "pregnancy dreaming."[29] Several told me of dreams they had during the later months of their surrogate's pregnancy. They were unable to recall the exact content of the dreams but remembered, upon awakening, that they had experienced a dream related to the pregnancy, to babies, or to themselves being pregnant. Rona, for instance, told me in the seventh month of her surrogate's pregnancy, "I feel like my mind is preparing me for motherhood. I have these dreams all the time where I am pregnant." What I found most interesting about such dreaming was the intended mothers' assertions that it is something pregnant women naturally "do." While studies have found that pregnant women may actually engage in a particular genre of dreaming,[30] what matters here is that intended mothers believed it to be true and that they viewed their own dreams as signs of the authenticity of their transitory state.

Intended mothers also engaged in practical preparations for bringing the baby home. Shopping for baby clothes, throwing baby showers, and preparing a nursery are ways many pregnant women in the United States pave their entrance into motherhood,[31] and it is not uncommon for intended mothers in the United States to follow suit. The surrogate sometimes even attends the baby shower as an honored guest. In a published essay on her surrogacy experience, one U.S. intended mother describes how meaningful participation in such practices was to her: "We went maternity clothes and baby clothes shopping. . . . It was a blast for me because I was able to experience everything that a pregnant woman experiences."[32]

Israelis, however, approach these practices with hesitation, preferring to wait until a live, healthy baby is born to indulge in them. Sered relates such behaviors to evil-eye beliefs and traditions passed down in Jewish communities for many generations.[33] Ivry has identified this type of hesitation with what she refers to as "the worst case scenario" type of thinking.[34] This type of cultural expectation contributes to the contemporary practices among Jewish-Israelis of not naming the baby until after the birth, postponing shopping for baby supplies until late in the third trimester, and paying for and taking the supplies home only after the birth. In this social climate, wherein pregnancy is overshadowed by a cultural ambiance of fear, intended mothers articulated excitement about performing the local pregnancy ritual of delayed shopping. Sarit, for instance, told me that one of her most exciting days during her surrogate's pregnancy occurred in its later months, when she "allowed" herself to go into a major baby supply store to choose furniture for the nursery. In the end, she did not buy or order anything, but she remembered that "I was moved just by the fact that I finally had the right and the privilege [*zchut*] to go in there." Similarly, Yael spoke about the transformative process of passing by baby stores and actually stopping to look:

> Before this, you would speak about children, but you knew what your situation was. But now, when you pass by children's stores, then you say, "Come look." Before, you would do it by yourself, not with your husband. Even when you would pass by the store by yourself, you would look at the baby clothes and think, "What if we had . . . ?" But now, you can do it together. He says, "Let's go buy this." I tell him, "No, not until he [the baby] is born."

Yael's words reveal that merely thinking about buying baby supplies or preparing the baby's room served as an important landmark for intended mothers in preparing themselves for motherhood. Natali, whose twins were born through surrogacy, told me that she had not "dared" to actually prepare the nursery before the birth but that she had spent days and nights planning the babies' room in her head. Her planning also included finding names for the twins before they were born, even though she did not share these names with anyone but her husband before delivery. She viewed these objects and abstractions as substitutes for not being "in" the pregnant body: "I couldn't rub a belly and feel, so my bonding with them was through things . . . through objects and through names and things that were more abstract."

These intended mothers' words reveal that their pregnancy practices achieve an ambiguous link to an abstract embryo/fetus/expected child and a hesitant transition toward a new role and identity. The "object of expectation"[35] may remain abstract, but the women's engagement in practices that mark their route to becoming mothers leads them to experience a progressively heightened expectancy. The sequence of medical events along this route adds to their claiming process as well, giving way to a sense of "carrying" some aspects of the pregnancy.

"CARRYING" MEDICAL RESPONSIBILITY

One of the main avenues for an intended mother to advance her claiming practices is through participation in the surrogate's prenatal care. This is enabled by the convergence of two factors. First, the fertility process necessitates that both women be treated by the same doctor so that their menstrual cycles could be synchronized. In this way, the eggs extracted from the intended mother's body on a particular date can be fertilized and transferred to the surrogate's hormonally prepared uterus within forty-eight hours of fertilization. Second, since fertility treatments for childless couples are subsidized by Israeli national health insurance, for all bureaucratic classificatory purposes, surrogacy is considered treatment for the intended mother's infertility. In line with the official guidelines of the Israeli Ministry of Health, procedures performed on both women's bodies (ova extraction from the intended mother's body and embryo transplantation in the surrogate's body) are routinely recorded in a medical file under the intended mother's name. Fertility medicines and medical referrals are also listed in her name, and the surrogate is represented by a page in the intended mother's file. This not only gives the intended mother access to all information regarding the surrogate's treatment but also makes her the primary patient during prenatal care—the one to whom all instructions and test results are reported.

The intended mothers found personal validation in the way medical files were handled. In a joint interview with Shahar, a surrogate, and Odelya, her intended mother, Odelya explained that her doctor had listed the pregnancy under her name from start to finish, crowning her the primary patient in the pregnancy: "All of the records were in my name except for the major ultrasound [skirat maarachot]. For that one he wrote her family name, dash, my family name. But the file [karteset] was in my name, and it says surrogacy. And all of her details are written there, and it says that she is my surrogate." This type of medical merging of the two women also served as a type of confirmation of their interchangeability with one another, a theme I pick up below. Here, however, I stress how this type of file management was interpreted by the women as shaping them into one "conjoined patient." Shahar explained, "He treated us both, like, together. . . . He treated us like one person. He put my file inside her file. . . . I didn't have a separate file and she didn't have a separate file. My file was in their file. And they were with me all the time, in the checkups." To this, Odelya added, "I was the one written down. I am her. It is the same one." Interested in whether physicians handling surrogacy cases also made this connection between files and personhood, I asked one fertility doctor who his pregnant patient was during a particular surrogacy case. His answer conveyed a similarity in thinking: "I would relate both to the surrogate and to the intended mother, both as individuals and as one together."

In most of the cases I followed, intended mothers were eager participants in the medical management of surrogates' treatment and prenatal care, handling all related documentation, scheduling, and information. Medical responsibility became a site for "carrying" some of the weight of the pregnancy and lightening the load for the surrogates. Surrogates usually viewed relinquishment of medical responsibility to their intended mothers as an additional vehicle of detachment: the less they had to deal with bureaucratic details related to the pregnancy, the easier it was for them to maintain their distancing techniques. They encouraged intended mothers to take on this intermediary role. Masha, for instance, took it for granted that her intended mother should be the first one notified of the pregnancy in Masha's body. She didn't want this news to be imparted to her until both of her intended parents had shared the news. When her intended mother phoned to tell her the positive pregnancy test results, she immediately scolded her for informing her before sharing the news with the intended father: "I said to her, 'Have you told Gavriel yet? . . . Don't call me back until you have told him!' I couldn't believe that she called me without even telling him yet that he is going to have a child."

As half of the conjoined patient, intended mothers often became mediators between physicians and surrogates; they would sometimes even visit the doctor alone at certain stages of the pregnancy to obtain prescriptions for the surrogate's treatment and to obtain referrals for prenatal diagnostic tests to be performed on the surrogate's body. They took responsibility for purchasing all medicines prescribed to the surrogate, delivering them to her, scheduling doctor's appointments, and dealing with any bureaucratic hassles along the way. Intended mothers repeatedly informed me that their scheduling and intermediary responsibilities made them feel as though they had an essential role in the pregnancy. Sharon summed up the quality of this role, saying, "I managed this pregnancy. . . . It is to manage a pregnancy in its entirety. To worry. To make appointments." Likewise, Natali noted that "all of the bureaucratic things went through me. . . . It was simply our pregnancy, and we carried her [the surrogate] with us." Natali's formulation of herself and her husband vicariously carrying the surrogate and the pregnancy is an oxymoron when one considers a surrogate is often called a "gestational carrier" in popular English and is called the "carrying mother" [em noset] in the Israeli surrogacy law. In a new take on their "carrying" roles, surrogates carried the baby, while intended mothers "carried" the documentation, artifacts, time-management responsibilities, and identity-generating potential of the pregnancy.

In most cases, intended mothers accompanied their surrogates to the embryo transfer, to all ultrasounds, and to delivery. However, many intended mothers also accompanied their surrogates to each and every prenatal care appointment. Eager to participate in any medical events that could give them access to the pregnancy, intended mothers would often travel for up to two hours to a surrogate's city to attend a doctor's appointment with her. Yael told me during the sixth month of her surrogate's pregnancy, "I go with her to every checkup. To everything. Not only does she want me to go, but I also want to. So that I can feel it too. I might not be experiencing the pregnancy [physically] but I experience all of the processes around it." She referred to carrying medical responsibility for the pregnancy as "a full-time job"; her husband also told me that Yael left her cell phone on twenty-four hours a day and slept with it at arm's reach, ready and prepared to rush out the door in case their surrogate called, which happened quite often because she frequently experienced bleeding during the pregnancy.

When something went wrong, it was also the intended mother who took responsibility for pursuing specialist information and making the tough decisions. In one case, an intended mother who participated regularly in the surrogacy forum shared the story of her quest for information after a routine prenatal diagnostic scan revealed a potentially serious fetal anomaly. It was she who conducted research, spoke to geneticists, took her surrogate for repeat scans and for second and third opinions, and finally decided, together with her husband, to terminate the pregnancy. Her surrogate, who was also a forum participant, remained an observer, encouraging her intended mother and sympathizing with her but not actively pursuing a medical solution. Although it was her body that was ultimately involved, she clearly delegated all responsibility related to the medical aspects of the pregnancy to her intended mother.

In addition to managing the paperwork, appointments, and medical worries related to the pregnancy, the intended mother was the main party interacting with the doctor during medical appointments, asking questions and listening intently to instructions, while the surrogate stayed relatively silent, symbolically stepping aside to enable the intended mother to play the role of the primary "pregnant patient." Masha, a surrogate, related that, during appointments, "mostly he [the doctor] would talk to her. I didn't really need to know." The direct inter-action of her intended mother, Tova, with the doctor during Masha's checkups intensified Tova's identification of herself as the pregnant patient, although she remained aware that this was a partially imagined role. She reported, "After every checkup I would tell my parents about it as though I was the one going through it, but I wouldn't get too into it, so that it wouldn't hurt." Odelya also indicated that her doctor made her the primary focus of doctor-patient communication:

> I am the one who he makes the appointment with and I am the one he gives the results to, not to her. . . . He behaved toward me as though I was preg-nant. I come with her, he speaks to me. . . . He speaks to me next to her, but his eyes are pointed at me. . . . If we were at a checkup and he would start explaining to her . . . then she would [also] say, "Explain to them; they are the parents."

The convergence of the surrogate's and the doctor's efforts to label the intended mother the *official* mother enhanced her confidence in her ability to claim the role, status, and label of designated mother in the pregnancy. Riki, for instance, reported that her surrogate's insistence that the doctor not begin his checkup without her was an implicit public confirmation of Riki's role. She reported that her surrogate "refused to let the doctor begin his checkup without me. Even when I was thirty minutes late one time, she made him wait. She said that this is Riki's baby and that she had to be here." The doctor's indulgence of the sur-rogate's wishes signifies his recognition of the social and psychological necessity of Riki's participation, since there was no medical reason for him to wait for her to arrive. This is especially notable when we remem-ber how rigidly structured doctors' time is in medical settings in which other infertility patients are lined up waiting for appointments.

In this framework, doctors play an important role as co-constructers and confirmers of the intended mother's transition to motherhood. It was the doctor's authoritative recognition of her role in the pregnancy that stirred the first inkling of a maternal identity in Sarit:

> I saw how they inserted the embryos into her womb, and that was really the first time that I felt like a mommy. I got there a little late, and they had already laid her down on the bed. Then the doctor said, "Here comes the mommy." And when he said that, I got very excited, because I really did feel right then like a mommy.

The physician's act of labeling the intended mother "the mommy" even as he conducts an embryo implantation procedure on the surrogate's body encourages the intended mother to identify with that social label and serves as authoritative confirmation of the women as a conjoined patient. Several intended mothers directly ascribed their doctor's personal interest in cultivating their adoption of the new social label to his or her familiarity with their prior reproductive history. After treating her for fertility-related issues, often for many years, the physician knew the intended mother well and had a grasp of the desperation that had led her to spend many years trying to become pregnant through assisted conceptive techniques. Although some may be quick to point out the potential for conflict of interest when a doctor treats both surrogate and intended mother, a doctor's knowledge of both sides of the surrogacy relationship can also help the women advance their common goals: to deflect responsibility for the medical aspects of the pregnancy from the surrogate onto the intended mother and to cultivate the intended mother's claiming practices. The doctor's support and cultivation of the intended mother's claim to maternity could even be considered a type of "healing" or caregiving practice performed in conjunction with the surrogate's care work toward the intended mother, discussed further on.

In general, the dynamic described here may be unique to the constellation of geographical proximity and social medicine that is particular to Israel. When surrogates and intended parents live great distances apart, as is the case in many U.S. and binational surrogacies, a couple may not be able to accompany the surrogate to all medical appointments. In addition, medical insurance providers may not allow the same lenience in medical signifying that characterizes the Israeli case, and may only allow a woman to attend particular doctors or clinics. These factors might lead a surrogate to visit her local obstetrician for prenatal care, who might treat her the same as during her previous (personalized) pregnancies and require that she manage all medical decisions and paperwork herself. Her doctor may have little contact with the intended parents or deliberately protect the patient's privacy from them, effectively dismissing the intended mother's access to participation in prenatal patienthood. A surrogacy agency may then step in to manage many of the tasks that intended mothers "carried" in my study; this can release the surrogate and the intended parents from these responsibilities, but it also denies intended mothers one of the central vehicles of identity construction that the Israeli women can access.

Importantly, although all of the surrogates I spoke with viewed this allocation of medical responsibility positively, it is by way of an exceptional case that we can grasp how much the medical system, surrogates, and intended mothers are all complicit in labeling the intended mother the primary patient. One surrogate, who was featured in national news reports, lodged a formal complaint with the Israeli Ministry of Health accusing the staff of a prominent IVF unit of mistreatment when they followed what I have discussed above as routine surrogacy protocol. A PhD and a birth educator (defying any typecasting of surrogates), she interpreted the hospital protocol as denying her respect. She felt sidelined by the doctor's treatment of her intended mother as his primary patient: "From the moment of the embryo transfer . . . I became as if invisible."[36] She had expected to be directly addressed by the attending physician and informed of every step of the embryo transfer process, but the doctor responded to her questions by referring her to the intended mother, whom he had directly informed of all the details.

This surrogate was equally taken aback by the file-naming protocol: "After the embryo transfer, when we received the printed records with the patient's information, I noticed that the details in it were not mine. . . . I looked further and saw that no sensitivities were listed to medicines. . . . The biological mother's name was listed on the page. . . . The embryos were inserted into my body and I did not exist on the patient log."[37] Later, the surrogate was astounded to learn that the doctor had informed the intended mother, but not her, of the positive outcome of the pregnancy test.[38] Her reaction to the discovery that her intended mother was being treated by the medical system as the primary pregnant patient brings the agency of surrogates who *do* comply with this categorization into sharp relief. Allowing the intended mother to assume this role is not just part of the surrogate's distancing repertoire but also an offering: an act of relinquishing control over a particular aspect of surrogacy in support of the intended mother's identity-building practices.

WORRYING AS KIN CLAIMING

While the practices discussed above may have helped an intended mother access a route toward claiming the maternal label, they often had little effect on her accompanying goal of creating emotional attachments to the fetus. In a few cases, intended mothers did feel that the fetus had become more tangible and that their actions had generated what they believed to be normative prenatal attachments. Olina wrote on the surrogacy forum website: "In relation to connecting to the child during the pregnancy, our dear surrogate is now pregnant (nine weeks) and I feel very attached to the child. I see the pulse on the ultrasound, I know what his dimensions are, how he is developing, I read a lot about child development during pregnancy and I know what he has in a certain week. I feel him." Natali similarly hypothesized that her accompaniment of the pregnancy from outside the pregnant body may have enabled her to connect with her fetuses in ways that she might not have "in the body." She suggested that she had bonded more than a "regular" pregnant woman does because her own body did not distract her:

> I think that I felt more than a regular woman, because . . . for me the pregnancy was very sterile, and there was just them [the twins], and I see them on the ultrasound and I know that "this is mine." The pregnancy isn't mine but what is inside is mine. I mean, the womb and the belly aren't [mine], but this is [the twins]. So I think that I did really bond with them. . . . In a regular pregnancy you might be angry at the fetuses because you have pain or something. But I only had the beautiful things to look at all the time. Only the positive things.

Even so, most intended mothers did not feel that such vicarious pleasure was enough to compensate for their inability to gestate. Much like the expectant fathers interviewed by Draper in England and the U.S. expectant mothers through adoption in Sandelowski's study,[39] intended mothers believed that the embodied experience of pregnancy was a central vehicle for "knowing" their child in utero and for transitioning to social parenthood. Prenatal and postnatal maternal-infant bonding and attachment have long been contested in anthropological scholarship as matters of choice rather than innate, instinctual, universal behaviors.[40] Nonetheless, the belief in prenatal bonding remained a convincing cultural convention among intended mothers, leading them to think that their inability to gestate their child left them shortchanged. Sharon, for instance, related,

> I think maybe because he didn't grow in my belly and that I didn't feel the fetal movements, that I didn't physically feel him, has its effects. I didn't become attached to the fetus. I was curious about what kind of child will come out, what he'll look like, that he'll be healthy, that the [prenatal] tests will be okay. I didn't develop feelings.

Sharon's testimony makes us stop for a minute and retrace our steps: are these the words of an intended mother or of a surrogate? Like surrogates, she describes a general interest in the health of the fetus but also a sense of emotional detachment from it. Moreover, she, too, views the body as central to the constitution of maternal-fetal attachments. However, whereas this assumption led surrogates to map, divide, and detach body parts to prevent the formation of so-called natural bonds, Sharon views her physical remoteness from the body as negatively affecting her emotional capacity to bond. Little does she know that her distanced attitude toward her fetus actually shows just how much she has in common with many other Jewish-Israeli pregnant women: postponing the development of emotional attachments until after the *fetus* is born as a live *baby* may be a Jewish-Israeli cultural norm.[41] Indeed, the assumption that being "in" the pregnant body makes it easier to form prenatal attachments is generally questionable in this age of prenatal diagnosis.[42] Instead of her position appearing stigmatic, then, Sharon's hesitancy could be interpreted as a normative sign of the transition to motherhood.

Nevertheless, most intended mothers had never been pregnant themselves and believed wholeheartedly that that the body and the experience of being pregnant were crucial to forming emotional attachments. The divisions they held between mind, body, and emotion reflected, in many ways, surrogates' distancing of the pregnancy. Riki, for instance, told me in the fifth month of her surrogate's pregnancy that "on the surface level, I am 'cool,' but I think that is simply because I haven't digested it yet, because I don't experience the pregnancy." She differentiated between the surface, mental level of her consciousness and the emotional level: "On the mental level, I know that it's mine, I know they [the twins] are supposed to arrive, I'm excited. But emotionally, it doesn't make me cry or have palpitations."

Like Sharon, Riki attributes her emotional distance to her disembodied position, but in addition, she notes that her apprehension is a self-protective measure: "It is both a defensive mechanism not to get hurt, because, G-d forbid, something could happen, but also because objectively I'm not pregnant and there are no sensations." Other intended mothers also expressed such culturally common fears. Their apprehensions were amplified by their past experiences with reproductive failure, as Yael expressed in the sixth month of her surrogate's pregnancy:

> I am afraid to become too attached because of what happened last time [miscarriage]. . . . I am afraid to even be happy. Afraid to bond and just afraid. . . . Every day that passes I say thank G-d that everything is okay. . . . Every time the phone rings my heart jumps. . . . Every time [the surrogate] calls, she says, "Yael, don't be scared, everything is okay, I just called to say . . ." There is this fear until he comes out into the world alive and whole.

Yael's fearfulness may sound extreme to the optimist's ear, or to some it might sound like a Jewish stereotype in line with the folk convention that Jews, particularly Jewish mothers, are prone to worry.[43] However, it is also not uncommon for non-Jewish intended mothers in the United States to embrace "worrying" about the pregnancy as a means of connecting with the process. Indeed, one of the themes that resurfaces in a collection of twenty personal stories of intended mothers in the United States is the central role that worrying took on in their lives as they grappled with their general lack of control over the surrogacy process. Their stories include descriptions of being cautious, anxious, afraid of disappointment, and careful not to "jinx" their good fortune. As one of the intended mothers in that collection imparts, "I started worrying: I obsessed about everything. To be honest, I don't know how Leanne [her surrogate] put up with me half the time."[44]

Like their U.S. counterparts, Israeli intended mothers worried that something might go wrong with the pregnancy more than they did about the surrogate potentially wanting to keep the baby. Still, there was nearly always an unspoken, lingering fear that the surrogate could renege on her agreement to give up the child. These doubts were amplified by occasional newspaper articles, television movies, and rumors that called attention to the uncommon yet much publicized cases of surrogates who changed their minds and chose to keep the babies. Even intended mothers who professed total confidence in their surrogate were taunted by friends and family who would ask, as one intended mother relayed, "Aren't you afraid she'll run away with the baby?" or who advised them, as another intended mother reported, "to get a court order preventing her from leaving the country." Subsequently, many surrogates found themselves engaging in a kind of therapeutic work with their intended mother aimed at allaying her fears, much of which concentrated on bonding the intended mother to the fetus.

SURROGATE CAREGIVERS

While intended mothers tried to use their abstract claiming practices to compensate for the privileged embodied knowledge of the fetus that they believed their surrogates possessed and they lacked, surrogates found themselves in ambivalent, complex positions as well. Surrogates, who believed that mothers and babies *should* bond during pregnancy, were sometimes troubled or disappointed by their intended mother's hesitancy to bond in their stead. As Sima said to me, "There was a point when I told her that no one was bonding with these babies." Surrogates thus found themselves calling attention to their bellies and personifying the fetus to facilitate intended maternal-fetal bonding, even as they distanced themselves from the pregnancy as part of their body-mapping protocol.

The bonding and calming efforts that a surrogate directed toward her intended mother included persuading the latter to touch her (the surrogate's) belly, lay her head across the belly, speak to it, and caress it. In a video recording that Rinat showed me of herself and her couple hours before the birth, Rinat encourages her intended mother, Sarit, to bond with the fetus, saying, "You are his biological mother. I am not. Feel him. Enjoy him." Sarit lays her hand on Rinat's belly and strokes it, commenting, "So cute." Rinat responds, "When I was in bed last night [in the hospital] you felt him, and you saw how he falls asleep and how he wakes up." Sarit smiles, answering, "He jumps, rides waves, does somersaults."

Whereas Sarit, so close to the birth event, seemed to accept Rinat's bonding attempts without difficulty, most surrogates noted the reluctance of their intended mothers to bond. The case of Shahar and her intended mother, Odelya, is a good example. Odelya told me that Shahar "was always trying to have me put my hand, but I was afraid to touch. . . . She'd press [the belly] and I'd say, 'Don't press! Don't you dare! So that nothing will go wrong!' . . . I was hysterical." To this, Shahar responded, "She didn't understand that when I press, I'm not hurting them [the twins], I'm just moving them. . . . It doesn't reach them, they just move and then she could have felt it." This hesitancy on Odelya's part persisted even after the birth, and instead of concentrating on what was happening to her own body in the immediate aftermath of the delivery, Shahar found herself focusing on Odelya and encouraging her to hold her newborn babies:

> Then they brought them to her all clean and tidy so that she would hold them. And I am still saying to her, "Hold them! Hold them!" and she didn't want to, that crazy woman. . . . She was afraid. She says to me, "No, I'm afraid." . . . He [the doctor] is fixing me up there in the meantime and I am telling her, "Hold them! What's wrong with you! I mean, wait a minute, what happened to you? Hold the big one at least." So they did give her the big one in her hands and they held the small one.

Connecting Odelya to the babies and coaxing her into the role of mother emerged as difficult tasks. In this case, as in many others, encouraging the intended mother to bond becomes a venture into folk psychology. Similarly, Orna told me that she spent much of her time as a surrogate trying to coax her reluctant intended mother to bond: "Every time I was with her, I would take her hand. I would say, 'Here is the foot, here is this, let's move him." And she'd say to me, 'No, no, don't hurt him.' 'I'm not hurting him, just so he moves. It's a sack, like a plastic bag that you move. It doesn't get hurt.'" She told another interviewer, "I felt that she needed me to connect her to the pregnancy. She wasn't looking to connect. She was taking care of me so that I would take care of him [the fetus]."[45] Drawing on a "folk model" of psychology,[46] she told me that when she was a surrogate, she "didn't need a psychologist. I was a psychologist for myself. And for the mother."

Surrogates seriously undertook such "therapeutic" conduct toward their intended mothers, and they considered it a weighty responsibility. In several instances, I heard surrogates describe their efforts like Idit did, saying that because her intended mother exhibited such reluctance, Idit "shared with her forcefully. . . . I made sure that she becomes attached. Because my role is actually to create the attachment between them. It actually strengthened me and my detachment from the child." Beyond merely facilitating a connection and allaying fears, Idit saw her role as "making a mother"—helping her intended mother move into her new identity: "I would teach her as a mother to a mother. I actually paved her entrance [hechnasti otah] into being a mother! I taught her to be a mother! I would always put into her head that 'your bachelor life is over; soon you are going to have a child, enough!'"

When I asked Idit a year after the birth if she wanted to be a surrogate again, her response did not surprise me: "I don't think I have the strength [koach] for it, and it is not worth the money. I don't mean the pregnancy. That is not the problem. . . . It is all of the psychological work I had to do with the mother. I was her psychologist. I don't have the strength to go through all of that again. It is difficult." Idit's lack of enthusiasm to repeat the experience has nothing to do with regret at having relinquished the baby. In fact, she doesn't mention the baby at all. Instead, she refers to the multidirectional emotion works[47] that she had to undertake as a surrogate that depleted her of her "strength."

U.S. surrogacy agency directors told me repeatedly that many of the surrogates they work with now prefer to work with gay male couples because they find the relationship to be less stressful. As one director put it, "Intended mothers who have not had a child before come with a lot of baggage. . . . There are more issues for intended mothers. The surrogate is doing something she can't do but thinks she is supposed to do, tried to do." The gay male couples, he observed, "come from a different place. . . . They haven't had years of infertility and they trust her more. They know they can't control her. They couldn't be pregnant and know that, so there is no compensating." While these generalizations about intended mothers may be critiqued for the gender stereotypes they convey, associating women with hysterical qualities and men with rational thought, they do shed light on a pattern that is similar to the one expressed by Idit and other Israeli surrogates: the strain of the emotion work they conduct vis-à-vis their intended mothers.

When surrogates refer to their role as one of providing the intended mother with "therapeutic reassurance," a picture emerges of the surrogate as a paid caregiver. The metaphors described in chapter 2, which emphasize the surrogate's nurturance and development of the couple's nature within her warm womb, similarly highlight the notion of "caring." Specifically, the surrogate's idea that she maintains warmth despite providing a neutral, mechanical environment for the fetus hints to the importance that she attaches to retaining the image of a caring woman[48] at the same time that she refutes any claim to being the mother of the child she gestates. The idea expressed in the metaphors that she is feeding her children, the couple's child, and the couple also signifies a central aspect of caregiving.

Warmth and caring are also conceptually linked to the women's self-description as babysitters, for babysitters care for other people's children without claiming maternal entitlement. Colen's study of migrant caregivers and their employers in New York also suggests strong parallels between surrogacy and caregiving.[49] Using the concept of "stratified reproduction," Colen illuminates the dispersal of motherhood among caregivers, which is similar in some ways to the surrogate's distribution of maternity. Colen's caregivers have traveled to another country to earn money to support their families, leaving their own children behind to be raised by others. However, in New York, they work as paid caregivers, raising other people's children, to whom they are "like a mother." Like the surrogates in my study, these paid caregivers and their employers distinguish between mothering care work and being socially labeled a specific child's mother. However, I contend that there is an important difference in the recipients of the caregiving in each case, for Colen's informants were caring for children; surrogates are also caring for other mothers.

This distinction can be further clarified by comparing surrogates to another type of caregiver—birth attendants, doulas, or midwives. Like midwives, surrogates expertly use their intuitive and embodied knowledge within a medical technological framework;[50] like doulas, they nurture and guide a (pseudo) birthing woman through the childbearing process; and like many activist midwives, they are experts in reproduction whose work is based on an ideology of helping other women become mothers, even if it is also compensated financially. Whereas midwives help women give birth to babies, however, surrogates help infertile women give birth to themselves as mothers. And while midwives concentrate on the childbirth event, surrogates emphasize the pregnancy. A main locus of the surrogate's caregiving work toward the intended mother was through the body and the "shifting" of the pregnancy, which created an embodied connection between intended mother and surrogate. This embodied connection can produce an intimacy that can have profound implications for the women involved and for the success of the whole process, as I explore in the following chapter.

CHAPTER 5

The Shifting Body

It is now clear that the intended mother's experience of surrogacy cannot be separated from her relationship with the surrogate. Surrogates play a central role in fostering the intended mother's goals, whether by allowing her to assume control of the medical aspects of the pregnancy or by actively trying to bond her to the baby. The story behind the surrogacy agreement, then, becomes less about the surrogate giving birth to a baby and more about how surrogates, like midwives, actively help other women give birth to themselves as mothers. In the following discussion, I address the surrogate–intended mother relationship from the perspective of the body. I look at the role that pregnant embodiment plays in the women's interactions with one another and at the way that intended mothers make efforts to encompass, symbolically attach, and experience the pregnancy through their bodies. I call this process "the shifting body" because it involves the shifting between the two women of social labels, identity-building processes, and embodied expressions of pregnancy; the very aspects of pregnancy that the surrogate has distanced, detached, and disembodied are channeled into the intended mother's construction of a "pregnant identity." I also address the emotional dimensions of the women's convergence throughout the surrogacy process.

CHEMISTRY, CLICKING, AND CONNECTEDNESS

The grounds on which the shifting body developed can be traced to a very early point in the surrogacy process. Specifically, the intended mothers I observed seemed to have been intuitively aware from the time of their initial search for a surrogate that they needed to find someone with whom they would be able to closely identify and with whom they saw the potential for a friendly, comfortable, and even intimate relationship. Although they kept the criteria of the surrogacy law in mind, they still mostly relied on their physical and emotional instincts to indicate compatibility. Surrogates, on their part, also felt it was necessary to have an intuitive connection, through the body, with the woman for whom they would carry the child. This was evident in the informal idioms of "chemistry," "connection," and "clicking" that surrogates and intended mothers alike used to define the affinity that they felt when they first met the surrogacy partner they were "destined" to be with.

These three notions represent degrees of attraction in Hebrew-language references to romantic love. Thus, what Sapir, a surrogate, describes below in relation to surrogate–intended mother relationships could easily be read in another context as dating advice: "If the two don't click from the beginning, then it is worthless to continue. . . . I don't have to fall in love with her and she doesn't have to fall in love with me. . . . There just has to be a sort of common language between us. . . . There just needs to be chemistry." Sapir does not see surrogacy partnerships as dependent on love at first sight—the kind of deep and enduring romantic love that begins with excitement, thrills, palpitations of the heart, and the partners' complete absorption in one another[1]— but she does see some degree of instant attraction between the parties as critical.

Chemistry was believed to be the defining element that could make or break a surrogacy arrangement. Lihi, a surrogate, noted, "Chemistry is something that you can't replace with anything else. It is like having chemistry with your spouse—you either have it or you don't. That's why I say, if I do it [surrogacy] for another couple, it won't be the same." With few exceptions, surrogates and intended mothers chose between two or more potential partners on the basis of instantaneous, intuitive recognition and familiarity, rather than concrete, objective considerations. Idit rejected a couple she had been matched with by a commercial agency because of the absence of such a connection, even though the two had agreed to pay her a relatively high fee and their file was ready for submission to the approvals committee: "Something told me not to do it with the couple they introduced me to. They aren't right for me. There is no chemistry. It is really important that there be chemistry." Sarit, an intended mother, confidently asserted that finding a partner for the surrogacy process with whom one has chemistry is

> the hardest part of the process. Because the minute that you . . . make a connection with the right woman, and the chemistry between the two sides is good, then you can go through anything together. Then the medical part doesn't look so hard. . . . The connection with the woman is the most important part. . . . The couple has to find the right woman, and the woman has to find the right couple for her.

Chemistry signified the extent to which the women felt "naturally" drawn to one another and able to communicate freely and openly on an emotional level from the start. With the idea of chemistry, the women called up the same nature idiom that surrogates used to distinguish themselves from the fetus and to establish their solidarity with their own kin. Whereas the surrogate claimed that she did not bond with the fetus because it was not created from her nature, the surrogate and intended mother both became instinctively, emotionally attached to one another through the "natural" affinity that they refer to as "chemistry." This "natural" connection that formed between them, as we shall see, is also expressed through particular body parts (eyes, heart) and substances (blood, tears). When the same relationship that surrogates withheld from the fetus becomes a necessary prerequisite for the women to achieve a mutually satisfying surrogacy experience, a triangle of connections and disconnections is established.

In most of the narratives, the women recognized that they were "naturally" and "chemically" in tune with one another when their bodies notified them of it. Surrogates described their need to feel this connection through the heart—a personalized organ of emotion and love in their body map. Tamar described her thoughts the night before her first meeting with her couple: "I wondered what kind of couple they were. . . . They have to be a couple that get into your heart a little. I am not saying that I have to fall in love with them at first sight, but that they should get into the heart." The chemistry that Masha felt with her intended mother, Tova, was signaled through the eyes: "The minute our eyes met, there was chemistry. From the moment that we began to speak, it felt like I was sitting with someone whom I had known for at least five years. I knew right then that she was the one." And Sarit, an intended mother, felt the "right" connection in her belly, the very organ in which the surrogate would eventually "hold" the baby: "When you see the right woman . . . you go by the feeling in your belly. . . . That is how I felt with her. . . . We had immediate chemistry."

Women saw these meetings as initiating a type of metaphysical link, a fated connection, as Riki described after meeting her surrogate: "The first time we met, I went to meet her with a friend, and my friend just cried and cried : . . she said that she could really see the bond forming between us, and it made her cry." Rinat, a surrogate, also emphasized the role of fate in the surrogate–intended mother relationship. She noted that, in her couple's long search for a surrogate, she "was their fifty-first in number. . . . But the others hadn't clicked; there was no connection like ours." She relayed how she had inexplicably recognized her intended mother, Sarit, from her distant perch at the window of her second-story apartment: "And they came in the car, and she was looking, and I said to her, 'Sarit, I am here.' As if I had known her from somewhere . . . and from then on, she decided that I would be her surrogate." The rigorous medical and psychological tests that they underwent to satisfy the surrogacy approvals committee, Rinat insisted, only served to strengthen what the two women already knew: "When we did the tests [for the approvals committee], right away they said to us, she is right for you."

The women often described their first meeting with one another as a sequence resembling romantic courtship. Miri described her first meeting with her surrogate as a "blind date": "The night before you can't fall asleep, and you think about what it will be like, and what she will say. You wonder if she will like us. . . . It is very similar to a blind date." Miri's surrogate, Tamar, described the first fateful encounter in these terms: "As soon as they came up the escalator, I said, 'This is the couple.' . . . And that was it. From that moment, we clicked. Just like that." This "blind date" usually evolved into a type of courtship that initially played out in public venues, such as a café or a mall. Masha said, "The first meeting was in an open, neutral place, where we could speak and clarify the things we had to talk about." She noted that "after we got to know one another and we were serious about one another" they transferred their meeting place to one of their homes, and after several months had passed, Masha introduced her intended mother to her family.

From the moment of that initial click, the intended father's presence fades into the background and the relationship between the surrogate and intended mother begins to take center stage. Much as Ragoné found among surrogates and intended mothers in the United States,[2] Israeli women defined surrogacy as "women's business." In most cases, intended fathers regarded this emphasis on *connecting* as trivial; as one man remarked, "If you ask my wife, she'll say that there was chemistry. I say that is female nonsense [*shtuyot shel nashim*]." When I asked another intended father if he had felt "chemistry" or "clicked" with the surrogate when first meeting her, he said, "Let's not exaggerate. Women, you know how they talk . . . but I looked at her, I thought the price is right, she looks nice enough, and I had no intention of meeting a lot of different candidates."

I was repeatedly struck by the way intended fathers, instead of focusing on cultivating a relationship with the surrogate, were focused on the end product of the agreement, tending to take a more businesslike approach to the surrogate-couple relationship. Intended fathers were involved in the negotiations over the contract, financial decisions during surrogacy, and the birth itself, but tended to step aside during other aspects of the process. There were exceptions, of course, but most men tended to remind, influence, or even pressure their wives to view surrogacy as a business agreement, as illustrated by one intended father, who interjected in the middle of his wife's "clicking-chemistry" narrative: "It isn't like we are marrying her. I see it as business like any other business deal [*esek l'kol davar*]." The men's marginality to the process signaled the exclusivity of the surrogate–intended mother relationship, in most cases, from the very beginning. Natali compared her own "chemistry" with her surrogate to her husband's distance:

> She [the surrogate] was a little shy with him [the intended father]. She and I were very friendly, very connected, and he was a little more distanced. . . . When he would take her home . . . she would say to me, 'Why is he so quiet?' I mean, she had nothing to talk about with him. . . . It is a forced situation, . . . two people forced to be together when they have no chemistry. The chemistry was more between us.

The women's use of clicking and chemistry to denote their coming together in the reproductive relationship is closely connected to the formation of the shifting body. When the women click, their two bodies are integrated into a composite ensemble. In this mechanically rendered connection, the pieces that click remain distinguishable, much like a jigsaw puzzle, in which the unitary surface retains the original outlines of the intersecting pieces. Chemistry denotes the nature of boundaries of this connection, for like a chemical reaction that occurs when two substances are mixed, the body and identity boundaries of the two women can become blurred through their union. The shifting body develops between these two poles of clicked integration and merged union. The two women join while retaining their sense of having individual, bounded bodies and mutually exclusive identities. At the same time, they converge and expand their personhood beyond the boundaries of the traditional individual, bounded body and experience temporarily merged identities.

PROSTHETIC CONSCIOUSNESS

Finding the right woman to connect with was only the first step toward developing the shifting body. Intended mothers were able to extend their own bodily boundaries and capabilities by way of the connection with their surrogate and to access the process of pregnancy through her. For some intended mothers, the ability to have children created from their own eggs and carried by a surrogate filled out a body image that they had considered defective, disabled, and not "whole" because of their missing uterine body part or otherwise compromised reproductive capacity. Riki, for instance, described feeling for over a year that her hysterectomy "was written on my forehead . . . like a scarlet letter. . . . I felt disabled. As if without an arm or a leg." Knowing that her eggs could produce babies with the help of a surrogate made her stop feeling disabled: "I can create life [*leholid*], that is the point. . . . That was my issue, [I am] not barren."

Rachel, who had lost her womb to cancer, recounted her surprise that her husband's family had accepted her so readily "despite what I represent. Because I represent an empty place [*makom shel ein*]. Because I have no womb, no potential to give him children." In contrast, when she spoke about the frozen embryos she had secured before her hysterectomy, she gestured outward with her hands as though encompassing a rounded belly and said, "From the moment that I knew that I had the embryos, I felt like they were right here. It was as though there was already a pregnancy." She conceptualized her surrogate, in turn, as the material site of her extension: "I see her as the part of me that is missing. She is my uterus."

Rachel's identification with her embryos generates an image of her surrogate's body as temporarily incorporating a part of her own body.

She imagines the pregnancy existing in a distanced yet connected space projected in front of her body and conjointly held by the surrogate. She visualizes the surrogate as an appendage—a living, breathing, active extension of her body. The image suggests a prosthetic limb, an analogy that one intended mother made explicit. May, who suffered from a blood-clotting problem that led to the loss of her leg after the traumatic delivery of her only child, compared her use of a prosthetic leg to walk with her need for a surrogate to have a second child: "I can't live without my leg. My prosthesis. She is not a prosthesis but . . . I could die if I get pregnant again. I need her to carry it." Careful in her wording, May still evokes the comparative function of her prosthetic leg and her prosthetic carrier. She also hints that both are necessary for her survival, or at least for her quality of life, for she cannot live without one and could die if she doesn't have the other.

Extending this analogy, we might conceptualize the intended mother as formulating a "prosthetic consciousness," a term Wilson defines as a "reflexive awareness of supplementation . . . what happens within the mind once . . . an unseen technological system entirely alien to all your previous bodily processes has been joined (whether integrated or merely appended) to your body."[3] This image also accords with Merleau-Ponty's formulation of the walking stick as an extension of the blind person's body.[4] The intended mother, in this sense, incorporates the surrogate into her own bodily schema as an appended extension, changing her embodied experience and extending her perception of the limits of her body.

Intended mothers who had unexplained infertility, who had no missing piece, so to speak, similarly conceptualized the limits of their embodiment beyond their corporeal boundaries to include the surrogate as a type of satellite site of their own reproductive efforts. Moreover, although this type of projection was more pronounced among intended mothers whose own ova were used in conception, even intended mothers who were not genetically linked to the embryo developed the perception that their bodies' boundaries and capabilities had been functionally extended during surrogacy. Indeed, the formation of a prosthetic consciousness had more to do with the intended mother's focus on the embodied experience of pregnancy and her desire to participate in the pregnancy process than it did with a genetic link.

Consequently, after realizing that she would need to resort to egg donation as well as surrogacy, Rachel explained that she still preferred surrogacy to adoption because it would enable her to vicariously share in the experience of pregnancy, including its embodiment, through the surrogate: "I know that the genes don't really matter, since it isn't my egg anyway. But I want the process. I want to go through the pregnancy with her. I want to be with the surrogate, to watch my child develop, to feel pregnant through her." Likewise, Malka, who had two children through adoption, nullified genetics as her reason for approaching surrogacy and emphasized, instead, her desire to experience the process of pregnancy and birth through her surrogate. When an agency set her up with a surrogate who lived over four hours away, she was not able to take part in the pregnancy as a full "partner," as she had hoped. She wrote in an e-mail, "I would never have done it if I had wanted another child through the mail. Don't misunderstand me. I did feel this pregnancy, but not enough. She lived so far away."

The intended mother's prosthetic consciousness was not antithetical to the surrogate's conception of her own body in surrogacy. Instead, it integrated seamlessly into the surrogate's body map, in which the belly was marked as a distanced space. Thus, the surrogate employed similar depictions of body as an appendage to or replacement for the intended mother's missing womb. This was particularly manifest in the way most surrogates chose to explain their role in surrogacy to their own children. Almost all of the surrogates I spoke to told their children that the intended mother had a "broken womb," a "broken belly," or even a "hole" in her belly that prevented her from keeping a baby inside. Put in plain words, they told their children that their role was to "hold" [lehachzik] the baby for the intended mother, to protect it and take care of it [lishmor alav] until it was ready to "go home."

The image of the surrogate's uterus as the intended mother's missing piece also accorded with the way surrogates consigned their belly area to a disembodied space during surrogacy. Shahar encapsulated her feeling that the belly module existed in such a linked but distanced space, saying, "It was as if the pregnancy moved alongside me." She directly described her role in surrogacy as providing the appended belly that her couple was missing:

> I am the part that she can't do. That's all. And that's how the doctor would treat me. I felt that I am the part that she can't do. I am the supplement [tosefet] to their relationship as a couple. I am the part they couldn't do. I am the appendage of the belly. I am this couple's appendage of what they couldn't do.

Like their intended mothers, surrogates also imagined the intended mother as virtually carrying the belly they had detached in a type of shared, disembodied space between them. Nina expressed this when we spoke during her fifth month,

> *Nina:* Everyone asks me how it is that I don't feel a connection [to the fetus], but I'm telling you, there is just a switch in the mind. It is like my belly isn't here [nods toward belly with her head]. It is like for this period that my belly is there, with her [nodding her head to where her intended mother stood, a few yards away].
>
> *Elly:* I wonder if she feels that your belly is with her . . .
>
> *Nina:* I don't know, but that is how it should be.

The body model depicted here can be viewed as a mirror image of the conflicting body model arising from Goslinga-Roy's analysis of a gestational surrogate and an intended mother whom she followed in California.[5] Goslinga-Roy interprets the surrogate as extending her body beyond its privatized, individualized limits, with the intention of making her body into a shared communal space with her intended mother. The intended mother did not reciprocate in this sharing, conceptualizing her surrogate as a borrowed womb. In my study, the extension of bodily boundaries was the domain of intended mothers; they were the ones to expand their perceived bodily boundaries with the intention of sharing in the surrogate's body as an offshoot of their own embodied selves. The surrogate was the one who was encompassed and appended, and who presented the intended mother her disembodied womb as a compartmentalized offering; she shared the body but still retained a very individualized perception of it within the lines of her body map, carefully orchestrating which parts of the body and the embodied self she was sharing and with whom. Nevertheless, underlying Goslinga-Roy's interpretation is an insight that resonates with my own findings: the openness and willingness of the surrogate to share the pregnancy with her intended mother, as I describe below.

CHANNELING PREGNANT EMBODIMENT

Surrogates' and intended mothers' idea that the pregnancy could exist in a space detached from the surrogate's body and attached to the intended mother's embodied space led to interactions between them that in turn led to the shifting of pregnant embodiment. These interactions were often initiated by surrogates as part of their own distancing techniques; they involved an explicit focus on bodily experiences once the surrogate was pregnant. Surrogates not only interpreted bodily symptoms nonemotionally, to neutralize them for themselves, but they also reported them to the intended mother, to defer them onto her. This communication pertained to any and all physical symptoms of the pregnancy, including nausea, vomiting, and cramping. This effort simultaneously aided their own distancing efforts and helped to promote connective emotions in their pregnancy partner (see figure 6).

Although the bodily channeling dwelled on physicality, many of these interactions occurred over the phone, without the women being physically present within the same room. Idit described how she would call her intended mother and tell her, "'Your fetus is moving, I have nausea, I feel this way' . . . everything that I felt, it was important to me to transfer it to her." Idit felt that her channeling efforts produced sympathy pains of a sort in her intended mother: "She felt it a lot! She felt it psychologically. Like when I had cramps, the moment that I had cramps, I would feel it and I would tell her and she would feel it, you understand?" Orna believed that along with bodily symptoms (nausea, vomiting) she must communicate any emotions she related to the pregnancy (fears, feelings):

> I passed her all of the feelings of the pregnancy, including the fears, the feelings, the nausea, and the vomiting. I told her everything that happened to me during the pregnancy. I would complain all the time how hard it was for me and explain to her every detail. She very much felt this pregnancy. I would call at late hours of the night and I would speak to her sometimes for the entire night.[6]

In comparison with the surrogate's often challenging efforts to bond the intended mother to the fetus, communicating symptoms of the pregnant body—separate from the fetus—was an easier task. Masha told me with a degree of humor about the depths of abject physicality this involved, for example, when discussing vomit: "I try as much as possible to give her the feeling that here, this is what I am feeling, try to feel it like I do. . . . I told her that I will let you know exactly when I am vomiting so that you can feel exactly what I feel [laughs]." In this way, she tried to encourage her intended mother, Tova, to "feel a little bit of what it is like to be a pregnant woman." Nevertheless, Masha remained constantly aware that all that she was able to share with Tova was mediated by words and by their collaborative imagination: "I know that she will never be able to give birth, so I just try to explain it in words to her. It's true that it is only through words that I can give her that feeling, but the mere fact that I demonstrate [elucidate] for her what I undergo

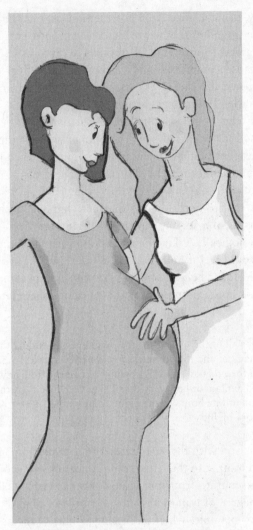

Figure 6. Illustration depicting the surrogate
and intended mother sharing information
and experiences regarding the pregnancy.
Originally appeared in *Lehiot Mishpacha*
magazine. Reproduced with the permission of
the artist, Danna Peleg-Segal.

[*mamchisha la et ma sh'ani overet*] is still significant for her." Masha conveyed her regret that, as much as she tried to share it, Tova could never, in her opinion, fully appreciate the pregnancy experience without experiencing it in her own physical body: "Sometimes it pains me that someone like Tova . . . can't physically experience the pregnancy and birth, because a woman who hasn't experienced it will never know how special it is."

Along with channeling physical symptoms, surrogates encouraged their intended mothers to use their own intuitive knowledge[7] to become more aware of the bodily experience of pregnancy. Masha relayed how she encouraged Tova to look toward her own embodied and intuitive knowledge to guess whether the embryo transfer had been successful: "[She asked me] 'Do you feel something? Do you think you are pregnant?' And I said to her, 'Do you? It is yours, do you think it took?'" In this manner, Tova began to increasingly identify with the pregnancy. Masha related that, as the pregnancy progressed, Tova would call her and seemingly "know" that the baby inside her had just kicked or that she was feeling cramps in the left side: "I asked her how she knew, and she said, 'What do you think? I feel it too.'" Tova, in a separate interview, explained, "I experienced the pregnancy in a natural way. . . .The minute that you live the pregnancy, then you are pregnant. I would ask her about her sensations when I would experience them."

In a follow-up interview with Tova and Masha together several weeks after Masha delivered Tova's daughter, Tova said, "I would wake up with cramps in my back, and I would know that she was having cramps. I suffered through this pregnancy with her." Masha confirmed this: "Elly, I am telling you, it was really like we had telepathy. She felt it too." The bodily sensations and telepathic thoughts shared between the women reached a climax as delivery time neared. Tova recounted her experience of Masha's delivery, marveling how she was so in tune with Masha by this time that she intuitively knew when Masha's labor began: "I felt the birth contractions on the evening of the birth, and I waited for her outside her house before she came down. And maybe it will sound a bit unreal, but I had milk and the doctors were in shock." As Tova related, the height of her identification with Masha's body occurred when her own breasts spontaneously secreted milk after she viewed her newborn babies. Like the stigmata of the Middle Ages—"miraculous" signs of the crucifixion that appeared on Christian women's bodies—Tova's miraculous milk production signified her full incorporation of the pregnant body and presented her with a validating sign that she was the "real" mother of the child. Even more so, it served as proof to both women that the body had shifted, since surrogates, including Masha, often interpreted their lack of milk production as a bodily sign that they were not the mothers of the children they gestated.

Intuitive knowing and intentional channeling of embodiment played a similarly powerful role in the interactions between Rivka and her surrogate, Orna. Rivka credited Orna's communication of the pregnancy to her as central to her own growing sense of embodied identification: "She passed everything she felt on to me. She didn't want to feel it. Not the pregnancy, not the nausea, not the vomiting. . . . She would call right away and transfer them to me." This channeling had a strong impact on Rivka, as she too gradually began to intuitively "know," empathize with, and internalize the pregnancy: "I felt exactly like her. And she gave me the feeling and the sensation that 'it is you—it is you!' . . . And you know, there were really common things between us. And neither she nor I knew. It was only when we would call and tell each other, then she would say, 'Wow, I am also like this and like that.'" For Rivka, this intuitive and embodied connection made her identify so intensely with the pregnancy and with Orna's body that she retrospectively acknowledged a sense of having been pregnant herself, not through a surrogate. She related,

> I want to tell you something that worked for me at least. I felt pregnant. I felt everything that she felt. On the same day that her belly hurt, my belly hurt. I [would] say to Orna, "My belly hurts." Now she, even when she had even the smallest [bout with] nausea, she would call me and I would feel it. I would say to her, "You know what, I feel like it is me." . . . The transferring part and the feelings, I felt exactly the same [as a pregnant woman]. Maybe that is what gives me the push to say, yes, I was pregnant, and not through a surrogate. Because I felt exactly what she felt.

The knowledge that their verbal channeling of the pregnant body had its limits did not stop the surrogates from trying to trigger a physical and metaphysical response in the intended mother's body, as though vicariously embodying and experiencing pregnant physicality could somehow help the intended mother to conjure a "pregnant identity." Miller defines "pregnant identity" as the identity a woman acquires when she is socially recognized as pregnant.[8] Distinguishing between this social component of pregnancy and what she terms "physiological pregnancy," Miller argues that the two are separate phenomena that do not always occur simultaneously. She refers to two instances in which social and physical pregnancy emerge separately: "false pregnancy" (pseudocyesis, or phantom pregnancy), in which a woman who is not physically pregnant may believe that she is and her body may manifest signs of pregnancy; and "undiscovered pregnancy," in which a woman's physiological state is not socially labeled as pregnancy because she is not aware that her physical symptoms signify gestation. Miller suggests that, for social and physical pregnancy to occur simultaneously, society exerts special efforts to label and socialize.

In the Israeli case, the surrogates exert special efforts to prevent what Miller calls "normal pregnancy" from occurring. They try to keep the social and physiological components of pregnancy separate by distancing any social labels of pregnancy from their physiologically gestational bodies. At the same time, however, when surrogates channel pregnancy symptoms to their intended mother, they are attempting to access the supposed transformative power of the body to help the intended mother to construct a pregnant identity. What the surrogate is shifting along with the physical symptoms of pregnancy is thus the supposed potential of the pregnant body to construct a pregnant identity and to gradually confer maternal status. It is this movement of the pregnancy across the women's integrated bodily connection that leads me to call this construction "the shifting body."

Before I settled on this term, I deliberated over other possibilities. At first I referred to the connection between the women as a "third body," because it exists in the women's imagination as a unit detached from yet also linked to both of their bodies, existing in a space in between their corporeal selves. I subsequently thought it might be best described as a "cyborg network," because the influence of technology is evident in all stages of the women's modular interlinking. However, I finally chose to call the ensemble "the shifting body" to conceptualize its function in moving social labels, identity-building processes, and even embodied signs of pregnancy between the two women's bodies. This is a shifting body rather than a "third" or "cyborg" body precisely because it is not static and because it is constructed via interaction between the two women and those around them.

EMBODYING THE PREGNANT IDENTITY

As part of their surrogacy experience, most of the intended mothers, including those who did not feel actual physical symptoms, described their sense of "feeling pregnant." Both intended mothers who had previously experienced pregnancy and those who had never conceived used this phrase. The sense of vicarious pregnancy often emerged from their general preoccupation with issues concerning the pregnant body and fetal development. Natali explained,

> I was very connected to the pregnancy, but I didn't feel physical things related to the pregnancy. . . . It was on my mind twenty-four hours a day. I mean, everything, as if I was going through a pregnancy, except for feeling [physically]. It really was. What's going on now, and what's this, and what do we do next, and what happens during the birth, and what after the birth. I mean, it kept me busy twenty-four hours [a day]. I couldn't, really, I almost didn't function. It was always right here behind my head. That was my connection. Outside of the physical side, I think that I felt everything. All of the psychological and mental parts.

Natali's idea of carrying the pregnancy "always right here behind my head" is a clever variation on her experiential yet disembodied pregnant state. The perception that the intended mother was vicariously "carrying" the pregnancy was strengthened when friends and family spontaneously recognized her pregnant identity. One woman who approached surrogacy abroad before Israel legalized it told a newspaper reporter of this experience:

> Across the sea, there is a woman that is swelling from month to month and carrying your child, while you are continuing with your life as usual. I felt pregnant and not pregnant. A friend told me that a baby was born with a birth defect. When I expressed my shock, he said, "Oh, sorry, I forgot that you are pregnant."[9]

This example calls attention to the impact of geographical proximity to and frequent communication, shared language, and face-to-face interaction with the surrogate on the intended mother's vicarious pregnancy experience. It also suggests one reason why the Israeli women's embodied experiences were more intense than those reported in other places where surrogacy is practiced. A significant number of intended mothers in Griswold's collection acknowledge that surrogacy is "as close as you can get to pregnancy without being pregnant yourself,"[10] but none of them described their participation in pregnant embodiment to the degree that the Israeli women did. Likewise, ethnographic data on U.S. surrogacy arrangements include some minor mention of this type of phenomenon, but to a far lesser extent.[11]

In contrast, among Israeli intended mothers, manifestation of pregnancy symptoms was more the rule than the exception, and it was not interpreted as an oddity but as an affirmation of maternal claiming goals. A wide range of physical changes were reported, including weight gain, sensitized nipples, aching breasts, cramps, stirrings in the belly, and hormonal changes. Intended mothers who had given birth before undertaking surrogacy experienced these vicarious symptoms but usually to a lesser degree than those who had never conceived.

Rachel, who was in her late forties and required egg donation in addition to surrogacy, felt a change in her body in the weeks after meeting her surrogate. She noted that she had begun to experience symptoms of menopause before she and her surrogate were introduced but that, in the weeks after their meeting, she felt as though the symptoms were abating. Two weeks after their meeting, she called me to tell me (because she knew I would be interested and would not mock her) that she had stopped having hot flashes, that her nipples ached and her breasts felt different, and that she felt stirrings in her abdomen, "as if I might ovulate. I know there's probably no chance that I will [ovulate] but I feel them, my ovaries." Sarit reported two distinct physiological marks of her vicarious pregnancy, one internal (cramps) and one external (a skin rash):

> I felt very connected to the pregnancy. I really felt pregnant. Sometimes I would really sympathize with her. I mean, during the period that she had cramps, I also felt them. There weren't many things that really physically happened to me, but yes, I did get a rash, a strange skin problem that I hadn't ever had before. Itchy skin. And I felt different, I felt like something was happening to me. Something felt different.

Similarly, Ariella, who spoke to me frequently during her surrogate's pregnancy, called me one day to share what she considered to be a particularly remarkable medical finding. It was during the later months of the pregnancy, and Ariella had decided to prepare more embryos to freeze for a second round of surrogacy in the future. As part of this effort, she had taken a blood test to assess her hormone levels, the results of which she excitedly reported: "When they checked my hormone level, the level was really high. . . . I mean, the hormones were really high, like a pregnant woman has." Ariella's hormone level, Sarit's rash, and Rachel's reversal of menopause symptoms constituted uncontrollable, almost miraculous signs of their bodies manifesting "natural" pregnancy. In Ariella's case, the uncontrollable mark of her body's "natural" embodiment of the pregnancy was further legitimated by the scientific measure provided by the blood test results.

External recognition of the vicarious pregnancy was highly significant for the intended mother's identity-building process. Ariella proudly reported how her colleagues at work had contributed to her pregnant identity by recognizing her "glow" and her "bulge": "Everyone told me that I got much prettier during this pregnancy. That I look prettier. That I glow. I even had a small belly, and you have seen me, I am skinny. You know, my breasts really hurt after she was born too. I bet you that I could have breastfed her if I had tried." Odelya also noted the impact of her work colleagues' reaction to her vicarious pregnancy: "I was glowing. And I am usually a serious woman. I mean, I have rough features in my face. . . . And suddenly at work people are saying to me, 'What a voice you have now, what softness.'" Importantly, these references to intended mothers' glow, heightened beauty, breasts, and softness of voice may be interpreted as positive affirmations of their femininity and womanliness.[12] These references hint at the notion that "gender work" is being undertaken during surrogacy, possibly reconciling some of the damage to women's gender identities that may have resulted from their experiences of infertility.

For some, such validations seemed humorous in retrospect. Miri recalled that a neighbor had stopped her while she was pushing her surrogacy-born infant in the baby carriage a few months after the birth: "She said, 'Now I understand. I thought that you had just gotten fat, but now I see you were pregnant.' I just smiled and laughed." However, in most cases, social recognition of the vicarious pregnancy strongly affirmed the intended mother's pregnant identity. Sarit provided what might be the most vivid depiction of a vicarious pregnancy being externally validated and the effect that it had on her:

> During the time that she [the surrogate] was pregnant, I took a course in bio-energy. The teacher was always saying to me, "Energetically, you are really pregnant. You have a really large belly," . . . she would say, "and it is amazing. I see such a strong connection between you, between you and your baby. You are together all the time." And when she said that, I became very excited, and it did strengthen my feeling that I really did feel very connected to him. Even if physically he isn't with me. I mean, there are so many levels. And she said that this is the first time that she has encountered someone doing surrogacy and that her baby isn't with her in her belly. And she said, "Your energies are of a pregnant woman. You are pregnant."

The phenomenon described here shares similarities with pseudopregnancy, or pseudocyesis, a condition that occurs when a woman who is not physiologically pregnant believes that she is pregnant and manifests bodily signs of pregnancy such as abdominal bloating, hormonal changes, and cessation of menstruation.[13] In some cases, pseudocyesis is attributed to social factors, such as the experience of prolonged infertility and the acute desire for pregnancy. For some intended mothers, many years of infertility may have factored into their heightened identification with their surrogate's pregnant body.

However, most discussions of pseudocyesis attribute the phenomenon to psychological factors (psychopathological delusions) or a medical condition (bloating and pregnancy-like symptoms caused by an abdominal tumor). In popular culture, the condition is usually associated with psychopathology. Discussing men's reports of fatigue, food cravings, vomiting, headaches, and dizziness during their female partners' pregnancies, Munroe and Munroe differentiate between the sociocultural phenomenon of simulated pregnancy and the involuntary phenomenon of spontaneous pregnancy-related symptoms.[14] The vicarious pregnancy of intended mothers may have included spontaneous, involuntary symptoms, but I suggest that they can be better understood as part of an ongoing process of embodied claiming than as delusion. The phenomenon is therefore less like the psychological phenomenon of pseudocyesis and more similar to the cultural rite of couvade, as I argue further on.

Understanding the spontaneous bodily signs of the vicarious pregnancy in terms of appropriation techniques can also explain their link to the intentional acts of some intended mothers to make sure that the pregnant body shifted onto them and that it could be externally recognized. In a handful of extreme cases, intended mothers wore pregnancy costumes throughout their surrogate's pregnancy and avoided telling even their closest family about the surrogacy. One intended mother had a theater company prepare a special pregnancy costume for her, similar to those it used in its productions. An opening in the costume allowed additional material to be added as the vicarious pregnancy progressed. In this special outfit, the intended mother "carried" the pregnancy until the moment her surrogate gave birth by cesarean. Two other intended mothers wore less sophisticated types of padding and kept the surrogacy a secret from all but a few select people. In several cases, intended mothers also underwent hormonal treatments to induce lactation and to enable them to breastfeed their newborns. Although their stated purpose for doing so was to facilitate bonding with their newborn, they may also have wanted to inscribe an additional marker on the body to be publicly identified as a birthing mother.

The intended mother's attempts to encompass the pregnancy by inscribing the symptoms that the surrogate channels to her onto her

own body might, from a certain perspective, be seen as a type of play
acting. In other words, we might easily conclude that these women are
playing at being expectant mothers, and that the best way to do this
is to simulate pregnancy. However, I would suggest that their behavior fits Handelman's description of crossing over "from simulation to
reality, from play to seriousness,"[15] because their interpretations and
definitions of what they are doing and feeling reveal that the vicarious
pregnancy is very "real" to them. They are not "playing" but seriously
adopting the practices of pregnancy and articulating identity through
those practices.

Vicarious pregnancy might also be viewed as a type of gender performance[16] through which intended mothers seek to portray a socially
desirable ideal of "femininity" that they have been heretofore excluded
from because of their inability to bear children. Drawing on essentialist
characteristics associated with Western ideals of femininity, they call
attention to the softness of their voices and the fullness of their breasts.
They engage in pseudopregnant embodiment, calling on pregnancy and
childbirth as experiences that are often socially constructed as standards
for proving "normal womanhood" and achieving feminine identity.[17]
Their attempts to form emotional attachments to the fetus express their
claims to being "good women" and "good mothers," and the exclusion
of their male partners from the relationship with the surrogate shapes
that relationship into a female domain. In this way, the shifting body
becomes a means of "doing gender."

VISUAL VALIDATIONS OF THE SHIFTING BODY

Alongside the intended mothers' testimonies about the public recognition of their vicarious pregnancy, some surrogates suggested that the
pregnancy had been publicly invisible on their bodies. In this sense, the
shifting body was externally validated for both sides of the equation,
reinforcing the surrogate's sense of detachment from the belly and the
intended mother's "pregnant identity." Surrogates recounted how their
social circles had sometimes failed to recognize their bodily changes—
such as increased body size and enlarged breasts—as signs of pregnancy
or that those around them affirmed that they did not look pregnant.

At one of the meetings of the surrogacy support group, Ravit, who
was seven months pregnant, sat next to me in a bulky shirt. Across the
table, another surrogate, Sharon, observed, "Ravit, you don't have a
belly at all. Where is the belly? We want to see." Ravit stood up, posed

to the side, and asked, "Do you see now?" The women at the table shook their heads. "It just looks like I am fat," she told her audience, "It doesn't look like I am pregnant." Indeed, I noticed that Ravit's hips, buttocks, and waist had thickened since I last saw her, but she did not have a protruding belly that could be immediately recognized as a sign of pregnancy. Her pregnancy actually could have gone socially unnoticed, even if that was not her intention. However, it was the other surrogates' affirmation that Ravit did not look pregnant that confirmed her distancing efforts.

The invisibility of the pregnancy was central to Sapir's construction of a nonpregnant identity. She told me that she was "lucky" that she is "a healthy kind of a woman, kind of fat, and I didn't have such a big belly. So it covered me until the ninth month." Turning to her friend, who had joined us during the interview, she asked for confirmation that she had not looked pregnant, and her friend asserted that she had not identified Sapir's fatness as pregnancy until Sapir informed her of the condition. According to Sapir, very few people "knew that it was a belly of pregnancy. But if you would see me, you would say, 'Wow, what a fat woman.' Even my walking was not like a pregnant woman. . . . I was regular. My breasts stuck out more than the pregnancy did—[I mean,] the belly."

Whereas surrogates could only call attention away from their gait, belly shape, and increased girth to a certain degree, most still made attempts to disguise the pregnancy by wearing their normal clothing rather than making the symbolic transition to maternity clothes. Sherry excitedly showed me that she could still wear her low-cut "hipster" jeans in her seventh month, saying, "From behind, no one can tell I am pregnant. I am still a fine catch [chaticha]." Other surrogates wore baggy clothes. Ye'ara, for instance, proudly reported that when she was "well into the eighth month," she surprised one of her clients by telling her that she would not be taking full maternity leave: "She looked at me and said, 'What? You are pregnant!?' Because you really couldn't see it if you didn't know. And I always wore big sweatshirts, so I looked normal." Other surrogates spoke of having obviously distended bellies but what seemed to be socially invisible pregnancies. In an online surrogacy forum, Nati reported having gone to a dinner at her boyfriend's family home, where those present had not been told about the surrogacy. Although she was nearing her sixth month of pregnancy and subjectively felt her condition to be physically obvious, Nati wrote that "no one even noticed that I was pregnant. Can you believe it?!"

Sharing her experience on a public Internet forum, where other surrogates and intended mothers would read it, enables Nati to further articulate and receive public confirmation of her nonpregnant identity. Other surrogates drew on the responses of those around them to *prove* the social invisibility of their condition. Orna, for instance, recalled that several men had asked her on dates while she was visibly pregnant because they could see that she wasn't socially pregnant:

> What courage a man has to ask me out when I am pregnant! Maybe I'm married? So they would tell me: "We asked you out, we courted you, because you gave us the feeling that it isn't you and that this pregnancy is not a pregnancy." I don't understand it, but it was transmitted to people . . . they told me . . . "You gave us the feeling that it wasn't you, dancing, happy, and you take the pregnancy like a sack everywhere. We could feel that you were divorced."[18]

When she receives no public validation of social pregnancy, despite her apparent condition, Orna is reassured that she is not "really pregnant." Lihi similarly told me that her pregnancy went unacknowledged by her youngest daughter, who failed to recognize her mother's naked belly, seven months pregnant with twins, as pregnancy: "I was in the shower with her one day . . . and I asked her, 'Why do you think Mom is so fat?' She looked straight at me and she said, 'Mom, you're not fat, you're skinny!'" Lihi added that, although her daughter had not interpreted Lihi's protruding belly as pregnancy, she had recognized a classmate's mother's rounded belly as pregnancy. Lihi explained, "She looked at it [my belly] and didn't see it. And also with others, they didn't see it like they would have if it had been my pregnancy." I asked Lihi whether this lack of recognition of the pregnancy had helped her to distance herself from the pregnancy. Lihi answered:

> Yes, I guess that it did, not just from her, but from everyone. No one made a big deal about it from the minute that they found out that it wasn't mine. And since they didn't treat me like I was the mother, it just strengthened my feeling that it isn't mine.

The shifting character of the body was particularly highlighted when descriptions of the surrogate's invisible pregnancy were juxtaposed with descriptions of the intended mother's visible bodily changes. Odelya told me that Shahar, her surrogate, had lost twenty-two pounds while pregnant with Odelya's twins. Odelya, who had gained eleven pounds, asserted, "I found what she lost." Likewise, Rivka told me that her surrogate, Orna, had gained minimal weight, which she lost immediately after the birth, whereas she herself gained twenty-eight pounds during the pregnancy:

> Let me tell you something that will really amaze you. During her pregnancy I gained a lot of weight. A lot, and I was also puffed up, in the way that . . . look, also from the tension I wouldn't even eat, and still I got fat. I was round, and when she gave birth, she lost weight. She returned to the exact same [weight]. . . . And I didn't lose it. I lost it after two to three weeks. You begin to feel—it is as if people saw you pregnant and you weren't pregnant. You understand. She let me feel that.

When I first interviewed Masha, she was seven months pregnant with the first child she bore for her couple. She turned her back to me and outlined her figure with her hands, urging me, "Look, from the back I don't look pregnant, just full-figured." In a follow-up interview several weeks after delivery, Masha's intended mother, Tova, told me and a notably full-figured but not overweight Masha of her intention to join Weight Watchers to lose the weight she had gained during the pregnancy. Masha excitedly exclaimed, "You see, Elly! She gained the weight instead of me!" To this, Tova responded, "You know, the neighbor down there doesn't know about the surrogacy. She saw me with [the baby] and didn't even think about it. People just think I was fat because I was pregnant."

Later on that afternoon, Tova showed Masha and me a video recording of the baby's naming ceremony. At one point, the camera focused on Tova, in a black pants outfit, dancing vigorously with her sister. Pointing to the screen, Masha said to me, "Look how fat she looks there. She looks like she just gave birth." Tova, smiling, humorously responded that one of her distant relatives had warned her not to dance so exuberantly because it could be dangerous for a woman who has just given birth. These two examples together demonstrate how emphatically the body becomes a marker of pregnant identity through the women's interaction: in both cases Masha notes how the pregnancy marked Tova's body instead of her own, thus designating Tova as the one who inhabited the "real" pregnant body.

Changes in body size, shape, and weight are common during pregnancy, yet it is often assumed that these bodily changes are of little or no consequence to pregnant women.[19] Earle's study of pregnant women in the United Kingdom reveals that taking on the characteristic shape of pregnancy was highly significant to particular groups of women who wanted to make their pregnant status publicly obvious, for example, women for whom achieving pregnancy had been difficult and over-weight women who viewed the social label of pregnancy as temporarily relieving them from the social label of fatness.[20] Bailey's conventionally pregnant British interviewees also viewed inhabiting greater than usual bodily space as enhancing their sense of being special and having additional cultural value during pregnancy.[21] It is therefore not surprising that weight gain was such a strong parameter of the shifting body in surrogacy. Just as being mistakenly identified as fat rather than pregnant reinforced the surrogate's nonpregnant identity, the social labeling of the intended mother's increased body size as due to pregnancy reinforced her pregnant identity.

INTERCHANGEABILITY AND SUBSTITUTION

These routine acknowledgments of the surrogate's absent pregnancy and the intended mother's experiential pregnancy led women to engage in a game in which they challenged those around them to identify who was who, ritually validating their interchangeability. This arose very clearly in my first interview with Tamar and Miri, while Tamar was five months pregnant with Miri's baby. A few hours into the interview, Miri's husband returned home with two little girls who were close in age, one of whom was Tamar's daughter and one Miri's. Miri had conceived her daughter on her ninth IVF attempt and had then undergone another seventeen unsuccessful IVF cycles hoping for a second child. The girls burst through the door energetically, ready to run to their mothers, when Miri commanded them to stop. The girls froze, and Miri challenged me, "First, guess which one is mine and which one is hers."

Surrogates and intended mothers depended on those closely acquainted with their surrogacy to validate their interchangeability through similar identification games. The medical arena, in which surrogates and intended mothers were often bureaucratically considered a conjoined patient but were classified under the intended mother's reproductive goals, became a major site for the women's experimentation with identification tests, using medical professionals as dupes or ploys in their game. Rinat noted that, when she had to be hospitalized because of pregnancy complications, she and her intended mother intentionally played an identification game with a nurse who didn't know about their surrogacy:

> And she [the intended mother] was with me in the hospital. On the week-end she stayed with me in the hospital. Thursday, Friday, and Saturday she was in the hospital. Next to me in the same room. Yes. They gave us a

room alone. And when a nurse came who didn't know about our story, she started to yell. So I said to her, "Who are you yelling at." Right away I said to her, "Do you see her? That is me." And she said, "But you . . ." and I said to her, "Do you see her? She is me." So she didn't understand what it was [all about] and she went to the head nurse and said to her, "In that single room, two women are sleeping." And she answered her, "Yes, I know. Those are two women who are one. They are two that are one." And then she sat down and explained it to her.

One common arena for this type of identification test was the ultra-sound examination. For instance, Yael noted that her surrogate had pre-tended that she was Yael while answering an unknowing technician's questions: "The nurse asked her, 'How many [children] do you have at home?' and she answered, 'None.' As if she was me. So she [the ultrasound technician] said, 'Well, you have a boy.'" Riki recalled the ultrasound tech-nician's confusion when he saw that Riki's name was on the referral but the ultrasound was to be performed on another woman's body:

> The doctor asked us, "Who is Riki?" And I said, "I am." Then he asked Yelena, "Who are you?" And we said, "We are together." He said, "This is a fetal ultrasound, right?" And we said, "Yes." "The ultrasound is for you [to Yelena] and you are Riki? I don't understand." Then we explained that it was surrogacy.

We might consider Riki's account as exemplifying a means by which the intended mother measures the extent of her interchangeability with her surrogate. When the technician expresses his confusion, Riki's sense that she is a replacement for Yelena, just as Yelena is a surrogate (liter-ally, a substitute) for her, is strengthened. Each time similar scenarios are enacted, the intended mother is made to recognize the differences and simi-larities between herself and her surrogate. Riki described how amused she was by these opportunities for identification tests and how they resulted in strengthening her sense of being connected to her surrogate:

> It was that connection, that sense of fate, I mean, it really amuses us. We go for checkups and so, it's like this, there are checkups that are because of me, like amniocentesis, and the whole genetic biological issue is mine.[22] And then, what name do we write down? We are always encountering that kind of thing and we laugh about it. Because, on the other hand, the pregnancy is hers . . . so we do it once under her name and once under my name. Or whatever we feel like. . . . It is her pregnancy, but my test.

However, alongside this play of overlapping bodies and selves and the compromise of alternately writing down one name and then the other, Riki seems to want to define her own presence in the body as the determining one ("the whole genetic biological issue is mine"). Likewise, she noted that when Yelena's name was attached to the ultrasound images of her twins, she could no longer accept their interchangeability and insisted that her own name be written on the photos:

> It is extremely complicated. At first, we did an ultrasound, and I said she is pregnant, so it should be under her name. And then on the ultrasound photos, it said her name on top. And then my mom was looking and I was showing her the pictures and boasting, "Look at the pictures" and everything. And then she said to me: "But that is her name!" Then it really felt strange to me and I said, "Wait, those are my fetuses!" And then it was as if the ultrasound was saying. . . . So I asked for my name to be on it. . . . It is she who is pregnant all the time and then the fetus is also under her guardianship. But that really stings, because then, wait a minute, what part do you have in it? Because of my age we did the amniocentesis and that was because of me, so that had to be in my name. And in the end everything is in my name and that is the end of that.

Riki limits the identification game when her blurring with her surrogate reaches the point of stirring up doubts or confusion about who the mother is, who "owns" the babies. In other words, Riki enjoys being interchangeable with her surrogate, but only as long it does not threaten her claims to the social label or the children. Thus, women's unification only pertains to the pregnancy and not to its outcome; it is constructed against the women's firm understanding that the intended mother already is, and will continue to be, the only mother to the child.

The limits of this interchangeability were also evident in the exchange of humor that symbolically expressed the fear that a genetic mix-up would signify the surrogate was the "real" mother or that the surrogate's boyfriend was the genitor. Sarit told me that she would often joke with her surrogate's boyfriend, who was of Yemenite origin, "My baby better not come out looking Yemenite!" These joking interactions that referenced the ethnic heritage of the surrogate did not convey a perception that the surrogate's womb might impress her characteristics on the baby. Rather, as described in part 1, ethnic heritage was understood as a mark of "nature" that identified the fetus with its ethnic origins, and the influence of the surrogate's womb on fetal outcome was consistently nullified. Thus, these humorous exchanges were used to ritually mark the boundary of the women's interchangeability, which was allowed only up to the point of a mix-up. This doubt-abating humor referenced not only ethnicity but phenotype as well, as I observed when

Dina, who pursued surrogacy in the United States, showed me a home video of the birth of her child to a blonde surrogate in California. At the moment that the baby's head appears, the doctor jokingly announces, "She's a blonde!" insinuating that the baby resembled the blonde-haired surrogate and not the dark-haired intended parents, whose initial shock turned to laughter when his joke was exposed.

MERGING INTO ONE BODY

The shifting body and the women's validated interchangeability some-times became so convincing that it led them to imagine their two bodies as interlinked or fused into one joint entity. The most popular phrase for describing this fusion was "we are one body" (see figure 7). Dalia described her link with her surrogate in these terms: "I felt that she, who is carrying my child, she is the closest thing to me. As if we were two halves of one belly that unifies us."[23] While women imagined the belly as a type of shared "third space" between their individual bodies, they conceptualized their integration in terms of two halves of one whole. Lihi likewise described sharing her body with her intended mother: "I really felt that when I was doing it [surrogacy], then during that period my body was not just my body, but it is also Danit's body, and that is natural." Lihi saw this linked body as seamlessly piecing together their personalities and understandings as well: "Her qualities [tchunot] joined 100 percent with my qualities and her comprehension [havana] joined 100 percent with my comprehension. So there is no room here, let's say, for cracks."

The women's integration, notably, drew on parts of the body that the surrogate had distanced from the fetus, connecting her emotionally and intuitively to the intended mother as "one mind," "one bloodstream," and "one soul." Ayala, an intended mother, related, "Her bad mood also affected me. It was transferred to me in a sort of telepathy, as if we were two parts of one body, of one soul."[24] Riki described how her surrogate intuitively "knew" Riki's emotional state. She said that when her father-in-law met her surrogate, he hugged her

and he said he really appreciates what she is doing for me. And do you know what? . . . She stroked my head when I had tears in my eyes without even seeing my tears! She just feels me. And this really isn't just some kind of perfect picture that I am drawing for you. . . . In this type of relation-ship, when everything is fine and you open up your feelings and the channel between you is open, then it is a very special type of relationship.

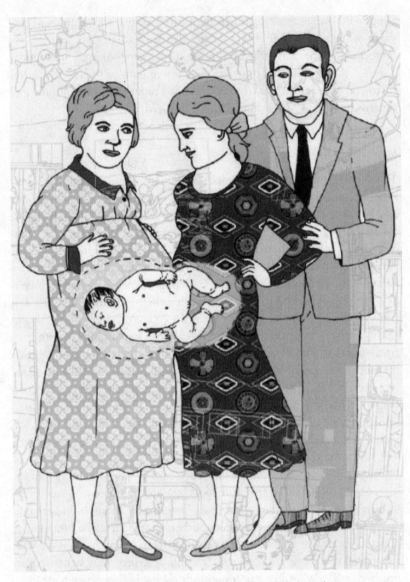

Figure 7. Illustration depicting the surrogate and intended mother as individual bounded bodies sharing a belly that connects them. The intended father supports the intended mother. Originally appeared in *Yedioth Aharonot* newspaper. Reproduced with the permission of the artist, Rutu Modan.

The women's integration conjured up imagery of similarity, merging, and simultaneous unity and duality. Often this was discursively referenced in a rhetoric of "we" to describe their temporary joint personhood. Surrogates and intended mothers commonly said things like "we are pregnant," "our pregnancy," and "we have a doctor's appointment." Sometimes this sense of "we" was also confirmed by doctors, nurses, and other medical staff, who used the plural feminine form for "you" [aten] instead of the singular feminine form [at] when giving medical instructions regarding the surrogate's body. For instance, Rivka explained that the doctor instructed her and her surrogate to "go eat, maybe while you [plural] eat, she [the fetus] will move."

Their two-as-one situation was also configured by observers' emphasis on how much they looked alike and by their use of kinship terms. Tilly repeatedly told me that people had commented on her resemblance to her intended mother, to the point of assuming they were sisters. Yael reported that she and her surrogate were misidentified as sisters at the clinic "because we even sort of look alike, we are quiet, we don't bother anyone." Lihi, who actually did, in my opinion, closely resemble her intended mother, told me that the two had been mistaken for twins. Twinship, according to Turner, highlights oppositions and complementarities: the equal and opposite aspects of duality.[25] In his analysis of Ndembu twinship rituals, Turner explains that imagery of twinship speaks to the process of uniting components of a dyad. In terms of the surrogate–intended mother relationship, twinship was linked to coupling, which Turner suggests is another expression of the same metatheme of duality and unity.

Women often used coupling and marriage imagery to describe their connection. This imagery directly links to the idea of two bodies becoming one: Genesis 2:21–24 states that man and woman "shall be one flesh" when they marry and enter a reproductive union. Repeatedly, I heard surrogates and intended mothers describe their relationship as a temporary marriage or as "just like any other couple relationship" [zugiut l'kol davar]. Aliza told me how badly she felt that her husband did not have much of a role in the surrogate relationship, suggesting that she had replaced him in the conventional structural role of an expectant father: "It is as though I am the husband and she [the surrogate] is my wife." Ayala suggested that the relationship between intended mother and surrogate was "in many ways more intimate than the relationship of husband and wife. My husband . . . knew from the beginning that my relationship with her would be more important because I am the one who must form a tight bond with her, who must enter into a close relationship with her, of woman to woman."[26]

In another play on this idea, the women included the intended father in their descriptions of their unity by fashioning themselves as his two-as-one wife. Along these lines, Rivka explained, "My husband was there for me, whatever I wanted he did. . . . I mean for me, in quotation marks, for her. Whatever I wanted to pass on to Orna [I would], so he would actually spoil two. Do you understand? It is something that can't be explained. It is two that are one. Today I say to Orna that it is like one body." Rivka described how she directed her husband to be a "good husband" to Orna, as if Orna *was* Rivka: "If he saw, G-d forbid, a laundry basket, he would lift it. As if she was me. We would go to visit her as if it was me. As if he is doing it for me. . . . He would do the things that a husband does for his pregnant wife. Period. A good husband." While Rivka viewed this construction as enabling her to play the role of "pregnant wife" vis-à-vis her husband, Orna too enjoyed temporarily "being" Rivka because of the attention she received from both of her reproductive partners. She told a newspaper reporter, "The husband was an attentive man, he was always spoiling both of us. He would buy us presents. It was as if he was married to two."[27]

As two-who-are-one, the women shared an intimacy with one another that they did not regularly share with other women in their everyday lives. Surrogates and intended mothers often talked openly about their love for each other and even exchanged short written statements, or "love notes," on the surrogacy forum for the entire online surrogacy community to read.[28] In some cases, this intimacy was also expressed to various degrees physically. Physical interactions included touch, nudity, and other behaviors that challenged heteronormative boundaries but that were normalized by the women as part of their shared embodiment. For instance, in some cases, intended mothers administered the surrogate's hormone injections, usually to the buttocks. The sexual overtones of these encounters were normalized through humor. When Miri told me in a joint interview with her surrogate, Tamar, that, after administering an injection, she would massage the area around the injection site, Tamar jokingly interjected, "You just wanted to get to know my ass!"

In most cases, surrogates were naked in their intended mothers' presence during medical appointments. Tilly, a surrogate, said, "I was totally naked in front of her a few times, and I didn't mind. When we went to the *mikvah* [Jewish ritual bath], I took off all my clothes and went in, and even in the beginning, during the embryo transfer, she saw how her daughter was put into my body." It was also common for surrogates and intended mothers to walk around publicly—on the street and in the clinic—with their arms intertwined or their hands tightly clasped. It was routine for them to hold hands during the embryo transfer, the ultrasounds, and delivery. Odelya, an intended mother, related,

> The "couple" becomes the surrogate and the mother. The connection is between the intended mother and the surrogate. I would go in when they put the camera to film the fetuses in the ultrasound. And she didn't say a thing. She sat there like this [with legs spread]. I would cover her from politeness, because she is like my daughter. I would caress [*milatefet ota*] her. I would sit and caress her skin and her belly. Just like that [shows me a picture of herself laying her head against Shahar's protruding belly and wrapping her arms around it], I would hug her, lean on her, sit with her on the bed.

Surrogates also routinely encouraged this type of intimacy. Sapir reported that she would spend hours lying on the couch with her head resting against her intended mother's chest while her intended mother caressed her belly under her shirt. When Miri's surrogate, Tamar, underwent an amniocentesis in her fourth month of pregnancy, she spent three nights at Miri's home. During that period, Miri asked her husband to withdraw from their marital bed so that she could sleep there with Tamar. Miri told me that while Tamar slept, she caressed Tamar's belly; all night, she spoke softly to the fetus in Tamar's stomach and watched over both of them, fearful of complications from the procedure.

In some cases, the women's unification also involved monogamous use of their bodies. Mutual abstinence from intercourse during the pregnancy was repeatedly the case, even though most contracts did not prohibit the surrogate from having intercourse during the majority of the pregnancy and there was no prohibition at all on the intended mother's sexual conduct. Calling the relationship between herself, her husband, and her surrogate a "triangle," Odelya noted that "the sex was altogether erased in this triangle. . . . I didn't have sex with him for the whole process almost, and she didn't with her boyfriend either." Odelya said that, even when her abstinence created tension between her and her husband, she could not focus on anyone other than her surrogate:

> And suddenly, she and I, we became addicted to one another. I mean, it was just her and I exclusively [*hi v'ani neto*]. I walk down the street, I think about her. I shop at the store, think about her. Sleep, think about her. I would fall asleep, and think about the process. . . . It was on my mind, I didn't have anything beyond it. My horizon line narrowed to [surrogate] and that's it. Nothing else interested me.

Whereas the emotional and physical homosocial associations are implicit in Odelya's comments, other women I spoke to explicitly connected the hugging, kissing, caressing, and hand holding that they engaged in with their reproductive partner to the interactions of lesbian lovers. Although none of the women identified themselves as lesbian, some jokingly spoke about how their interactions could be misinterpreted as such.[29] Tilly repeatedly described to me during her pregnancy how her intended mother would "feel her up" [mizmeza oti]. In an interview a week before the birth, she said that her intended mother "loves my body so much. She is always touching me, feeling me up. Even my breasts. She is always hugging and kissing me. People who see us in the street or in the clinic think that we are lesbians! But I don't mind, because I feel so close to her. I really love her."

Whether they are "lookalike" sisters, merged lovers, or two women symbolically sharing one body, the underlying theme of these formulations is that the women are so similar, so merged, and so interchangeable that they can replace one another. The ultimate goal of surrogacy, which, I reiterate, literally means "substitution," can then be achieved: the surrogate is pregnant but it as if she is the intended mother; the intended mother is not physically pregnant but it is as if she is the surrogate.[30] From the intended mother's perspective, it is only by manifesting this sameness that her fantasy of being vicariously pregnant through her surrogate can come true. By finding a woman with whom she clicks and with whom her initial chemistry can develop into a telepathic, twinned, merged union, she can transition to motherhood by way of encompassment and identification and ultimately experience the pregnancy *in the surrogate's stead*. The surrogate may thus be a "substitute" for the intended mother, but the surrogacy process itself entails the intended mother becoming a substitute for her surrogate.

Stacey's concept of "feminine fascination" is particularly relevant in this context.[31] Stacey noticed that heterosexual women in the 1930s and 1940s reported adoration for their favorite female Hollywood film stars that bordered on homoerotic love. In her discussion of this adoration, Stacey suggests that the female admirers were undergoing a process of feminine identity formation through their identification with the actresses and their film roles. Much like the intended mother in my study, the admirer in Stacey's study would find some similarity between herself and the star despite her conscious knowledge that it would disappear after the film had ended. Although the fans acknowledged the impossibility of their achieving the ideal femininity of the star they admired, they nevertheless underwent a transformation in their own feminine identity because of the temporary fluidity that their spectatorship allowed.

The intended mother's infatuation with her surrogate and her identification with the surrogate's body can be interpreted in analogous terms of feminine fascination. The intended mother knows that she herself will never be able to physically embody the pregnancy or be the star, so to speak. However, like Stacey's spectator, the intended mother's intense identification with her surrogate contributes to her formation of a pregnant identity and to her claiming practices. The surrogate's role can also be compared with that of the star, for her body represents the fertility and femininity that the intended mother (and the admiring film fan) wants to acquire. The attention that the intended mother lavishes on her surrogate makes the latter feel special, needed, and loved. It also amplifies the surrogate's feeling of power when she realizes that, although the intended mother may have surpassed her in terms of marriage, career, educational, or financial success, it is she who is the object of desire. Finally, it enables her to distance herself even further from the fetus by making pregnant embodiment more about sharing and intimacy with her intended mother than about gestation.

ON BOUNDEDNESS AND ENCOMPASSMENT

Thus far, I have focused on the general development of the shifting body in surrogacy arrangements. It is important, however, to understand the two extremes between which this form of interactive body and identity work is usually conducted. At one extreme, the shifting body can give way to attempts by the intended mother to completely encompass, append, and overtake the surrogate. At the other extreme, the intended mother's lack of participation in the shifting body can leave the surrogate without sufficient support to maintain her disconnections. In the first scenario, intended mothers may identify so strongly with the pregnancy that they view their own selves as dominant within the merged body. For instance, Ayala described feeling the pregnancy in her body so intensely that she wondered whether her surrogate had felt pregnant to the same degree as *she* had:

> From the very beginning, I felt pregnant. From the minute they inserted the embryos, I felt like it was my body going through it. What's more is that I have already experienced the feelings of pregnancy so I knew what it was like. Not only on an emotional level but also on a physical level it

affected me. I really had the same feelings she did—I felt it. It was really like they say, a man whose wife is pregnant goes through it. I too really felt all the nausea when there was nausea and the heartburn when there was heartburn. I don't know about her, but I really felt what she was going through. . . . Outside of the feeling of responsibility and pains on an emotional level, I felt really connected to her.[32]

Ayala's strong identification with the pregnancy blurs the hierarchy of selves she sees inhabiting the pregnant body. She simultaneously positions herself as the secondary partner in the pregnancy ("like they say, a man whose wife is pregnant"), and promotes herself to the primary partner ("I don't know about her, but I really felt what she was going through"). In a televised documentary on their surrogacy process, Ayala yet again positions herself as the main occupant of the pregnant body, even failing to mention that her surrogate is the one who is biologically pregnant:

The fact that we live near each other and are together all of the time, I think, is a very important part of the process. What she goes through, I also go through. . . . And we speak a lot about these things, and she is a partner in this, we are together; we are one body together now, that is what I want to say. We are one body together that is pregnant with twins.[33]

Ayala's description of her surrogate as a partner in *her* pregnancy calls attention to the precarious balance necessary to enact the shifting body. Unlike the clear boundaries of ownership of the body that the surrogate offers through her body map, Ayala's description suggests her perceived total convergence of the two women's bodies into an inseparable unit in which Ayala's selfhood is dominant (see figure 8). Her depiction reveals the very fine lines that separate the various degrees of the shifting body. If the boundaries of each woman's individual body remain conceptually clear to the intended mother throughout surrogacy, and if it is clear to her that it is the surrogate who is sharing the pregnancy with *her*, then the women's engagement in the shifting body and in interchangeability remains mutually respectful. In this case, the intended mother extends her own bodily boundaries to encompass the pregnancy only to the point permitted by the surrogate, and she merges with her surrogate without stifling her. The shifting body, then, serves both women's interests by simultaneously supporting the surrogate's detachment techniques and the intended mother's appending practices. However, if the intended mother's perception of the boundaries between her self and her surrogate blurs these limits, she may expand her reach beyond the sur-

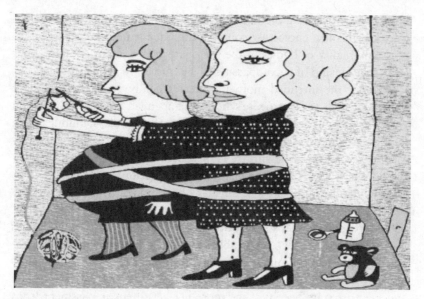

Figure 8. Illustration depicting the surrogate being encompassed by the intended mother in a suffocating relationship. Originally appeared in *Yedioth Aharonot* newspaper. Reproduced with the permission of the artist, Rutu Modan.

rogate's "red lines" and try to overtake the surrogate's entire person. It is in such scenarios that tensions arise between the "choked" surrogate and the colonizing intended mother. This was the scenario that played out in Sima's story, related in part 1.

The fine lines marking the shifting body can be conceptually understood by countering the theoretical notion of encompassment with the surrogate's body map. Encompassment, a concept frequently applied to the analysis of colonial projects, was developed by Dumont from his analysis of the caste system in India[34] and his reading of Hertz's theory of right-handed dominance.[35] Dumont defines encompassment as a situation in which two contraries are recognized as opposites (such as the right and left hands) but one (the right hand) is considered to be hierarchically whole, or elevated, and the other is seen only as a part of, or subordinated to, that whole.[36] Encompassment is thus the hierarchical absorption of one entity by another so that one category hierarchically includes the other, as in the encompassment of minority groups by a state structure.[37]

The surrogate's approach to the shifting body is nearly always based on the strong sense of personal space that her body map enables her to

retain, so that sharing the body with her intended mother is an orchestrated, controlled choice. By contrast, the intended mother's perception
of the mutuality of bodies in the surrogate arrangement is often closer
to a "relationship of encompassment" because of its whole-to-part construction;[38] the intended mother perceives her body as the dominant
body to which the surrogate's body is appended and the connection
with the other woman as servicing her own goals. As Dumont's term
implies, the intended mother's encompassment of the surrogate involves
a perceived unity at the surface (superior) level that covers up the distinction between units at the hierarchically inferior level.

The intended mother's assessment of her embodied relationship with
the surrogate can have divergent effects on the women's relationship.
If the intended mother's perception of the mutuality of the two bodies
remains respectful, then she is able to engage in the shifting body without infringing on the surrogate's sense of bounded individuality. However, the more blurred her perception of the boundaries between herself
and her surrogate becomes, the more her act of encompassment leans
towards colonization. In these terms, the surrogate temporarily forfeits
her ownership of the belly area of her bodily territory and connects
parts of herself with her intended mother with the understanding that
they will be held in a reciprocal relationship with the intended mother.
When this does not happen, the surrogate can experience a sense of loss
and even bodily repercussions, as I describe below.

ENCOMPASSMENT AS HOLDING

Maintaining a semblance of the shifting body proved to be a necessity
for ensuring a successful surrogacy outcome. Surrogates did not want to
be subsumed and encompassed to the degree of colonization, but they
did want their intended mothers to be engaged in vicariously "holding"
the pregnancy with them. For instance, some surrogates expressed disappointment and frustration when their intended mothers were hesitant
to take on medical responsibility for the pregnancy.

Although they were the exceptions rather than the rule, a number of
surrogates I spoke with complained that their intended mothers had not
been involved enough in the pregnancy, leaving them to manage organizational tasks that, as part of their distancing strategies, they would have
preferred to avoid. Lihi noted that when her second intended mother did
not take on the responsibilities that Lihi had expected her to, it resulted
in Lihi having to stand in lines at hospitals and pharmacies and to travel

to appointments at awkward times. She constantly compared her second intended mother's withdrawal from these tasks to the way her first
intended mother energetically took them upon herself: "Danit [the first
intended mother] would come with her datebook, and she would know in
advance if we are doing a test here, a test there, how it will be organized,
how it will work out. . . . Danit was concerned that nothing should worry
me." In comparison, her second intended mother "left it up to me."

Lihi also noted that the doctor in charge of fertility treatments and
prenatal care during the second surrogacy treated her with disrespect.
His attitude insulted Lihi and created tensions between her and her
intended mother when the latter, who had friendly relations with the
man, her longtime physician, did not reproach him for his behavior
toward Lihi. When Lihi spontaneously miscarried in the nineteenth
week of her second couple's pregnancy, she compared her body's difficulty in carrying that pregnancy to term with the relatively easy time she
had carrying her first couple's twin pregnancy. She blamed her inability
to complete the second (singleton) pregnancy on her intended mother's failure to assume the responsibilities that Lihi expected her to, as
well as on the failure of the relationship between herself, her intended
mother, and the doctor. She supported her contention by noting that the
intended mother and the doctor during the first surrogacy had praised
her body for its sturdiness and strength because it had accomplished the
difficult task of carrying twins to the end of the gestational period.

Lihi's assumption that dysfunctional relations and unfulfilled expectations between the intended mother, the surrogate, and the doctor can
result in pregnancy loss recurred in various formulations in my interviews with other women. Three surrogates who had not conceived after
multiple embryo transfers told me they believed the lack of success was
attributable to their intended mother's disengagement from the process
and to the strained relationship among those involved. One of these
surrogates went on to conceive in her sixth attempt after she and her
intended mother had reestablished their trust in each other. Another left
her first couple after eight failed attempts and went on to conceive after
the first embryo transfer with her second couple, who were much more
engaged in the process.

Another surrogate, Batya, asserted her belief that her intended mother's
disinterest in and failure to "hold" the pregnancy with her were to blame
for Batya's body "pushing the pregnancy out" in the twenty-eighth week
of gestation. Batya, who was only thirty-one but had birthed five children before she became a surrogate, had established a close relationship

with her couple during the eighteen months it took for them to receive the surrogacy committee's approval to proceed. Yet as soon as she underwent the embryo transfer, her trust in her intended mother and doctor was lost; without her knowledge, the intended mother had coaxed the doctor into implanting the embryos that remained after Batya's transfer into her own body. In a twist of fate, Batya and her intended mother both became pregnant. However, instead of the intended mother accompanying Batya to doctor's appointments and trying to experience the pregnancy through her, Batya found herself alone and secondary:

> The whole pregnancy she didn't pay any attention to me. She went to [a famous professor] for checkups and I went to the local clinic. . . . I didn't even know if she was happy, to tell you the truth. She was already pregnant, so what does she need me for? . . . She feels her own pregnancy, she doesn't need to feel mine too! . . . If I had been pregnant alone, then it would have been different. I know that her attitude would have been different. . . . I felt so . . . like she doesn't need me.

In the twenty-eighth week of gestation, she experienced bleeding and was hospitalized. In contrast to other surrogates whose intended mothers stood by them throughout, Batya lamented that her intended mother did not visit her during the week she was hospitalized, or even after she was rushed into an emergency cesarean operation. When Batya commented that she had carried her own five children full term, I asked her why she thought that her body had ejected the surrogate baby early. She responded matter-of-factly, "She [the intended mother] didn't help me hold it! And it fell!"

Batya's idea that the intended mother's disinterest in jointly "holding" the pregnancy led to the preterm birth is closely connected to the psychological model of "holding" proposed by Birman and Witztum in their study of integrative therapy methods to support women's experiences of pregnancy following infertility.[39] They proposed that a type of therapeutic intervention they call "maternalizing," which involves frequent therapeutic meetings, could create a framework for helping the previously infertile woman to "hold" the pregnancy. Their approach focused on building a dense fabric of support for the woman, generated through therapeutic interaction centered on understanding, empathy, warmth, communication, containment, hope, and faith. They contended that this strong support of the pregnant woman metaphorically creates "an external nest, a containment system" that is able to "contain the internal nest" of the pregnancy.

Taking the idea of containment or holding out of the context of its specific therapeutic and psychological implications, I suggest that, as a metaphor for a certain type of relationship, it can shed light on the support network that surrogates come to expect during surrogacy. The surrogates I interviewed made attempts to involve the intended mother in the pregnancy, to shift the body and to encourage the intended mother to participate in "holding" the pregnancy. The intended mothers did not necessarily have to append the belly through pseudopregnant embodiment, but surrogates expected them to show an active interest, accompany them to medical events, interact with them on a routine basis, and be their "partners" in the pregnancy. When the intended mother was hesitant or refused to help "hold" the pregnancy, as in Batya's case, surrogates believed that they had a more difficult time carrying the disconnected pregnancy.

The holding metaphor thus reveals that the surrogate's strategic orchestration of the disconnections of the body map is dependent on her ability to maintain connections with her intended mother: the surrogate cannot disembody the pregnancy and distance the fetus without the intended mother's reciprocal embodiment; metaphorically, if this is not forthcoming, the pregnancy will "fall." This idea is also closely connected to the insights Benjamin and Ha'elyon derived from their analysis of Israeli IVF users' experiences.[40] They argue that their interviewees were able to cooperate with the IVF treatment only as long as they related to their bodies as machines, emotionally dissociated themselves from the physical and emotional "pain" of treatment, and detached their bodies from their "souls." Maintaining detachment was possible as long as the painful experiences they went through were considered meaningful. When the pain was linked to motherhood, it was tolerable, but when it lost this crucial link, it was fully felt and detachment could no longer be sustained; "the powerful emotional experience reconnected body and soul."[41] It was after such a powerful emotional event or turning point that some of the women in their study decided to stop treatment.

We might understand the shared "holding" of the surrogate pregnancy in these terms. For surrogates, maintaining divisions between the personalized and distanced parts of the body map was crucial, but it required reciprocal encompassment by the intended mother. Much like the IVF patients described above, when the surrogate's detachments lost their meaning and no longer contributed toward making a mother, then the surrogate could no longer maintain them. Her "exit point" from the process was manifested somatically when the pregnancy "fell."

SURROGATE COUVADE

For intended mothers, the birth was the culmination of identification with the shifting body to such a degree that some felt that they were giving birth themselves. In many cases, as the birth became imminent, the intended mother mimicked the behavior of a pregnant woman. In the eighth month of her surrogate's pregnancy, I spoke on the phone to Elana, who worked as a therapist. She was distracted: "Elly, I am so manic. I am trying to finish everything off before I go on maternity leave, but I can't concentrate. Patients need my attention, but my mind is somewhere else." In addition to inability to concentrate, the intended mother's mode of expectancy includes other body-centered behaviors such as sleeplessness and "nesting"—the impulsive preparation of the home for the new arrival. Several intended mothers told me that they hardly slept at all during the last few weeks prior to the birth.

Mali wrote daily messages on the online surrogacy message board during the last two months of her surrogate's pregnancy, often in the middle of the night—a testimony to her sleeplessness. She described restless behaviors such as constantly lining up her cell phone, her husband's cell phone, and the house phone by her bedside each night and repeatedly checking that they were in working order in case the surrogate called. She described how she stayed close to home—"I don't leave the house, don't leave my town, not even to the neighboring cities"—as well as sleeplessness and frequent urination: "For a week already I haven't slept, I get up to pee four times a night, like someone who is nine months pregnant!" Mali also described feeling an internal sense that the birth was nearing, culminating in a sudden urge to prepare the baby's room the night before her surrogate's water broke: "I came home like a gust of wind and within two hours the room was ready. . . . I had emotional contractions every half-minute. . . . Friday night I checked the hospital bag a million times. I must have known. . . . Something bothered me and I didn't know what. Ruti [her surrogate] was calm as usual, but I was walking on needles already. A mother knows. . . . That's just how it is."

Her sense of tension was so high that when the phone did ring and her surrogate announced that her water had broken, Mali sat on the floor and burst into tears. She described walking into the hospital with her surrogate, who was calm and collected despite having regular contractions and leaking amniotic fluid: "I jumped upon her with the intention of picking her up and helping her walk. In the end it was the opposite—

she held me up so I wouldn't fall. Like I said, I had emotional contractions." As in Mali's case, intended mothers often had strong reactions
to the news that their surrogate had gone into labor. Pnina humorously
reported that when her surrogate called to tell her she had begun to
have contractions, Pnina peed her pants: "Later I told everyone that *my*
water broke."

The scenarios the women described during the birth itself were
equally significant in terms of the shifting body. Ayala described how
she and her surrogate prepared their interlinked bodies for delivery:
"She and I pressed our bellies together. We hugged each other hard and
kissed. It was as though we were transferring the feelings to one another,
and giving one another strength."[42] In a televised documentary of the
hour surrounding the birth, Ayala is depicted nervously sitting outside
the operating theater where her surrogate is undergoing a cesarean section. When the filmmaker asks her why she refuses to take a mood
relaxant, she replies, "Because I want to be awake, with all of my senses
working. I don't want anything to dull it."[43] In an interview three years
after the birth, Ayala describes how she performed a couvade-like birth
simultaneous with her surrogate's delivery:

> They gave her [the surrogate] an operation [cesarean section], and I sat
> outside, and I got up, and sat down, and at one point I fainted. I lost con-
> sciousness and collapsed on the floor for eight, nine, ten minutes. And it
> ends up that exactly at that same moment they extracted them [the twins]
> from the womb. And everyone said to me, "Here, you gave birth to them
> just now." And at that very second I hadn't known what was going on
> inside, and she had gone in already at 7:30. Eight, nine, ten minutes. They
> elevated my legs and extracted our fetuses; I mean, they took our babies
> out, while I was still on the floor. And two women took me to a side room
> and brought me the children, and I burst out crying.[44]

Ayala constructs a narrative of the shifting body delivering the twins by
emphasizing the simultaneity of the events occurring inside and outside
the operating room. Yet this construction is not hers alone; the medical
staff witnessing her birthing rite validated Ayala's vicarious delivery. Such
a dramatic reconstruction of the delivery was not uncommon. Unlike
Ayala, who had to remain outside the surgery because her surrogate was
being operated on under full anesthesia, most intended mothers were
present during the birth. When the surrogate had a cesarean with local
anesthetic, the intended mother would usually sit or stand next to her
head, hold her hand, and witness the delivery from the surrogate's visual
perspective behind the surgery divider. Eva, a surrogate who delivered

twins by cesarean, described the birth in almost mythological terms. As Eva was being operated on to extract the twins, her intended mother stood by her side holding her hand. In back of her intended mother stood the intended father, holding his shaking wife so that she would not collapse from the excitement. The situation Eva depicted recalls a scene from Margaret Atwood's *The Handmaid's Tale,* in which Janine, a handmaid and human incubator in a nightmarish futuristic society, gives birth on a double-seated birthing stool while her commander's wife sits framing her from above and behind, as if giving birth herself. It also parallels the scene in Genesis 30:3 that influenced Atwood, in which Rachel appoints Bilhah to be her surrogate, telling Jacob, "She will bear a child on my knees and through her I too may have children."

Like Eva, most surrogates encouraged their intended mothers to take an active part in the birth. For instance, Rinat described how she squeezed her intended mother's hand with each contraction so tightly that she left a mark on it. Sarit confirmed that she had felt an ache in her belly while Rinat was in labor. Rivka also detailed her vicarious experience of her surrogate's conventional delivery: "When she had contractions I felt it. I felt horrible. . . . Her goal was that I feel everything that she felt. And I did feel it. . . . When they induced, you know, she feels pain. I looked at her, and I also felt pain." Odelya reported that her reaction to the cesarean operation was even more extreme than her surrogate's reaction, even though it was the latter who was being operated on: "I think that during the birth itself, I shook more than she did. I stood next to her, holding her hand, and I was shaking. She was trying to calm *me* down. They are opening her up and she is calming me. I had Parkinson's [shaking] all over my body."

The idea of the surrogate birthing the baby on her intended mother's "knee" was played up by surrogates and intended mothers alike. Rena, whose surrogate, Tanya, delivered the baby after a long period of labor, told me that near the end of the vaginal delivery, the surrogate was so exhausted that she could no longer push. Trying to help her, Rena held the oxygen mask to Tanya's nose, rested a hand on her belly, and rhythmically encouraged her to breathe and to push. Tanya credited Rena with enabling the delivery: "She told me that without me she couldn't have done it. She said that I helped her give birth." Tanya herself reported that she experienced the delivery as the height of her union with Rena, a moment of intimacy in a shared body that was highly emotional for both of them:

We both cried in the delivery room. We were really together. Like one person. . . . The whole time the mother held me in her arms. And when the delivery began she cried with me and she held my hand and she was really with me . . . and she didn't know what to do . . . and then the baby was born . . . and I looked, and the mother saw the baby, and she cried, and she hugged me.[45]

The more that the intended mother identified with the pregnancy, experienced a phantom pregnancy, and had a couvade-like experience of the delivery, the more she was likely to tell me that she felt she had given birth herself. Rivka, for instance, confidently stated that she had birthed her daughter:

Two hours later she gave birth, [corrects herself] we gave birth, [corrects herself] I gave birth. . . . And I had never seen what a birth was like. . . . And here it is you, it IS you, I felt like it was me, it WAS me, I really felt it. . . . Yes, in the end, it was my delivery and my experience. It was my personal [experience], and I stood next to her and encouraged her a lot.

Here, Rivka vacillates between claiming the birth for herself and acknowledging that it was Orna who physically delivered the child. Several times during our interview, this pattern repeated itself, with Rivka narrating the pregnancy in the first person, saying "while I was pregnant" and "after I gave birth." It was only after I called her attention to the use of the first person that she retorted, "But I did give birth to her. . . . I remember giving birth to her." Her assurance of this "fact" was so adamant that for a moment I believed that she did.

Sarit also fully incorporated her vicarious embodiment of the pregnancy and delivery into her experience:

I guess that . . . today I don't even remember that I didn't give birth to him. I mean, my body, if I would have given birth to him I would have felt the same thing happening. . . . I feel as though I did give birth to him. I don't have, I mean, it is not like every time I look at him and that I think about him and talk with him, that there is this picture stuck in my head that I am not the one who gave birth to him. Because . . . that is the past. It is like a stage that has disappeared.

The incorporation of the experience, embodiment, and social identity of pregnancy had been so strong in her case that her body reacted to the birth with an emotional windfall that Sarit identified as the normal response to childbirth:

Also from a mental perspective I responded as though I had given birth. . . .
After I came home I had ten days of a very intense emotional state. I would
cry a lot. I cried for all of those years, you understand. Also from joy, and
also from mourning. . . . And I didn't know what was happening to me. I
didn't want to eat either. . . .You also have to let go of all of the sadness
of your life. . . . There were many years of sadness, and the air goes out
slowly, slowly, slowly.

The vicarious pregnancy occurs at the same time that the intended
mother, for cultural and other reasons, hesitates to bond with the developing fetus, so her development of a pregnant identity may conflict with
her hesitation to believe that she is going to become a mother. Thus, at
the surface level, the vicarious embodiment of the pregnancy does not
appear to further the two aims of the intended mother's claiming practices: claiming kin ties with the fetus and claiming the label of mother
to the child. Instead, it functions in a vacuum in which the fetus and its
distinct connotations for each woman is delegated to a separate sphere,
and in which the distinct social label that the intended mother strives to
be associated with after the birth remains in a liminal stage.

The women's discursive and embodied exchange does further both of
the women's goals through its strong parallels with the couvade ritual,
a phenomenon described in the anthropological literature that closely
resembles what the medical and psychiatric literature view as pseudocyesis. Anthropologists use the term couvade to discuss the development of symptomatic behaviors of identification, such as behavioral and
physiological changes, among men during their mates' pregnancy and
birth. The majority of anthropological studies of the subject look at
couvade in nonindustrialized societies, including men's observation of
food taboos, restriction of ordinary activities, and even seclusion during
their mates' pregnancy, delivery, or postpartum period.[46]

The shifting body can be viewed as a variation of this premodern
practice that occurs, surprisingly, in the most highly technologized,
modern (or perhaps postmodern) context. I find that two of the many
interpretations in existence of the couvade are most informative in this
case. The first is that of Paige and Paige, who explain that couvade often
occurs in societies where women have intercourse with multiple partners, so it is necessary for a husband to use ritual tactics to gain social
recognition as father to his wife's offspring.[47] A man performs couvade
to dispute paternity claims of adulterers and to convince his community
that his own paternity claims are legitimate. These customary rites are so
central to the social recognition of paternity rights that a man's refusal

to perform them is interpreted as a sign that he does not want paternity rights to a woman's child. The second interpretation of couvade derives from Middleton's analysis of Karambola society, in which couvade is undertaken by a husband partly to counter the excessive preeminence claimed by his wife's agnates in the act of creating the child.[48] Through the couvade, the husband documents his own consubstantiality with his wife and child; he shows how he "gives life" to his child.

These approaches to the couvade are demonstrative of the centrality of the body in surrogacy to the formulation of identity, kinship, and paternal/maternal rights. Much as in the scenario described by Paige and Paige, in which there is more than one possible father,[49] in surrogacy there is more than one woman who can hypothetically claim maternity rights. In this respect, the intended mother's vicarious embodiment of the pregnancy can be read as an expression of her desire to be socially recognized as the mother. Likewise, as in Middleton's account,[50] the intended mother's vicarious pregnancy can be interpreted as her statement through her body that she has contributed more to the creation of her child than merely half of the gametes. By emphasizing her sameness to the surrogate, she also figuratively equalizes their positions and counters the surrogate's supposed privileged embodied knowledge of the child. In summary, the intended mother's couvade-like behavior becomes a tool in the claiming process; it is a way for the intended mother to mark her territory, to claim the child, and to claim the route of production of the child as her own. As the culmination of her pregnancy practices, it retrospectively positions her entire pseudopregnancy as part of a continuous couvade-like process.

GESTATION, BODY, AND IDENTITY

As I have shown in this chapter, surrogates and intended mothers make efforts to resolve the ambiguous connotations of surrogacy through both individual and collaborative efforts. Each woman, pursuing her own personal goals, undertakes an individual "project of the body."[51] The surrogate's body project involves ensuring that her maternal and familial identities remain untouched by surrogacy through embodied strategies of distancing, transferring, and attaching the pregnancy to the intended mother. The intended mother's identity work involves incorporating the pregnancy identity through vicarious embodiment.

Significantly, the women in this study undertake these comprehensive attempts to resolve the categories of mother and family through their bodies in the context of a state-approved, contractual agreement that secures the intended mother's legal right to the child. Nevertheless, neither she nor the surrogate seems to feel that this authoritative endorsement is enough. Instead, they ritually legitimate the intended mother's maternal and kin claims by drawing on couvade practices—a premodern script for establishing kinship and paternity. Their efforts reveal how much is at stake for them in keeping kin categories clear; they also reveal how intolerable the confusion of the basic categories of body, nature, motherhood, and family is to them. Women do not ultimately resolve the anomalies of surrogacy, but they constantly work them out through their cognitive and embodied efforts throughout the surrogacy process.

The collaborative interweaving of the women's individual body projects is also significant.[52] Within the scholarship on the body as a project, the focus is often limited to the individual. In the shifting body, we witness a form of collaborative, cooperative, dual body work that depends as much on the interactions between the two women as it does on their individual efforts. Each woman's self-project is advanced through her body-centered interactions with the other; the body is engaged as a tool in the distribution of identity between them. Through the surrogate's practices of disembodiment and the intended mother's vicarious embodiment, the two women jointly highlight the way that interactively making the body absent or present can affect identity. The same body that is made absent for the surrogate is channeled into making a pregnant identity present for the intended mother, extending her sense of embodied selfhood beyond her physicality. These collaborative efforts thus illustrate a case in which identity is not just constructed through the body[53] or through interaction with others,[54] and is not merely an individual pursuit but a "joint body project."

A final observation can be made in regard to the significance of gestation itself. Throughout my discussion of the surrogate's body-mapping techniques, I have stressed the women's readiness to disregard the impact of gestation on fetal outcome. I have suggested that this may reflect the strong influence of genetic kinship paradigms on their biomedically influenced way of making sense of pregnancy; a reaction to their awareness that Judaism views the birth mother as the "real mother"; and the influence of a particular culture of pregnancy in Israel that downplays the significance of gestation. However, the practices that the women engage in surrounding the shifting body give testimony to the idea that, while biological gestation is nullified in the surrogate's distancing practices and in the women's privileging of genetic kinship paradigms, the simulation of gestation by the intended mother is crucial. It is not enough for the intended mother to have a genetic connection; instead, she has to engage in a pregnancy by proxy, to embody the gestational environment "carrying" her child, and to "replace" her surrogate in a prosthetic process of "pseudoprocreation."[55] Whereas Firestone once envisioned the replacement of pregnancy by artificial womb simulators as the possible solution to gender inequality,[56] the shifting body divulges that women may not be so willing to forgo the access that embodiment through gestation offers them in pregnancy-identity construction.

PART THREE

Separating

IN THIS PART OF THE ETHNOGRAPHY, I explore the post-birth period. Chapter 6 looks at the return of state intervention in the immediate aftermath of the birth and at the rites of categorization undertaken by hospital staff during that period. The directed separation that occurs accords, for the most part, with the intended mother's desire to seal off her new identity from her surrogate and to incorporate it as her own. It is also revealed as a classifying strategy that upholds the expectations of the contractual basis of the arrangement; from this perspective, the surrogacy arrangement can be viewed in terms of the intended mother's consumption of the surrogate's services. Chapter 7 explores the surrogate's experience of the postpartum period, including her reaction to separation from the intended mother and her expectations related to reciprocation of her efforts in gifting terms. I examine degrees of acknowledgment of the surrogate's gift in the actions of intended mothers and suggest that the degree of acknowledgment can predict the future of the surrogate–intended mother relationship.

CHAPTER 6

Rites of Classification

To this point, women's personal experiences have taken center stage; the state, as noted in the introduction, does not actively pursue an interventionist role after screening applicants and sanctioning the agreement. Once the contract has been approved, the surrogacy approvals committee's job is completed; no state representatives have any contact with the contracting parties during the conception process or during the early months of the pregnancy. Following brief contact in the fifth month, when the couple phones a state welfare officer to notify the state of the pregnancy and the anticipated due date, the parties do not interact with state representatives until after the baby is born. The direct opposition between the state's strict interventionist approach before contract approval and its absence throughout the actual surrogacy process is puzzling: if the state goes to great lengths to screen parties involved in surrogacy and to sanction their contracted agreement, why does it then leave them to experience surrogacy in a vacuum?

Even more puzzling is that the state attempts to uphold strict legal classifications of maternity and family and to make sure that surrogacy does not challenge national and religious boundaries, yet within the void created in the state's absence, the women engage in many boundary-challenging practices. They produce a type of linked and sometimes merged subjectivity during the pregnancy that they liken to figures that defy classification: twins, interchangeable persons, the conjoined patient, two in one body, two-who-are-one. They engage in an exclusive union of female-only reproduction in which fathers are sidelined, making surrogacy into a type of "virgin birth" that challenges the patriarchy.

One might speculate that this temporary form of "conjoined life" that the surrogate and intended mother dyad represents would be intolerable to the state; as Shildrick suggests, the idea of conjoined twins functioning as a merged unit threatens the masculine, Western discourse of singularity, corporeal and mental autonomy, separate personhood, and bodily self-determination.[1] Moreover, as Davis-Floyd has argued in regard to childbirth rituals in hospitals, technocratic societies and Western medicine are generally uncomfortable with cultural anomalies of this kind.[2] Indeed, studies have shown that hospital staff tend to prevent anomalous relationships from forming between organ-donor families and recipients by instating strict rules of anonymity between parties.[3] Yet the merging of the women into one body in the case of surrogacy is co-constructed and supported by the women's doctors and fed by the bureaucratic classifications of the medical establishment. How is it possible for the state to tolerate the intensification of the anomalies of surrogacy and for the medical establishment—as an agent of the body politic—to participate in their construction?

The state's tolerance of the women's intensification of these anomalies can be understood precisely because it occurs in the state's absence—it occurs in a liminal time frame and space. As Turner's theorization of the structure and anti-structure of ritual suggests, "the paradoxes of classification can only exist in the liminality of ritual."[4] Developing Van Gennep's model of the "rite of passage" and expanding on the transitional phase, Turner contends that a cultural realm outside of ordinary space and time is created during the separation phase. This liminal "space" exists "in between all times and spaces governed . . . by the rules of law, politics and religion, and by economic necessity. Here the cognitive schemata that give sense and order to everyday life no longer apply but are suspended, even reversed or dissolved in ritual symbolism."

Applying Turner's concept in a metaphorical sense,[5] we might view the process through contract approval as the separation phase, after which surrogates and intended mothers enter a liminal period of ambiguity. The surrogacy committee's selection and approval process generates the time-space framework of the cultural realm in which the women intensify the anomaly. During the liminal phase, surrogates and intended mothers behave like any of Turner's other "ritual subjects" would.[6] They set their former statuses and attributes aside (social and economic hierarchies). They elude classification and blur conventional distinctions (body/self, mother/pregnant woman). They are reduced to a uniform condition and are indistinguishable from one another (interchangeability, one body). They undergo ordeals. They are educated by their "ritual elders" (the body politic, the medical institution). They develop an intense camaraderie with one another. They engage in liminal activities, explore alternative structures, and are playful and subversive in their ambiguity. And finally, they reverse dominant symbolic binary oppositions of Israeli society, including individuality/duality, heteronormative/homosocial, material body/imagined body, embodied selfhood/vicarious embodied selfhood, nature/culture, and nuclear family/fictive kinship.

Yet I would argue that their subversiveness is tolerated by the body politic because, as Turner suggests, overturning the conventional social structure is part and parcel of the liminal phase. A temporary type of community, which Turner calls "communitas," emerges in the liminal realm. It is in this deeply creative, necessarily subversive incubation period that persons engage in playlike recombinations and inversions.[7] Turner contends that symbolic inversion actually serves as a means of ensuring transformation and that cultural resistance during the liminal period does not develop into a real alternative to the status quo. A Turner-inspired interpretation would thus maintain that the intensification of the anomaly does not represent a threat to the social order so long as reintegration subsequently occurs at all levels. We shall observe this reintegration phase below.

MEDICAL SEPARATIONS

As Scheper-Hughes and Lock remind us, the medical establishment can be viewed as an active agent of the body politic, carrying out the ideological aims of the state.[8] It is in this role that the medical system begins a regimen of separation between the parties as soon as the child is born. In contrast to its former complicity in the women's interchangeability, the medical staff now ritually differentiates the surrogate and intended mother by clear categorical labels of "mother" and "not mother." The medical staff is instructed to hand the newborn immediately to the intended mother and not to lay the newborn on the surrogate's belly to cut the cord.

In the surrogacy guidelines of one major Israeli hospital, the midwives are instructed not to show the surrogate the baby but to ask the intended mother for permission to do so. In all Israeli hospitals, both the intended mother and the surrogate receive identity bracelets with the newborn's temporary identification number, and the newborn is fitted with a bracelet on each arm, one with the intended mother's name and one with the surrogate's name. Only the intended mother, identified by her arm bracelet, is entitled to enter the nursery. The nurses are instructed to prevent the surrogate from entering the nursery without the intended mother's permission, a rule that they strictly enforce. A state welfare officer arrives within forty-eight hours of the birth to formally intermediate between the surrogate and couple by officiating at a meeting in which the surrogate signs a form stating her official relinquishment of custody. With ritualistic efficiency, this regimen of closure, containment, and individualization brings the life, so to speak, of the conjoined patient to an end, and clear and distinct boundaries are erected between the women as two separate patients in two separate wards.

The surrogate is hospitalized in the gynecological ward, while the intended mother is usually hospitalized in the maternity ward. This practice has become part of the regular protocol for surrogacy births in all Israeli hospitals since the Ministry of Health disseminated a brief establishing it as such in 2005. However, not all hospitals give the intended mother a room and hospitalize her, since the Health Ministry recommends but does not finance this practice. Some hospitals absorb the expense of the intended mother's hospitalization as both a humanitarian gesture and a marketing tactic that adds to their reputations and draws additional surrogacy births to their delivery wards; maternity is a lucrative business in Israel, and hospitals continuously find ways to attract more women to birth in their delivery rooms.[9] One intended mother who went through surrogacy in the early years of the law told me that her hospital's public relations director was so interested in garnering public attention for the hospital's role in this novel reproductive feat that he offered to hospitalize her in her own room on condition that she and her surrogate agree to be interviewed by a national newspaper. Other hospitals request that the couple pay for this service. The cost is usually a relatively small amount, roughly the equivalent of 100–150 U.S. dollars per night.

Likewise, all hospitals abide by the Ministry of Health's recommendation to hospitalize the surrogate in the gynecological ward or some other ward than the maternity ward. Before this protocol was officially established in a brief, most central hospitals already employed it. As a social worker involved in multiple surrogacy cases in a northern hospital in the early years of the law informed me, this rule was implemented for two reasons: to ensure that the surrogate was not mistakenly identified as the baby's mother, and to prevent her from experiencing emotional ambivalence at seeing other birthing women around her who would go home with their babies.

Another social worker at a central hospital proudly informed me that she had been the first one to institute this policy and that it had been so "successful" in her hospital that other maternity wards had quickly adopted it. The same social worker conducted a clinical trial in her hospital to test the effect of the intended mother's hospitalization on her ability to bond with the baby. The medical staff at the hospital coauthored an article that reported that hospitalization "might at least partially compensate genetic mothers in surrogate pregnancy arrangements for the possible damage caused by the lack of a natural pregnancy and delivery."[10]

A critical reading of this report reveals the extent to which the authors intuitively resolve the question of motherhood in their actions. Their explicit hypothesis was that certain hospital procedures could provide "an opportunity for early bonding" and "help raise the self-esteem of the genetic mother and strengthen her parenting functions."[11] Basing their assumptions on the psychological literature on maternal-infant attachment, the authors proposed that the intended mother's "natural," innate prenatal bonding capacity would be impaired because she had not gestated the baby herself. They proposed that enabling the intended mother's presence in the delivery room, handing her the newborn directly after it emerged, and giving her sufficient time after the birth to bond in solitude with her baby would enhance maternal-infant attachment. The intended mother was subsequently hospitalized in the new mothers' ward, and the staff was instructed to treat her just like any other new mother, "following to the greatest extent possible the procedure for natural mothers."[12] Intended mothers were subsequently observed for "normal" attachment behaviors. One of the two intended mothers who participated in the study was even encouraged to breast-feed her baby, which she did with the aid of hormone therapy.

This policy directly designates the intended mother as the one and only mother of the child, and not only is she encouraged to accept this social label, but her adoption of normative maternal attachment behavior is also verified through direct surveillance. She is even encouraged to perform the role of new mother by undertaking the routine symbolic actions associated with Western medicalized socialization into this role:[13] putting on a hospital gown, wearing a hospital identity bracelet, staying the night (or several nights) in a hospital bed, participating in the hospital's "rooming in" program, and, in at least one case, breastfeeding.

In comparison, the intended mother in Blyth's study of surrogacy in the United Kingdom was usually passed off as a friend of the surrogate, who, for her part, presented herself to the hospital as any other birth mother and did not necessarily notify the hospital of the surrogacy.[14] The U.K. surrogate and couple whose intrafamilial surrogacy agreement I observed also reported facets of their experience that were different from the Israeli case. Jenny, the intended mother, reported that she did not receive maternity leave from her job, unlike the Israeli intended mothers. She was not hospitalized, and only after her husband argued with the hospital staff to let her spend the night in the hospital with her newborn son was she allowed to stay the night on a cot in her sister Daniella's (the surrogate's) room. In the United States, there is no national protocol for the management of surrogacy deliveries, and I have yet to hear of an intended mother who was hospitalized or institutionally labeled as Israeli intended mothers are. The U.S. example that most closely resembles the Israeli case is one in which the intended mother was given permission to sleep on the sofa in her surrogate's room.[15] In her ethnography of assisted conception in the United States, Thompson argues that doctors and other clinicians orchestrated IVF in a way that validates the intended social labels of kinship.[16] However, the Israeli medical system's attempt to symbolically classify the intended mother as *the* mother seems to go even further in institutionalizing this process.

CLASSIFICATIONS AND IDENTITY

Although not the explicit intention of hospital policy, the medical staff's encouragement of the intended mother to perform the gendered role of a newly delivered childbearing woman facilitates and reinforces the claiming practices that the intended mothers themselves pursued throughout the surrogacy process: to claim the social label of "mother" and to bond with the expected child. Moreover, the hospital rituals accord with the intended mother's identity articulation by marking her body as a birthing body. She wears the clothing and the bracelet of a childbearing woman; she occupies the spatial territory of a childbearing woman by lying in a bed in a hospital room; and in the case of the lactating intended mother, she can even nurse if she chooses, an act that distinguishes newly delivered mothers from other women in a public setting. The hospital's symbolic recognition of the intended mother's new role is amplified by her reception of the birth grant and maternity leave from the National Insurance Institute, just like any other new mother.

Nearly all of the intended mothers I interviewed for this study chose to stay at the hospital, although some preferred to stay at the "maternity hotel" adjacent to the hospital, when available, rather than in the maternity ward. Those intended mothers who were hospitalized in the maternity ward told me how the medical designation rituals had affected their incorporation of their new identity and social label. Natali told me that she was "treated well" by the hospital, given "a beautiful room . . . a real suite" in the maternity ward: "They gave me the option of staying or, if I wanted, to go . . . so I stayed, because I wanted to get up for them [the newborn twins] at night. I was a new mother!" Maya, whose surrogate gave birth during the early years of the law, told me how she negotiated a deal with hospital staff, who had no prior experience with surrogacy births, because it was so important to her to be hospitalized:

> I demanded a room. . . . I wanted a room so that I could be hospitalized with the baby. It can't be that the baby will be there and I won't be there. And the law says nothing about that. The truth is that we made a lot of trouble over that. They told me to stay with friends and come. I said, "I refuse! I live far away, I want to be hospitalized!"

In the end, her demands reached the director of the hospital, and he agreed to give her a room in exchange for a small payment. After she was hospitalized, she was instructed by the nurse in charge of the ward to act like any other new mother would, wear a hospital gown, and not walk around too much. Maya recalled how the nurse warned her, "You are not going to walk around here in clothes. You are hospitalized, so you are in the hospital in a hospital gown like everyone else. So I wore a gown, and people came to visit me." Concerned that the two hospital bracelets fixed to her newborn son's foot signified that he had "two mothers," she described how she had symbolically secured her social label as the child's only mother: "I said, 'Why does he need two bracelets?' So I took hers [the surrogate's] off."

Maya also recalled how her status was kept so confidential that, at one point, "a nurse came in to take my temperature. I told her, 'Leave it, leave it; I don't need it.'" She also benefited from the perks that new mothers receive from marketing agents: "I also got all of these extras in the room—a pile of baby clothes and diapers in the room." The confidentiality surrounding Maya's medically cultivated birth-mother status was actively protected by a member of the hospital staff when other patients challenged it:

> When I left the hospital, I left in jeans, so everyone asked me, "How did you get [your body] back so fast? How did you return to your size so quickly?" Lucky for me, there was a nurse there who said, "There are some [women] that are just like that."

Intended mothers who were hospitalized, like Maya, were usually coaxed by the medical staff to play the part of a birth mother. Miri, for instance, told me that she had wanted to return home with her husband at night, but she was informed by the medical staff that the hospital's insurance could not cover that and she would have to spend the night in the hospital bed they had provided for her. Several intended mothers took full advantage of the leeway that their hospitalization gave them to play the part of a birthing mother to the fullest. Rivka was excited that her hospitalization enabled her to play her designated role in front of family members who did not know that a surrogate had birthed her child: "People came [to visit]. My husband's uncle came [and] he didn't know. He came to see me in the hospital."

In a separate interview, Orna, Rivka's surrogate, also informed me how Rivka's hospitalization had enabled her to publicly validate her recently vicariously pregnant and now newly maternal identity: "She had a room in the new mother's ward, as a birth mother herself. No one knew that she didn't give birth. Everyone thought that she had." When I responded that it must have been difficult to convey this impression, because Rivka's belly was not swollen, Orna replied: "You think people notice? She has a baby! Did anybody see her before? No. No one knew."

Orna added that it had struck her as simultaneously humorous and logical that, while she was on her feet, dressed in jeans, and running about within hours of giving birth, Rivka was dressed in a hospital gown, lying in a hospital bed, and receiving visitors: "Everyone thought she had given birth. . . . I even went to visit her and brought her flowers!" When I interviewed another intended father who was friendly with Rivka and her husband, he told me how tickled he had been when he witnessed this role reversal: "We went to visit her [Rivka] thinking that the surrogate would be recovering from the delivery. But we went in the room and there was Rivka lying in a hospital gown and surrounded with flowers!"

In most cases, the intended mother did not play the part of a physically childbearing mother as intensely as Rivka did. However, most
intended mothers did make subtle public statements that they had personally birthed their child. Sometimes they articulated this simply by
not calling attention to the fact that they had not physically birthed
their child or by responding ambiguously to questions about how they
had lost their "pregnancy weight" so quickly. In this way, the intended
mother's pregnant identity continued to be confirmed in the years following surrogacy as a sort of absent presence that had accompanied
her child into the world. The quintessential example of this is Sara's
response to a nurse at the well-baby clinic [tipat chalav] who remarked
that she had never seen a mother of twins regain her figure so quickly
after childbirth. Sara wryly responded, "I call it pregnancy, the 2004
edition" [herayon model 2004].

THE GLASS WALL

Whereas the medical categorization of the intended mother as the one
and only mother was embraced excitedly by most of the intended mothers I interviewed and supported by the surrogate, the surrogates were
usually more ambiguous about the roles they were assigned in the hospital setting. First, those surrogates who gave birth in hospitals with no
prior experience of surrogacy complained to me that the hospital staff
did not always know what to do with them. Ye'ara, for instance, found
during her first surrogacy that while her intended mother was hospitalized in the maternity ward and given her own room so that none of the
other new mothers would ask her questions, she was left in the hallway of the delivery ward for several hours before the staff could decide
where to put her.

Later, she was upset by medical personnel's change in attitude toward
her after the birth. Up to that point, she had described her experience
as "fun": she had enjoyed the friendly banter that she, her common-law
husband, and her couple had all engaged in with the medical staff during the labor and delivery. However, she felt angered and insulted when
she was finally transferred from her liminal position in the hallway to
what she considered to be a second-rate room without a private bathroom. Instead of the warm reception she had received in the delivery
ward, the nurses in the gynecological ward asked her invasive questions
about her "coldheartedness" in relinquishing the baby, and one nurse,
especially, treated her harshly: "She wouldn't help me get up from the

bed to go to the bathroom and I wet the bed in the end. Then I had to sit there until they changed the sheets."

Other surrogates lamented that hospital staff's strict enforcement of their separation from their intended mothers immediately after the birth was awkward and upsetting. The alteration in the positions of the surrogate and the intended mother following the birth is relatively extreme. Whereas the surrogate carried the fetus in her body for nine months, feeding it internally and mediating all of her couple's contact with it, she is suddenly required to ask the intended mother for permission to see the baby through the mediation of the nurse, hospital social worker, or state welfare officer. It is the intended mother who now holds, feeds, and is responsible for the newborn, and the surrogate is dismissed from her intermediary role. This change in the direction of their relations and the part played by the medical institution in generating their separation was vividly portrayed in a video recording that Rinat showed me of the hours following her delivery of Sarit and Reuven's son. The video shows the couple standing inside a glass-walled room while Rinat watches from behind the transparent boundary that divides them. Inside the room, a nurse instructs the new parents in how to handle their newborn child. At one point, Rinat attempts to open the door to the room for a closer look or to take part in the demonstration, only to be told to remain outside. She watches the couple, gesturing through the glass and attempting to share in their excitement. Her exclusion contrasts strongly with her constant and necessary presence at all of the medical procedures and during each stage of the pregnancy. Having been the main source of embodied knowledge for the couple regarding their child, she now witnesses a representative of the medical staff relaying information not merely in her stead but, for the first time, out of her presence.

The glass wall symbolically replaces the transparent medium that was present throughout the pregnancy—the ultrasound screen. Whereas only ten hours earlier, it was Sarit who peered through Rinat's skin with the aid of the ultrasound mechanism, now Rinat peers through the clear glass at Sarit with the newborn child. The boundary has shifted, and where it once separated Sarit from the fetus in Rinat's womb, it now keeps Rinat out of the closed room where Sarit tends to her baby. The nurse who prevents Rinat from entering the room exhibits her gate-keeping role as newly appointed intermediary between the surrogate and the newly formed intended mother–infant dyad that has replaced the women's prior, unmediated relationship. In this role, the medical professionals ensure the final shifting of the mother/child boundary and seal off the intended mother's body with the child attached.

Medical gatekeepers play a similar role in securing clear boundaries in the case of organ donation and transplantation. As Sharp's work on "organ transfer" in the United States documents, transplant coordinators and physicians, as well as transplant organizations, go to great lengths to separate the parties involved.[17] Unlike the surrogacy arrangements described here, in which this boundary work begins only in the postpartum period, organ transfers are consistently managed so that donor families and organ recipients remain anonymous to one another, with medical staff treating any communications between them as dangerous. Such types of behaviors among medical staff can be interpreted as "boundary marking mechanisms." In her analysis of the paradoxical behavior of physicians during grand rounds in an Israeli hospital, Weiss employs this term to describe how physicians defend themselves from threats to their status and counteract structural breakdown created by their entry into hospital territories that represent pollution (death, waste, sex).[18] In these terms, the hospital's ritual segregation of surrogate and intended mother can be viewed as a vehicle for the maintenance of structural order, as well as an effort to redefine the statuses of the surrogate and the intended mother so that only one of them is categorically labeled the baby's mother.

THE RETURN OF THE STATE

Alongside these medical rituals of separation and categorization, the post-birth period is marked by the state's resumption of its role as intermediary and gatekeeper of the agreement. In a final intermediary measure, the state secures the dismissal of any possibility of custody claims by the surrogate and officially bestows parenthood on the intended parents. Within twenty-four hours of the birth, the state welfare officer arrives at the hospital and secures the signatures of both parties on official papers relating to the surrogate's relinquishment of the child. The surrogate has virtually no rights to the child following the birth; her opportunity to revoke the contract is limited to the seven days following the birth. During this time, however, the surrogate cannot contest the contract on the grounds that she wants the child herself, but only on the grounds that she thinks the intended parents are manifestly unsuitable to raise the child.[19]

When the surrogate's relinquishment of the baby has been secured, the state welfare officer becomes sole legal guardian of the baby. This means that, although the intended parents can immediately take the newborn home in their custody and serve as his or her caregivers, any major surgery or decision regarding the child requires the welfare officer's permission. With neither the surrogate nor the couple legally recognized as the child's parents, the child is essentially "parented" by the state for the first weeks of its life. The couple applies to the family court for a parental order seven days after the birth, and the child receives a temporary identification number and a temporary birth certificate until the parental order is issued. It is only after the court approves the parental order (usually up to three weeks following receipt of the application, but sometimes as long as two months later due to bureaucratic delays) that the child is given a new, permanent identification number, issued a new birth certificate in the intended parents' names, and recorded in the intended parents' identity cards as their child. This intervention can be interpreted as a symbolic act in which the body politic claims the child as its own; the state is revealed as having ultimately commissioned the child's birth itself.

The intervention can also be viewed as a final measure to ensure that the social label of "mother" is distanced from either of the potential mothers until the state officially recognizes the intended mother as the one and only mother. This official recognition is also evident in the state's grant of maternity leave to the intended mother. The surrogate is also offered maternity leave, but few surrogates claim their right to it because the majority fear their government aid stipend will be withheld for the duration of the leave. Most surrogates are, however, compensated directly by their couples for "sick leave," recovery time lasting two weeks, or more if the surrogate has undergone a cesarean delivery. The intended mother and the surrogate are each awarded a maternity grant [ma'anak leda], which is a one-time monetary sum paid to new mothers by Israel's National Insurance Institute. The birth grant has a long history as an award paid to mothers for their "contribution" to the nation, and the sum granted increases according to the number of children a woman has birthed.[20] In this way, the state simultaneously rewards both women for "reproducing the nation," and both women accept this honor, even as the surrogate's refusal of maternity leave benefits symbolically singles out the intended mother as the only mother of the child.

To appreciate the significance of the administration of these rites of categorization on a procedural level, it is useful to compare Israel's practice with the way that the British government relates to surrogacy.

In Britain, the intended mother is given neither maternity leave nor any new mother's benefits. Moreover, the child's parents are considered to be the surrogate and the surrogate's husband or legal partner until the court issues the intended parents a parental order. In contrast, the Israeli system makes every effort to categorize the intended mother as "mother" from the beginning, withholding that label from the surrogate. This comparison demonstrates the sharp contrast between governments that do not intervene in natal policies and those that do, like Israel; it also marks the extent to which surrogacy is constructed as a collective issue in Israel and a private, individual issue in Britain (and the United States).

What is revealed by the Israeli state's role after the birth and its classificatory practices is that surrogacy, ultimately, is made to uphold state interests. Its labeling practices and post-delivery interventions ensure that surrogacy does not disrupt the traditional concepts of motherhood and family. Surrogacy emerges not only as a site for the body politic to symbolically, if not numerically, promote its pronatalist ideology but also as a locus in which the body politic can set an example of clear classifications and rigid boundaries precisely because it has legitimacy to bureaucratically control the process. In an era of reproductive technologies, alternative family formations, rising divorce rates, and other changes to the traditional ideas of family and motherhood, surrogacy emerges as what we might call "the last remaining outpost" in which the state can order, monitor, control, and distribute childbirth, children, and maternity.[21]

INTENDED MOTHERS AND RITES OF INCORPORATION

This official institutional protocol of separation seems to accord with intended mothers' own aims of finalizing the parental claiming process. Separation from the surrogate facilitates the elimination of the surrogates' symbolic threat to the intended mother's sole occupancy of the maternal category. The shifting body is finally disengaged entirely from the surrogate and shifted completely onto the intended mother; having encompassed the shifted body in totality, she no longer needs the surrogate to mediate access to her child, for she now *carries* the child herself. Neither does she need the surrogate to interactively co-construct her pregnant identity and social label, for she is now officially recognized as the one and only mother of the child. Even if surrogates made their intentions to achieve this goal very clear throughout the pregnancy, intended mothers often felt suddenly threatened after the birth by the possible competing claims that the surrogate represented. This perceived threat prompted most intended mothers to limit the surrogate's contact with the baby after the birth. Yael, for instance, claimed that she felt "relieved when they [the hospital staff] told her [the surrogate] that she couldn't see him [the baby]. She came to me and told me, and I was just quiet. I said that I had no influence over the hospital rules."

In some instances, intended mothers reported their ambivalence about the sudden symbolic "glass wall" mediation of professionals who came into contact with them after the birth. Dana, for instance, reported that the state welfare officer's advice to break off all contact with her surrogate immediately after the birth was contrary to her own instincts. She related that she had become so attached to her surrogate that she did not want to lose her as a friend and felt that this professional advice displayed the welfare officer's lack of sensitivity toward surrogate–intended mother relationships. In another case, Maya told me that, just after delivery, the nurses had advised her against showing her surrogate the baby, but Maya did so anyway on her own initiative, reasoning that "she carried him for nine months. She must want to know what came out."

Still, many intended mothers also expressed a need to distance themselves from their surrogate after the birth to finalize their claiming process and to fully assume their new identity, status, and role. During hospitalization, the intended mother usually visited the surrogate every day, but after the intended mother returned home, the intensity of their relationship usually began to taper off. Riki told me one week after her twins were born, "We were with her in the hospital that whole week. But now I don't really want to see her. I need time with my girls alone." This distancing had the effect of finalizing the claiming process. But it also reflected the intended mother's absorption in a new, all-consuming relationship, which took up all of the emotional resources she had invested earlier in the surrogate. Rivka noted, "There was a period, a month or two, when we weren't in contact, and then we got in touch again. It had just been so intense. I needed a rest."

However, beyond these two motivations lay the stark reality that the intended mother no longer had a vested interest in cultivating a close relationship with her surrogate. Rivka admitted as much, saying, "You have to separate between things. Here I had something very dear to me by her. So it was natural that all of me was hers. Because she was pregnant. But after the birth . . . it did die down a lot if you look at it. We were in day-to-day contact and then suddenly not, but it's natural. It's a very natural thing." I commonly heard similar descriptions of the relationship losing intensity as a "natural" outcome of surrogacy's end.

This need for separation immediately following the birth is often just as jarring a surprise to the surrogate as the medical staff's sudden change in protocol from support of the shifting body to institutionalized separation. Ragoné suggests that separation from the surrogate was not as pronounced a decade ago when traditional surrogacy, in which the surrogate provides the ova, was the common practice.[22] Indeed, she was surprised in her later fieldwork by the displays of unkindness directed toward gestational surrogates by their couples in the immediate postpartum period. Whereas in traditional surrogacy arrangements, the surrogates had been shown gratitude for their efforts, gestational surrogates were often not afforded that same kindness. Gestational surrogates who bore twins for their couples were shown even less kindness, presumably because their services would not be needed again.

Ragoné found that gifting language was much less prominent in gestational arrangements. This, to Ragoné, was a reflection of the primacy of the "blood tie" in U.S. kinship: when the traditional surrogate births a child of her own egg, the couple realizes that the surrogate has given "part of herself" and acknowledges this as a "gift of life." In gestational surrogacy, Ragoné contended, the surrogate is seen as merely having "carried" the same child that would have resulted if the intended mother had been able to give birth herself. In terms of lasting ties between the parties, the couples who would be raising the genetic kin of the surrogate could not deny her ongoing contribution to their family. As one intended father remarked to Ragoné about his traditional surrogate, "I realize now that what Jane [the surrogate] gave was a part of herself; that's fairly profound."[23] In gestational surrogacy, it seems, the ability to deny the surrogate's role in creating the baby is both easier and more tempting: if the intended parents believe the outcome would have been the same with or without her intervention, the urge to "erase" her immediately after the baby is born can be overwhelming. In the next section, we shall see that intended mothers often feel such a need to encompass in a singular occupancy the role, status, and identity of mother to their child that they engage in rites of integration that end up downplaying or entirely eliminating the surrogate's role.

DEFINITION RITES

The intended mother's distancing of herself and her newborn from the surrogate are part of a set of ritual practices and narrative techniques that she uses to elicit social recognition of her new identity and social status. These are rites of incorporation aimed at finishing off what her prenatal claiming practices began. Turner suggests that, in the reintegration phase of a rite of passage, the initiate must assume rights and obligations of a clearly defined and structural type.[24] Since there is no formal script for the rite of passage of a woman who becomes a mother through surrogacy, intended mothers engage in what Rubin, Shmilovitz, and Weiss describe as unconscious "personal definition rites," those of individuals undergoing identity changes that depart from the regular cultural corpus of life cycle events.[25] Much like Rubin and colleagues note in the case of formerly obese persons who undergo drastic weight loss and change their identity from "fat" to "thin," intended mothers perform an array of "rites of integration" to complete their identity change from "childless woman" to "mother." These rites include one common among "regular" parents, validating the child's resemblance to the parents, as well those common among persons who become parents through assisted conception or adoption, such as formulating a narrative of fated events[26] and presenting the child's origin story in a photo album.

The first of these techniques, validating resemblance, is a common practice among parents of newborns. However, in a situation such as surrogacy, in which not only technology but also another woman enters into the reproductive effort, the underlying fear that the child might really be the surrogate's is inevitably present. Accordingly, surrogates and intended mothers seem to almost obsessively emphasize to themselves, to friends and relatives, and to me, that their child looks nothing like the surrogate and exactly like the intended parents. I have noticed that, whenever I interview an intended mother or phone to congratulate her after the birth of her child, she tells me who the child looks like: herself, her husband, or another member of their family. Surrogates, by contrast, nearly always mention during such conversations that there is no resemblance between themselves and the baby and how happy the parents were that the baby looked like one of them.

This preoccupation with the resemblance of the child to the intended parents seems to voice a retrospective fear that the baby could have mistakenly been the genetic offspring of the surrogate or that the surrogate could somehow have "shaped" or affected the baby while it was in her womb. In a video recording of the moments after Tamar gave birth to Miri's daughter, the validation theme was especially prominent. The video, directed and filmed by the excited intended father, shows Miri, the intended mother, dressed in a green hospital gown sitting on a chair. Her face red and swollen with tears, she holds her newborn daughter. Miri's eight-year-old daughter Shiri, whom she gave birth to herself, is coaxed into the frame to stand next to her mother with her head positioned near the baby's face. The intended father's voice emanates from behind the camera, pronouncing their resemblance: "An exact copy. It is the same face." Then a large photo of Shiri as a baby is aligned parallel to the newborn's head. The father-director frames the shot so that the viewer sees the newborn, the baby photo of her older sister, and the older sister's face in one horizontal lineup of genetic characteristics, as kinship is ritually validated through their resemblance.

Through a second rite of integration, the intended mother assembles a photo album narrating the story of the child's entrance into the world. As Ben-Ari illustrates in his analysis of a rite of passage in a Japanese commuter village, the choice to take particular photos and to present photographic records in a particular way can influence how an event is later remembered.[27] As Boquet also reminds us, recent studies of kinship often focus on "new" reproductive technologies, but there are still many "old" reproductive technologies, such as photography, that are used to articulate kin ties.[28] Boquet posits that the conventions of family photography, in particular, transform relations into recognizable kinship forms.[29] Different kinds of photography can be used to constitute kin ties. Sontag imagined families as using photographic chronicles of themselves to memorialize, symbolically restate, and bear witness to their connectedness.[30] The act of photography and what one later does with the photos thus involves making connections between people. Through such conventions as making and showing albums or excluding certain photos from an album and instead consigning them to a drawer, family photography can be used to constitute kinship.[31]

In this light, intended mothers' photo albums frequently document their own participation in their child's birth as though they were the ones who actually gave birth. During an interview with Rivka one year after the birth of her daughter, she showed me an album filled with photos of the child immediately following the birth. The album contained only one photo of her surrogate, Orna. She is shown sitting among a group of people in Rivka's home at an informal gathering and is indistinguishable as having had any connection to the birth of Rivka's child. The majority of photos in the album told a narrative of Rivka herself as the birth mother. In a set of photos taken in the hospital right after the birth, Rivka is pictured wearing a hospital gown, her face beaming, and clearly exhausted. Pointing to the photos, she prompts me, "Don't I look like I have just given birth?" I answer, "Yes, you have that aura. You are glowing." Rivka continues, "But look at my face. At my expression. I look like I have just been through childbirth." I look at the photo, in which she does indeed appear a bit swollen in the face, and agree with her, "You do; you look like you've been through a difficult delivery."

Later, Rivka retrieved a small envelope of photos from her nightstand drawer in her bedroom. "These pictures I keep in my drawer," she tells me. The pictures show a very pregnant Orna smiling for the camera. In one photo, she is with the doctor, in another with Rivka's husband, and in a third, Rivka and Orna are shown embracing one another, both dressed in hospital gowns. The symbolic removal of the photos of the surrogate from the baby photo album was common among most intended mothers whose albums I was able to look at. The baby albums usually had the same structure: they began with the ultrasound photos, then progressed to photos of the newborn immediately after the birth, and then to photos of the newborn being held by each parent and other family members. When I asked if the intended mother had a photo of the surrogate, she usually responded that she did not, or else she produced one from a "hiding place," from a drawer where it was tucked away.

Mali was the only intended mother I encountered who actually had professional photos taken of her surrogate's belly. In the photos, Mali and her son are shown reading to the nine-months-pregnant disembodied bare belly, laying their heads on the surrogate's lap under the belly, and encompassing the belly with their hands. The surrogate's face is never shown. Under the photos, which Mali uploaded to the forum website, she wrote, "One of the reasons I did this is for my baby, so he will understand that even if I was not able to carry him myself (and that makes me very sad), I loved him, and I was there, and the surrogate was there, and we all protected him and spoke to him and waited for him. And there was a pregnancy and there were photographs and it was not in my body, . . . but we were there all the time. I want him to know when he grows up that we all loved him, even then, from outside the belly."

Some albums fortified the child's origin story with additional signs that the intended mother had been the birth mother. For instance, one album included several photos of the cesarean delivery, in which the newborn is shown being extracted and lifted above the surrogate's open belly. Whereas the surrogate's insides are graphically exposed, her face is hidden behind the surgery divider. The photos are followed by a series of shots of the intended mother in a hospital costume, sitting on a chair with a red, puffy face wet with tears as she holds her bundled infant. Anyone unaware of the surrogacy context would assume that she had given birth herself.

MIRACLES AND DESTINY NARRATIVES

These image-based narratives of the child's origins and the intended mother's role in the child's birth were supported by "miracle stories" in which intended mothers told of the fated, destined circumstances surrounding their surrogacies. These "it was meant to be" narratives are common among persons who become parents through adoption as well.[32] In these stories, intended mothers ascribed the success of the technology to their own determination and faith, identified "signs" that had revealed to them that surrogacy was their intended path, and usually emphasized how their surrogacy story had succeeded "against all odds." The surrogate was often positioned in these stories as a type of messenger or cosmic helper, sent to them by G-d to help them complete their destiny.

Several intended mothers connected the beginning of their surrogacy story to a symbolic death. Sometimes this "death" was surgery for cancer or gynecological complications that led to the removal of their uterus. Other women spoke of having fallen into a coma or having "died on the table" during a routine IVF procedure, usually after having undergone multiple attempts (ova extraction is carried out under full anesthesia and involves risks such as hemorrhage). Following this symbolic death, they received a sign that they would have a child through surrogacy. One intended mother told me that she could overhear the conversation between the doctors while she was unconscious during the emergency hysterectomy she underwent after her first child's birth: "I heard one of them [the doctors] saying, 'Now she can't have another [child].' Then the other one said, 'But she can do surrogacy.' When I woke up, the doctor told me that surrogacy was my option now, and it was as if I already knew."

Intended mothers also described meetings with their surrogates as signs of the destined nature of their surrogacy path. Nitai, unlike most intended fathers, even adopted this "destiny" rhetoric himself when he described the fated connection his wife and he had with their first surrogate: "We really fell in love with this woman, and I don't believe in mysticism and all that, but her son was born on the same date as my daughter was, and after we met, I said to Yaffa [his wife], 'If this isn't a sign' . . ." Riki drew mystic support for her transition to motherhood through surrogacy from the strange alignment of events that it corresponded to. She had married a widower with three young children when she experienced a late miscarriage that ended in hysterectomy. When her surrogate was five months pregnant with twins, she retrospectively considered the events that led her to surrogacy. The mother of her husband's children lost her life at age forty-two to cancer, and Riki was raising her children for her. Riki lost her womb at age forty-two and needed a surrogate to carry her babies for her: "It was like I had to lose my ability to give birth so I could raise her kids and someone else could take care of mine." These coincidences were reinforced when she arrived to sign the surrogacy contract in front of the surrogacy approvals committee and realized that one of the committee members was the doctor that had performed her emergency hysterectomy.

Most intended mothers' narratives also included a dramatic, miraculous point that proved to them that G-d had wanted them to have a child. Odelya's was the most dramatic miracle narrative I heard. During her twenty-second IVF attempt, she fell into a monthlong coma following the ova extraction procedure. When she awoke, she learned that her mother had passed away, that she could not endanger her life with additional IVFs, and that she had only four remaining frozen embryos to use if she wanted to try surrogacy. She met her surrogate, Shahar, by chance at a local gym and, against all odds, the surrogate became pregnant with twins on the first try with the last two embryos that had survived thawing. Odelya noted that this was particularly miraculous because the eggs had been extracted when she was forty-four years old and had been frozen for four years. Several months into the pregnancy, her surrogate visited her at work and dramatically let out a scream when she recognized the photo of Odelya's late mother hanging over the desk. It turned out that Shahar's own mother had been Odelya's mother's caregiver, which neither of them had known. Odelya interpreted this coincidence as proof that she had been destined to meet Shahar and to become a mother through surrogacy: "It was as though the minute I decided, G-d sent her." Looking at Shahar as we sat together with her after the interview, she said to her, "I told Elly my [late] mother sent you."

CONSUMPTION AND THE STAKES OF THE GIFT

In some respects, the intended mother's regimen of separation and individuation from her surrogate in the postpartum period might recast the entire surrogacy arrangement in terms of consumption, or the buying and using of goods and services. The surrogate, after all, was contracted to supply a particular set of services in exchange for monetary payment. Money has a divisive quality;[33] the exchange of money for a set of services leaves the buyer and the seller with no mutual obligation because the exchange expresses a relationship of otherness, a lack of relationship. Familial obligations are not the outcome of monetary exchange; families are popularly believed to give to one another out of love, not money.[34] From the perspective of consumption, both the intended mother's fascination with her surrogate and her encompassment of the shifting body might be recast as parts of the consumption process; the caregiving, closeness, and intimacy shared throughout can be retrospectively compartmentalized as a whole set of "extra" services that the surrogate supplied to the intended mother.

From this perspective, the Israeli state is cast in the surrogacy agreement in a position similar to that of the private market in U.S. surrogacy arrangements. As arbitrator of the agreement and as an explicit agent in the parties' separation, the state makes sure that the agreement distributes maternity in a one-directional, bounded, neatly categorized manner. The surrogate is, then, merely an instrument; maternity is distributed by the state to the intended mother by way of borrowing the surrogate's womb. This type of separation can result in the surrogate feeling used, like a commodity. Whereas many U.S. commercial surrogacy agencies explicitly formulate the contractual agreement in terms of a business contract and "educate" their surrogates to view surrogacy as a paid job, with the expectation of separation and a program for separation instilled from the start, in Israel, the state's lack of intervention in the "vortex" period leads to confusion when this institutional separation is suddenly imposed.

Yet as we shall come to see in the next chapter, these neat separations are not so ontologically secure as they might have been intended. As the process unfolds, the surrogate's expectations gradually develop into those appropriate to gift relations. It is by counterpoising the surrogate's gift logic with the regimen of consumption and separation that the "messy" dynamics of the post-birth period are revealed.

CHAPTER 7

The Surrogate's Gift

Whereas intended mothers often felt the need to distance themselves from their surrogate after the birth, surrogates often viewed a couple's abrupt change of attitude toward them as insulting. When I visited Belle in her hospital room two days after she had given birth, her couple arrived to say good-bye to her before they were discharged home with the baby. The intended mother initially entered the room, and the intended father remained at the door holding the baby seat with the baby in it. The room was filled with visitors from the surrogacy Internet forum, and we all excitedly urged the couple to show us the baby. The intended father moved inside the room, and we surrounded the baby with vocal "oohs" and "ahs." When Belle, lying in the hospital bed after cesarean surgery, asked to see the baby too, the intended father moved toward her hesitantly, keeping the baby seat at a distance from her. Belle then tried to look more closely, and he awkwardly extended his arm toward her but still kept the baby too far away for Belle to see.

When the couple left, Belle noted how strangely they had been acting toward her since the birth and how hurt she was by this behavior. Ravit, one of the surrogates present in the room, commented in response, "They acted as if from your bed you might grab the baby and run." The episode became a central topic of conversation at the next face-to-face gathering of the surrogacy Internet forum. One of the participants reported that Belle had not seen or heard from her couple for the remainder of her stay in the hospital or for two weeks after she returned home. Another surrogate commented to me, "It is not like we suddenly become monsters." An intended mother who was friendly with the couple reported to the group that they had only done what the social worker had instructed them to do. Belle's experience gave rise during that gathering to discussion among those present of how couples should and should not treat their surrogate after the birth.

As Belle's story imparts, surrogates often expect that the alliance formed with their intended mother during the pregnancy will represent the beginning of a lasting friendship or kinship bond. For some, these expectations complicated the post-birth period because their couple had contrasting expectations. Surrogates nearly always expressed anxiety over the approaching birth because they feared their intended mother would abandon them after the baby was born. Sapir described the birth as a highly emotional episode:

> When I gave birth, I became anxious and sort of depressed. Not because of what's-his-name, the baby or something, but because the whole thing was over. . . . I was really afraid that I was going to lose her. . . . So I started to cry in the [hospital] room, because it was over. Look, I was the center of everything for a year. And when I was hospitalized, I cried. I would cry at night, until the next day. . . . I cried over Shoshana, not the baby. So the next day Shoshana came when the welfare officer arrived, and Shoshana said that she didn't want to break it off and that calmed me down. . . . I can no longer imagine myself without speaking to Shoshana at least once a week. And it calms me down that I have permission from her to call her whenever I want, and even to visit her.

Like Sapir, other surrogates routinely informed me of their apprehensions about losing the relationship with their couple. Tsila told me two weeks after she gave birth that "the next day I cried a lot because I thought that I was losing a friend." Likewise, Sherry was noticeably upset when I called her shortly before her scheduled delivery to wish her luck. After repeatedly expressing during the pregnancy how close she had become with her couple—"They are like a mother and father to me now"—she was "preparing for the worst," that she would go on alone. When I spoke with her two weeks after the birth, she sounded much more positive, telling me proudly that her intended mother frequently phoned her because she missed her so much and that she even asked for her advice on parenting since Sherry was the more experienced parent.

Tamar described this particular type of anxiety as "emptiness": "Emptiness is the fear of the surrogate that it's over. Let's say the mother will suddenly be with the child and won't care about her [the surrogate] anymore." She explained that emptiness begins with a twinge of doubt: "There is a kind of 'twinge in your heart.' It is not because you are parting from the baby. It is because there is the fear you might lose the mother." Tamar notes that, in contrast to her relatively neutral separation from the baby, the thought of separating from her intended mother affected her *heart*—the personalized seat of the emotions in her body map—because Miri was a "part of" her and the baby was not: "Look, the whole pregnancy, the baby hasn't been born yet, and it isn't my egg and my embryo, but Miri was with me the whole time. We were best friends . . . and the intimacy. Miri saw me naked. I felt throughout the pregnancy that Miri was part of me."

ON CONTRACTS AND GIFTS

The surrogate's expectations of a lasting bond with the intended mother after the baby is born reveal a tension between two divergent perspectives on their relationship: contractual exchange versus gifting. Contracts were signed between the parties in all of the surrogacy agreements in this study; money was exchanged in all cases. Yet the monetary incentives were nearly always matched, if not superseded, at some point before the birth by the surrogate's commitment to her couple. Lihi articulated this change, noting, "Surrogacy begins with the money but it doesn't end with the money." In this respect, although the surrogacy arrangement began as a commercial exchange, surrogates came to shift their understanding of it as a gift exchange. One popular vehicle for expressing this sentiment was to confirm their loyalty to their "mission" even if they were offered twice the money by another couple or if they suddenly became wealthy. Eva related, "From a certain point onwards, even if I had won the lottery I would have continued, because the money stopped having the same meaning that it did in the beginning."

This shift in the surrogate's understanding of the relationship differs from the attitudes of U.S. surrogates studied by Ragoné, who, from the start, downplayed their financial incentives and stressed instead their altruistic motivations for entering surrogacy agreements.[1] Ragoné's findings are supported by Almeling, who found that the majority of compensated egg donors in the U.S. agencies she studied stressed altruistic motivations and did not even mention money among their motivations.[2] Both authors conclude that such sentiments enable surrogates to comply with the gendered cultural image of women/mothers as selfless, nurturing, and altruistic and to prevent remuneration from detracting from that image.

The Israeli surrogates, conversely, were up-front about their motivations being primarily economic; nearly all also expressed the desire to help a childless couple, but altruism was not considered a strong enough reason to motivate them to become surrogates. Indeed, accepting compensation for their surrogate role was not as stigmatized an issue among the Israeli surrogates as it seems to be for their U.S. counterparts, and I did not find the same attempts to justify their payment or restate their altruistic motivations that other studies found. This difference may perhaps stem from the religious background of the Israeli surrogates and the general lack of moral and ethical opposition in contemporary Jewish law to compensation for the donation of biological material.[3] It may also stem from the organizational structure of surrogacy: whereas U.S. surrogacy and egg donor agencies will sometimes refuse to accept a candidate who expresses overly strong financial motivations,[4] the Israeli surrogacy approvals committee legitimizes monetary payment by prohibiting solely altruistic arrangements and maintaining that surrogates should receive at least the standard compensation rate. If anything, the Israeli surrogates were less concerned with downplaying the money they received than they were with not being socially judged *freiers*. *Freier*—a key cultural concept in Israeli cultural discourse—can roughly be translated as a "sucker," an unwitting victim or dupe.[5] A surrogate might be deemed a *freier* if she were to accept too little money or if the amount she was paid was seen as not worth the effort.

I suggest that the surrogate's development of a gift rhetoric during the process is directly related to two elements of her experience: the body map and the closeness with the intended mother. I suggest that these elements contribute to a shifting of the surrogate's perspective over the course of the agreement, from viewing it as a contractual exchange to viewing it as a gift relationship. First, gradually, throughout the pregnancy, the surrogate learns to define the contours of her body map; by way of this exercise in self-definition, she comes to comprehend exactly what she has and has not invested in surrogacy. While she may never have considered the baby to be "part of her" and may distance the belly throughout, she comes to understand the enormity of her investments in the intended mother: her caregiving, identity-building, and bonding efforts as well as the camaraderie and sharing of the body she offers her throughout. Her efforts to make her counterpart into a mother are not part of the distancing protocol; these are personalized, intimate parts of the surrogate's heart, soul, and self. Second, the close and intimate relationship that develops between the surrogate and her intended mother also contributes to her comprehension of the relationship in gifting terms: the women may have started out as "business partners," but from the surrogate's perspective, they have become friends.

In contrast to contractual expectations, giving a gift is the maximum expression of non-otherness,[6] and in contrast to the exchange of commodities, gifts establish enduring connections between people.[7] Hence, when the surrogate says that the idea of the gift eventually superseded the monetary exchange, she is implying that her relationship with the couple has passed from otherness to relatedness. Gifts are invested with the giver's identity and thus create social bonds, in contrast to commodities, which can be alienated without tying seller and buyer to one another socially.[8] While the scholarship on the gift in reproductive contexts has stressed the power of the rhetoric of the "child as gift," the surrogate's body mapping ends up differentiating the gift from the child to some extent. By understanding the baby as originating in its parents' genes, the surrogates see themselves only as carrying the child and not as giving the child as a gift; since they did not believe that any part of their personal self was invested in the child, relinquishing it was not enough to generate expectations of reciprocity. Yet the surrogate's caregiving, bonding, and identity-building efforts conducted toward her intended mother did come from her self. She interprets her close relationship with the intended mother and the connection she feels with her as investments strong enough to serve as grounds for establishing a lasting social bond with her.

Occasionally, a surrogate expressed a willingness to forfeit the money to prove to her intended mother how much she loved her. Gali, a surrogate I met in the support group, shared her fantasy of surprising her couple after the birth by refusing to accept the final payment. The only such fantasy that actually did materialize among my informants was in Masha's case. After birthing one baby for her couple, Masha vowed to be their surrogate again without reimbursement. Having failed to convince the approvals committee to allow her to be their surrogate a second time solely altruistically, she contracted with her couple for a minimum fee. Two years later, after she birthed their twin girls, she refused to accept this pay. When I spoke to her several weeks after the second (cesarean) delivery, she said, "This time, when I did it without the money, it is something else. This time, I am really able to say that I did it from my love for Tova [her intended mother]. We have such a beautiful relationship."

The power of the surrogate–intended mother intimacy to shape the contractual relationship into a gift relationship is also expressed in the surrogate's personal commitment to the couple, even when it clearly went beyond the contracted commitment. The "tyranny of the gift"[9] coerced the surrogate to do things out of commitment to the alliance she perceived between herself and her couple that she would never have done in the context of a mere contractual exchange. For instance, Sima noted how she was apprehensive to undergo the embryo transfer and almost refused to submit herself to it until she looked at her intended mother and felt she could not forsake her: "I saw how I was an anchor for her."[10] She later told me that she ended up staying on as her couple's surrogate because of this sense of alliance: "The more I got to know her, the more I felt like I wanted to do this for her. Because she made me, in the way she treated me, feel close to her. . . . I said that I felt a kind of shared fate with her. She made me feel that way. She got to me, as you say. So I did it for her, let's say."

In extreme cases, this commitment transformed the gifting logic into one of self-sacrifice for the benefit of her alliance with and investment in the intended mother. For instance, Osnat, who was lauded in a national newspaper for her heroic commitment to her couple, continued to try to bear them a child even after they had made the decision to terminate her first two late-term pregnancies when fetal abnormalities were detected. Since the majority of the payment arrives only after a live birth, Osnat was paid only small sums for these terminated gestations; still, she told the reporter that she was determined to undergo additional embryo transfers for her couple, stating, "My goal in life—and this is not an obsession, like someone said to me—is to bring Dalia and Gilad a child. And that is what will happen."[11] During the years of her involvement with her contracting couple, she became involved with a man she planned to marry and with whom she hoped to have another child of her own. Still, she was willing to put her own life on hold in favor of her commitment to making her couple into parents:

> It is already the third try . . . and financially it hasn't paid off for a long time, but I love them and I want to help them bring a child into the world. . . . I don't regret it, it is worth all of the tests, the running around and the pain, because to give parents a child that is their own is a wonderful thing and I am willing to undergo it for them. I am giving them something that is flesh of their flesh.[12]

The notion discussed here, of a gifting logic gradually entering into the surrogate's conceptualization of surrogacy, tempers the idea of the dichotomous opposition of gifts and commodities through which surrogacy is so often discussed. Such dichotomous depictions of surrogacy in the popular and academic literature have tended to frame the entire relationship in terms of gifting (which risks romanticizing it) or in terms of commodification (which risks reducing it to a relationship of exploitation). My findings suggest that it is only by counterpoising the logic of contractual obligations with surrogates' development of a gifting logic that we can come to understand the complexities, tensions, and divergent expectations that both contracts and gifting generate in surrogacy relationships.

Moreover, the development of a consciousness of giving among surrogates at different points within the surrogacy arrangement tempers the perceived opposition between love and money than can be found in Euro-American societies[13] and in the scholarly literature more widely.[14] The surrogate's sentiments reveal that market reasoning does not necessarily subtract from the gift.[15] Rather, her sentiments reveal that gifts and commodities, and love and money, can be functionally and sequentially linked together and that one or the other can be privileged depending on the social context.[16] Surrogates perceive the exchange as contractual initially but ultimately as a gift. The payment does not eclipse the gift. This is similar to an idea Valerio discovered among the Huaulu people of Seran, Indonesia; Huaulu men claimed that they bought their wives for costly sums, yet this did not contradict their assertion that they did not sell their daughters or sisters but gave them away as gifts.[17]

Finally, the surrogate's understanding of her efforts in gifting terms tempers scholarly discussions of gift giving in reproductive contexts as they have been theorized until now. Specifically, anthropologists of reproduction have primarily discussed the role of the "child as gift" in reproductive contexts in the United States.[18] As I have described in this chapter, the child is not necessarily the most important gift, or the primary gift, that the Israeli surrogate gives; instead, the most personalized and important gifts she sees herself as giving surround making another woman into a mother. By broadening our focus beyond the "child as gift," we discover that, in some reproductive contexts, the most meaningful gifts that a person may see herself giving go beyond the child. In addition, as Layne has noted, the rhetoric of the "gift of life" and its association with the idea of the "child as gift" are closely associated with the New Testament;[19] these Christian inflections of gift rhetoric are pervasive in U.S. popular culture. The different emphasis we see in the Israeli surrogacy context on the nature of the gifts being given may open us up to thinking about the ways in which reproductive gifts are formulated in cultures in which non-Christian religions have more influence.

EXPECTATIONS OF RECIPROCATION

The entrance of a gifting logic into a surrogate's thinking starts to change her expectations regarding reciprocity for her gift, leading her to look beyond the payments for acknowledgment. As Marcel Mauss's theory of "the gift" has taught us, in contrast to commodities, which are bought and sold in a one-time transfer of ownership, giving a gift generates the expectation of reciprocity: one gives, another receives, and then, in acknowledgment of what is given, reciprocates.[20] Surrogates want acknowledgment equivalent to what they have given.

These expectations of reciprocity invariably potentiate misunderstandings, disappointments, and tensions between the parties to the contract. Surrogates expect that the couple not mention the money involved in the arrangement and that the surrogate be treated as a generous, important *giver*. This means the couple should not keep tabs on every extra shekel spent on the surrogate. It means they should pick up the tab for any expenses she may incur while engaged in activities related to surrogacy—for example, cab fare, a babysitter, and the bill for an outing at a café after a doctor's appointment—even if this is not stipulated in the contract. It means showing an interest in the surrogate's own well-being and not just in the baby she is carrying, showing that they think of her as more than just a "human incubator." For instance, the surrogate may expect the intended mother to phone her on a regular basis, especially after medical appointments. If the couple asks her to take a two-hour bus ride to a medical appointment in her third trimester rather than driving her there, the surrogate may interpret the request as degrading and as evidence that the couple does not appreciate her.

During the pregnancy, some intended mothers also come to understand this gifting logic as it begins to manifest in their surrogate's perceptions. In such cases, intended mothers shower their surrogate and her children with material gifts during the pregnancy as a form of "counterprestation"—return gifts that are given to secure the best gift possible from their surrogate. For every medical appointment, no matter how far away they live from her, they drive to pick up their surrogate, accompany her to the appointment, take her out to eat afterward, and drive her home. In this light, intended mothers who give of themselves to the surrogate during the pregnancy by "carrying" medical responsibility and actively sharing in "holding" the pregnancy might be viewed as making efforts to secure the surrogate's gift of sharing the pregnancy.

Other intended mothers view the surrogate's expectations as "necessary costs" of the surrogacy relationship. They find it difficult to dismiss the many extra expenses they encounter and describe what surrogates consider to be reciprocal debts in terms of a burden and an unfair price they have to pay for their surrogate's services. Intended mothers described to me how they had "spoiled" their surrogate but said that she had never thanked them for anything, only seeming to expect such attention; that their surrogate was overly demanding or took advantage of the situation; that the time and emotions they were investing in the relationship were "emotionally draining"; and that their surrogate was unfairly exercising power over them. However, the line between counterprestations and "necessary costs" was not always clear, and both types of sentiments could be expressed by the same intended mother during different periods of the agreement.

The strongest tensions that develop from the surrogate's expectations of reciprocation develop in the period surrounding the birth of the child. The surrogate expects the couple to acknowledge her gift forever as a debt of life. Whereas commodity exchange would mean they would part ways when she has finished her temporary "job," the surrogate expects her gift to create a shared future and a bond of enduring solidarity.[21] This ultimate form of acknowledgment of the surrogate's gift is not simple for the intended mother, because it confuses the clear-cut separations that she needs to fully bind and incorporate her new identity. Much is at stake for the intended mother if she recognizes the surrogate's contribution as a gift. First, as Mauss argues, the gift retains properties of the giver's identity, moving the image of the giver into the consciousness of the recipient in some substantial way, so that even if the gift has been abandoned by the giver, it still contains part of him. Accepting a gift is therefore to accept some part of the giver's "spiritual essence, his soul";[22] it is to integrate an element of the giver's identity into oneself.

Expanding on this idea in the context of Melanesian gift exchange, Strathern suggests that "the gift, as an appendage of the person who gives it, transfers part of that person with it."[23] Whereas the commodity model draws firm boundaries of contracted ownership of the child and unquestionably designates the intended mother as the only mother of that child, the gift symbolically continues the surrogate's possible "competing claims." And even though from the surrogate's perspective, the baby might be secondary to the other gifts she has given her intended mother, the intended mother does not always understand that initially. For the intended mother, acknowledging the surrogate's gift might constitute recognizing the surrogate's continuing symbolic hold over the child and over her own maternity. This might threaten the intended mother's claiming practices, making it more difficult for her to incorporate the child and the social label as her own.

In addition, if the intended mother acknowledges the surrogate's contribution as a gift, she is essentially agreeing to be bound to her in a debt of life for this priceless gift. As Douglas writes in her foreword to a more recent edition of Mauss's classic book, "A gift that does nothing to enhance solidarity is a contradiction."[24] Mauss maintains that every gift creates a connection, or link, between people, not only because accepting the gift constitutes agreeing to hold a part of the giver, but also because every gift holds the expectation of a return gift, linking giver and receiver in common ties of reciprocity.[25] When the intended mother acknowledges what she receives from the surrogate as a gift, she is agreeing to a long-term relationship with her. And this is not necessarily something she is prepared for. As Hyde warns us, "Because gifts do have the power to join people together, there are many gifts that must be refused."[26]

Finally, acknowledgment of the surrogate's contribution as a gift has the power to mediate the power hierarchy involved in the surrogate-couple relationship; it has the potential not only to serve as a leveling device[27] but also to endow the surrogate with the upper hand. As Mauss has famously noted, by giving the gift, "the giver has a hold over the beneficiary."[28] Giving a gift creates indebtedness and obligation; the recipient is required to reciprocate, so the definition of the exchange in gifting terms establishes a state of continuous indebtedness.[29] When the surrogate defines her gift as "priceless," then her couple can never fully reciprocate; she therefore symbolically has a hold over them for the rest of their lives.

Negotiations over the acknowledgment of the surrogate's gift come to a head in the hours, weeks, months, and years following the birth, in which a hierarchy of acknowledgment appears. The high stakes for the intended mother in acknowledging the surrogate's gift lead to various degrees of acknowledgment along a continuum between two extremes that I call "momentous acknowledgment" and "denial of the gift." As we shall see in the next section, acknowledgment could cement the surrogate–intended mother relationship, consecrating vestiges of their intimacy in their future relationship and revealing that the relationship was not all contractual. Denial of the gift, conversely, could lead the surrogate to experience a deep sense of betrayal.

FORMS OF ACKNOWLEDGMENT

I refer to *momentous acknowledgment* as the singular moment when the intended mother suddenly realizes the pricelessness of the surrogate's gift, and the women's temporary bond is suddenly transformed in her eyes into a heroic alliance. It is at this juncture that the intended mother's interests, fascination, and encompassment behaviors are suddenly overwhelmed by her realization that she really *does* love her surrogate as one loves any mythic comrade-in-arms.

When I phoned Sara several weeks after the birth of her twins, she told me that she had imagined herself running to grasp her babies in her arms the moment that they were extracted from Eva's womb. However, when the moment arrived, she realized that she would rather remain with Eva until the cesarean operation was over: "I just couldn't leave her there alone. I really only saw the babies afterwards." Sarit recalled that at the moment Rinat gave birth, she too was overpowered by her commitment to her surrogate: "Suddenly, the birth . . . I sort of expected that she would interest me less, like I would focus only on the baby. [It was] the opposite. During the birth, I understood how much I cared about her and how attached I had become to her." She described the hours of labor, emphasizing that she was more committed to Rinat's welfare than concerned about the well-being of her newborn:

> I really worried about her at first. I worried terribly. I mean, there was this thing where they took the baby to treat him, a first treatment kind of thing, and they had to scrape out the placenta that didn't come out [of Rinat]. And I felt very uneasy. I mean, until I knew that she was completely all right, I was not calm. Just don't let there be some kind of complication in this birth [I thought]. I mean, I couldn't stand the thought that, G-d forbid, she would be damaged from this birth, from the birth of my son. I really, really worried about her. I mean I had one eye on the child and one eye on her. As excited as I was that I suddenly had a child, I don't think I really even let it sink in then, but I was really with one eye, with one-and-a-half eyes even, on her.

Rinat, for her part, was touched by the knowledge of her importance to Sarit. As we viewed a video recording of the hours surrounding the birth, Rinat turned to me and said, "Soon you will see a part where Sarit is crying, because she was so worried about me. I didn't know she was crying that way; I only saw it for the first time on the film." Soon after, Sarit appears onscreen, standing in the hallway, only a few steps away from her baby in the mobile crib. Sarit's face is turned away from the camera, and her husband, Reuven, tries to comfort her. As the nurse enters the frame and begins to roll the baby away, Sarit does not follow but remains still, weeping in her husband's embrace. Next to me, on the sofa, Rinat says, "Do you see how hard she is crying? They took me in for a little operation after he was born. The placenta didn't come out fully. And she was worried about me. She didn't calm down until she saw that I was okay."

These moments of momentous acknowledgment can be understood as a form of symbolic sacrifice in which the intended mother chooses the surrogate over her new baby. Nili called me from her cell phone several hours after her surrogate gave birth by cesarean section. She sat on a bench outside the intensive care unit, worried because her surrogate had still not been moved to a regular room and no one would tell her why. She could not fully be with her newborn daughter until she knew that Tilly was all right. One intended mother who was interviewed in a national newspaper even expressed her momentary willingness to forgo having children in exchange for her surrogate surviving possible complications from the pregnancy: "At one point they took her to the operating room, and at that moment I prayed to G-d that she would be all right. I said to [G-d] that I don't care if I don't have children, the main thing is that she comes out okay."[30]

Many intended mothers express overwhelming gratitude and love for their surrogate that they only fully realized in the wake of the delivery. Miri recalled that her first thought the moment her baby was born was about her surrogate, Tamar: "Suddenly I understood how much I love this woman. I was filled with love for Tamar." In a phone conversation a few days after her child was born, another intended mother, Dana, said emotionally of her surrogate, "I can't imagine not speaking to her anymore. I called her this morning, and when I heard her voice, I started to cry. I love her so much. I feel like we are now connected by blood." Even Mali, who documented her struggle with jealousy of her surrogate throughout the pregnancy in messages to the surrogacy forum, found that contrary to her expectations before the birth, she suddenly found herself in its aftermath even more attached to her surrogate than she had been during the pregnancy. It was Mali, rather than her surrogate, who was the one to pursue a continuing relationship.

For surrogates, the moment when the intended mother acknowledged their gift became their *trophy moment,* the moment that they recalled in their narratives as the most moving moment in their surrogacy experiences. Orna recalled how her intended mother "chose her over the child" immediately following delivery: "Right after the birth, she didn't even go to the girl. She just strangled me with joy and hugs and kisses and everyone was crying." Rivka's instinctive action was interpreted by Orna as evidence that her image had truly seeped into Rivka's consciousness,[31] that the "part of herself" she had invested in the relationship was being held carefully by Rivka and reciprocated in her devotion. This is the ultimate sign of acknowledgment. The intended mother's reciprocal sacrifice "proved" to the surrogate that her intended mother really did care for her and retrospectively validated the "realness" of their relationship. Lihi reflected on her intended mother, Danit, in this regard:

> During each stage of the pregnancy, from the beginning to the end, from the first month to the ninth month, the most important thing to her was that I would be okay. For everything she would come and ask [the doctor], okay, the kids are okay, "but what about Lihi?" At every stage. . . . When [the doctor] told us that we would probably be hospitalized, when my blood pressure escalated . . . the first thing she said was: "Who will be with Lihi's daughters?" She says, "Do you have groceries at home?" . . .
>
> After the delivery, she was with me in the room to help me before anything else. She left her children and she was with me. That is Danit. . . . She did more than necessary. The first week, right after we left the hospital, that same night she called me. She had a mess at home and they [the twins] didn't eat and she didn't know what to do with them, but her first phone call was to me. Even more, the first Sabbath she told me, "You are coming over." I said, "I'm not." She said, "I won't take no for an answer." It was for the circumcision ceremony [brit]. She said, "I am going to tell you when and where and you will be there." And we were a little late and they waited. As if I am so important.

Not all acknowledgments of the gift took such dramatic form as the momentous acknowledgment, but other, more nuanced forms were also meaningful to the surrogate as validations that her gift was appreciated. One such form of acknowledgment occurred when the surrogate witnessed her couple's faces when they saw their child for the first time. Many surrogates called this moment "the best part." Masha, like many other surrogates, was struck by the profound significance of what she had done when she saw her gift register in her intended father's expression: "All I could look at was Gavriel's face. I will never forget it as long as I live. And when I saw Tova and Gavriel's excitement in the delivery room, I knew that there is nothing more wonderful than to give them this gift."

As Masha's words convey, it was often particularly significant to the surrogate to see the intended father's face on first sight of his newborn, since intended fathers often remained distant during the pregnancy;

their emotional response was therefore even more meaningful. This was especially true for Ye'ara, whose intended father (in her second surrogacy) had criticized her for being ill throughout the pregnancy and had repeatedly reminded her that "pregnancy is not an illness—my mother had ten children and never complained." After Ye'ara underwent an emergency cesarean, it was the verbal "thank you" from the intended father that became her most important validation:

> I know that at some stage . . . I remember that I woke up, and he stood there at the door, and he said, 'Ye'ara, I don't know how I can thank you. Thank you.' As if suddenly, I think during the birth, that in those moments, and afterwards when he had a baby in his arms, suddenly he understood the difference between what he had done all of those months and reality.

Couples' appreciation was also expressed in written form. The "thank-you letter" from the intended mothers to the surrogates usually became a cherished memento. The surrogates often framed them and hung them on the wall or kept them in their purses. Several times during interviews, surrogates brought out their letters and showed them to me proudly, much like trophies they had won. New mothers also read thank-you letters out loud to surrogates on several occasions I observed. For instance, Odelya read her six-page thank-you letter, which she had written out on parchment paper, aloud to Shahar in front of a crowd attending her post-surrogacy party. Similarly, Miri read her thank-you letter to Tamar at a surprise party she organized for Tamar a few weeks after the birth. I will never forget how Miri read out loud while sitting on the sofa close to Tamar, their heads leaning together and tears running down their cheeks:

> Dear Tamar,
>   I am sitting here to write a few words in an attempt to somehow summarize something that cannot be summarized in words. . . . Tamar, you gave me the greatest gift in the world. A special gift, a priceless one from such a priceless and special woman. I know that these words won't be able to express the true gratitude that you deserve. I love you my dear and thank you for this wonderful year, for your patience, endurance, kind ways [no'am hahalichot], and for trying to relieve me when you saw what stress I was in and for heroically enduring [amad't begvura] this unique process.
>   I love you, Miri.

Acknowledgment also took the form of the intended mother announcing the pricelessness of the surrogate's gift in public. For instance, in addition to reading the thank-you letter at Tamar's surprise party, Miri also made a speech in front of hundreds of guests at her baby's naming ceremony about her daughter's path into the world. Her voice broke during her speech when she mentioned Tamar, whom she praised, saying, "My Tamar . . . who with her rare courage of heart, in her kind ways, in the admirable conduct that she displayed all along the way that enabled this unique process."

In the four years that have passed since then, I have seen Miri express her appreciation of Tamar's gift in several appearances on television and on the radio. In one televised interview seven months after the birth, Miri was asked if she was still in touch with her surrogate. Miri's answer was bold and clear: "Of course. We just celebrated Independence Day together. I love my surrogate, a true love, and I am so grateful to her for what she did for me." Public statements of this nature are also popular on the online surrogacy forum, where intended mothers acknowledge that "there is no price for what she did." Although somewhat formulaic and very sentimental, these public thank-you messages were heartfelt and very meaningful not only for the surrogate and intended mother but also for the entire online surrogacy community. The post-birth message to her surrogate that Mali posted on the forum succinctly expressed that the "gift of life" she was acknowledging was not just the "child as gift" but many gifts: "What you have given us is not just nine months of pregnancy but an entire life afterwards. . . . It is the air we breathe, our happiness to wake up in the morning." Then, addressing all of the surrogates participating in the forum collectively, she added, "You are not just birthing children, you are birthing new mothers and new and happy families."

MATERIAL GIFT EXCHANGE

The forms of acknowledgment discussed above were accompanied in some cases by the material exchange of gifts between surrogate and intended mother after the birth. Ragoné found in her study of U.S. surrogacy in the early nineties that material gifts were so regularly given to surrogates by couples that the practice actually became incorporated into the recommended protocols of some surrogacy agencies.[32] Like Ragoné, I found that intended mothers often fantasized about the material gifts they planned to bestow on the surrogate after the delivery. Riki told me in the fifth month of her surrogate's pregnancy of the gift she planned to give her surrogate:

I am always saying that I hope she will give me two diamonds [twins], but
she is really the jewel of the crown. And I think about it and I really want
to make her a chain with a crown and a jewel in it. It is something that I
think about, I haven't planned it yet. But when I imagine it and I say how I
want it to be, then it is the jewel in the crown, yes. She gave me the crown
of motherhood and she is the jewel in it.

By comparing her surrogate's gift to precious stones, Riki is acknowledging the pricelessness of the surrogate's gift. Significantly, Riki
acknowledges her surrogate as an integral center point within her own
"crown of motherhood." Ragoné similarly notes that U.S. couples often
give their surrogates gifts of jewelry featuring the child's birth stone,
which she suggests memorializes the surrogate's connection with the
baby: "Worn on the surrogate's body, it symbolizes and validates the
special intimate bodily connection between surrogate and child."[33] Conversely, in Riki's case, and in the Israeli case more widely, the gifts of
jewelry memorialized the surrogate–intended mother relationship, with
much less symbolic reference to the child.

After the birth, many intended mothers chose to give their surrogates
expensive jewelry that symbolically represented their alliance. Roni gave
her surrogate a locket with her surrogate's birthstone on it, engraved
with the words "G-d bless you." The surrogate reciprocated with a pair
of earrings containing the same birthstone, telling her intended mother
that, wearing them, she would never be able to forget her. Another
intended mother bought an expensive jewelry set and gave her surrogate the ring and the bracelet while keeping the necklace herself. Still
another intended mother gave her surrogate a necklace with a charm
on it in the shape of a small heart within a big heart, explaining that
because her child's name, Libi, literally meant "my heart," the charm
represented her baby inside the surrogate and the surrogate's enduring
place inside the intended mother's heart.

The heart motif was common in many post-birth exchanges. Sarina,
for instance, gifted her intended mother with an art object she had
crafted herself in the shape of a heart. Since the heart was a personalized
organ of the body map, Sarina's gift represents a part of her personal
self for the intended mother to keep. When an intended mother gives
her surrogate a heart-related gift, it symbolically connotes her acknowledgment that the surrogate invested her personal self in their relationship. As Riki told me regarding the exchange of hearts in surrogacy:
"Nothing can translate into what you receive. Nothing. A contract is a
contract, but not here. It's not. It is the heart here—the heart, and if you

come with a full heart, you will get a full heart." It comes as no surprise that intended mothers who acknowledged the enormity of their surrogate's gift sometimes gave their babies gift-related names, such as Shai ("gift") and Matan ("gift" or "giving").

Material acknowledgment also took the form of gifts that the intended mother knew the surrogate would particularly appreciate: Sara took her fashion-conscious surrogate on a surprise shopping spree and told her to choose several new outfits at Sara's expense. Tilly's couple gave her money to pay for a vacation with her son. Other couples gave surrogates gifts for their whole family, such as a new computer or television. Most of the time, the surrogate understood the gift as one that the intended mother had personally invested thought in giving, so it was representative of their commitment to one another. Conversely, Maya told me how her surrogate was disappointed by the gift Maya gave her after the birth: a relatively uninspired set of dishes that testified to the relatively distant relationship they had shared during surrogacy.

Significantly, after the birth, surrogates also gave gifts to their couple, usually connected to the latter's transition to parenthood. Thus, the gifts were either clothes or toys for the baby or items that symbolized the surrogate's acknowledgment of the intended mother's status as sole mother to the child. Two surrogates, Tsila and Tilly, gave their intended mothers personal journals in which they had recorded all of their thoughts, feelings, and experiences throughout the pregnancy. And Sapir symbolically gave her intended mother an especially important token of recognition: the birth grant payment she was given by the state. In transferring the grant, which constitutes the state's recognition of childbearing women's contribution to the nation, Sapir relinquished her last remaining ties to the official title of mother to the child and crowned the intended mother as the one and only mother.

ENDURING SOLIDARITY

The surrogate–intended mother relationship forms the preconditions and infrastructure for a long-term relationship in the years following surrogacy. Whether this relationship is maintained depends on many variables: the intended mother's acknowledgment of the surrogate's gift, the type of relationship that the gift establishes between them, common interests, and geographical proximity. However, even when contact is not maintained through shared activities, in many cases, as I discuss below, the "enduring bonds of solidarity" still remain.[34]

In the most common scenario that I have witnessed in the years that I have followed surrogacy relationships, the intended mother's acknowledgment of the surrogate's gift creates what Kaplan calls a "heroic friendship" that follows the romantic model of friendship.[35] In other words, if the surrogate's gift is adequately acknowledged by the intended mother, and the intended mother actually does recognize the pricelessness of the surrogate's gift, then both tend to glorify their relationship as an important one that they nostalgically remember years later, even if they have not met or spoken for a very long time.

Kaplan identifies the heroic friendship as usually forming from male camaraderie in military settings and consisting of an exclusive bond between two men.[36] Many of the characteristics of the heroic friendships he describes parallel those of the surrogate–intended mother bond. The men in the romantic model have an intense encounter in which they experience an instant connection they describe in terms of "clicking" and "chemistry." They form an exclusive, intense bond that they equate with "love" or "marriage" and that they cultivate in an intense incubation period that is detached from their everyday lives (again, usually in the military). Kaplan argues that the men deliberately create an imagined shared past in anticipation of a shared future, even though their experience together is brief.

In one obvious parallel to Kaplan's model, the surrogate–intended mother bond is constructed exclusively between the two women. All other participants in surrogacy, including the intended father, the doctor, the surrogate's children, and the baby that the surrogate gestates are excluded from the surrogate–intended mother partnership. Moreover, just as the male heroic friendship primarily results from military encounters, the surrogate and intended mother view themselves as heroines in a military-like drama. As I further develop in part 4, in discussing surrogates' accounts as "quest narratives" of soldier-like heroines, the surrogates and intended mothers who conform to the romantic model view themselves as having jointly undertaken a mission in which the stakes for both of them are very high and in which they show courage, perseverance, and strength. Their camaraderie establishes a bond that endures even if, after "the mission" ends, they do not see one another for long periods of time or ever again, recalling the former military buddies Kaplan studied or the reserve soldiers studied by Ben-Ari.[37]

In later years, the heroic friendship shared during surrogacy usually dissolves relatively quickly into the memory of a bond forged during what they retrospectively view as a significant "life-event."[38] This dissolution occurs because of geographical distance or because, with the surrogacy over, they no longer have much in common. Shoshana, who had been extremely close to her surrogate during the process before she moved abroad, told me how their relationship tapered off afterward:

> A week after the birth, I told her that we were coming to visit, because I thought that it was very important that we don't just suddenly disappear. She did for me the best thing I have in my life; I won't just dismiss her. Afterwards, we left to go back abroad and the relationship continued through the computer—e-mail, a few phone calls, and then we lost touch. Not because something happened. . . . I actually feel like calling her and I will, to see how she is, because I believe that we will still be in touch in the future, just because for a few months we haven't been in touch. . . . I believe that we will still meet. . . . I think about her all the time. She is like a part of me. . . . You know, I can't forget her. She is great and she did such a great thing for me. . . . It tapered off because of the [geographical] distance. If I was in Israel, it might have continued.

Even if they do not keep in regular contact, the women give a mythic meaning to their relationship, creating a localized mythology;[39] this is the mythical bond established between them when they were "together in this quest." Over time, just as myths often do, the women romanticize the story of their bond to the point that they exclude mention of the tensions, injections, disappointments, and the monetary exchange between them. The narratives that I heard in the years following surrogacy thus became increasingly romanticized, and those, like Shoshana, who expressed intentions of reigniting the relationship did not often follow through.

In another scenario, the surrogate and intended mother do see one another on a regular basis, some once or twice a year and others every few weeks. At one end of this continuum, the surrogate and intended mother engage in an ongoing symbolic gift exchange. For instance, two years after her surrogate gave birth to her son, Yael told me, "I don't see Tali often, but I make sure to take her out to a restaurant on her birthday and to bring her flowers every holiday. My commitment to her isn't over just because [my son] is here." When I asked her how she would define Tali's relationship with her, she responded, "I feel like she is my sister, I swear I do." The ongoing interaction and the ascription of kinship terms to one another accords closely with an important quality of gift exchange—its potential to socially transform the relationship between persons into one of lineage or family.[40] Thus, when the gift is acknowledged by the intended mother and the intended mother continues to reciprocate with material gifts and social solidarity over the years, the relationship gradually transforms into a type of non-genealogical relatedness.[41]

This type of relationship conforms to Kaplan's model of the familial friendship, another popular type of long-lasting close friendship that is maintained by relating familial qualities to the relationship, since the family is understood in terms of lifelong relationship.[42] Accordingly, those surrogates and intended mothers who continued to be in regular contact in the years following surrogacy frequently reformulated their relationship in terms of "sisters," "mother and daughter," or simply "family." When I attended Lihi's wedding four years after she birthed twins for her couple, I observed that Danit, her husband, and their four-year-old twins were all seated at the bride and groom's personal table—the table reserved for their immediate family. And throughout the five years that I have known Lihi, she has referred to her intended mother as "Danit, my sister" [Danit achoti] and regards her as her closest friend. When Lihi experienced a late miscarriage for the couple she next con-tracted with as a surrogate, Danit sat by her side in the hospital along with the other intended mother.

Likewise, three years after their surrogacy contract ended, Rinat defined her relationship with Sarit in familial terms: "She is like my sister now. In some ways, closer than a sister. . . . She misses me a lot. She says that we have become like family." During the school vacation nearly half a year after she gave birth to Sarit's son, Rinat took her five children to stay with Sarit's family for several days. While Sarit and Reuven took Rinat's children to the mall and to the zoo, Rinat stayed at their home looking after their son. Of this exchange, Rinat told me, "See, they still only trust me to babysit." For Shahar, whose intended mother, Odelya, was seventeen years her senior, the surrogate–intended mother relationship transformed into a mother-daughter kin connec-tion. Three years after birthing twins, Shahar told me: "Odelya treats me like I am her daughter. . . . Look, I am a young woman, and she is more motherly towards me. And I treat her as a mother. A mother and a friend. If I have a problem, I turn to her." When I asked Odelya how she relates to Shahar now that surrogacy is well in their past, she responded in the same way: "Her mother and I are the same age. . . . And she said [about me], 'I relate to her [to Odelya] more than my own mother. What she has done for me, my own mother never did for me.'" It did not sur-prise me to hear that Odelya had walked Shahar down the aisle at her wedding in place of Shahar's own ailing mother four years after Shahar delivered Odelya's twins.

When the surrogate and intended mother remain close, the surrogate is incorporated into the intended mother's extended family. Rivka told me two-and-a-half years after Orna gave birth to her daughter that during the Sukkot holiday, Orna had phoned her to ask if she could join Rivka's family for the holiday, rejecting her own extended family's invitations to celebrate with them:

> She loves me very, very much. . . . On Sukkot, she didn't want to do Sukkot with anyone, only with me. She said to her mother—her own mother! . . . Her family really wanted her to come to them, and she said, "No, no, no. The truth is that I really feel like being with Rivka." . . . So she called and I invited her. . . . And my sisters-in-law, they give such a good feeling, that she is part of us. . . . [They consider Orna to be] Rivka's friend, a member of the household [*bat bayit*].

When the surrogate–intended mother bond becomes a familial friendship, it is often described in terms of kinship idioms that are pseudo-genetic in nature. For instance, one week after Sherry had given birth to Dana's baby, Dana reported feeling as though they were "now connected by blood." Interestingly, Dana's idiom overrides the lack of a traditional blood connection to the child by either woman, for the embryo implanted in Sherry was created by means of anonymous ova donation. Still, the symbolic blood that connected the two became a way of ascribing kinship to one another. Similarly, Roni described how she felt about her surrogate a year after the birth, saying: "We are like one bloodstream now." Since the Jewish-Israeli Roni, whose parents immigrated to Israel from Morocco, did surrogacy in the United States with a Puerto Rican Catholic surrogate, the symbolic kinship bond between the two women crosses even more boundaries. Yet again, the bloodline that runs through her and her surrogate seems to eclipse the child completely.

Acknowledgment of the gift, then, generally results in positive experiences for all concerned. An entirely different scenario occurs when the gift goes unacknowledged.

THE DENIAL OF THE GIFT AND MISCARRIED RELATIONSHIPS

To this point, I have discussed relationships in which the intended mother eventually acknowledges the surrogate's gift and "enduring solidarity" is cemented between them, even if only mythically. However, the opposite scenario also occurs, in which the pricelessness of the surrogate's gift is never acknowledged. In such cases, the surrogate's narrative is recast in terms of a lament over an unfair business deal and an unreciprocated gift. If she already feels unappreciated at the beginning of the contract, the surrogate might leave her couple, even if they have already passed the state screening process and made several embryo transfer attempts. If acknowledgement is not forthcoming while she is pregnant, she might rebel against her couple. For instance, in one case that I followed, the surrogate became angry at the couple for constantly citing the contractual agreement and for what she perceived as their lack of financial generosity toward her in regard to unforeseen expenses she had incurred because of surrogacy-related medical appointments (bus fare, babysitters). Midway through the pregnancy, she began to "punish" her intended mother by refusing her entry to medical appointments, including ultrasounds. She ultimately excluded her couple from the delivery by going to a different hospital than the one where the delivery was planned. She hid the fact that she was a surrogate from the medical staff and phoned her couple with news of the birth only several hours after the baby was born. In this way, she denied her intended mother many of the gifts that other surrogates had given—including the gift of the process of becoming a mother through her.

Sometimes the gift is never acknowledged. I have seen this scenario only in a relatively small percentage of the cases I have followed over the years, but when it occurs, the repercussions are extreme. For instance, Sima, who saw herself as a gift giver and felt committed to her intended mother's happiness throughout most of the pregnancy, retrospectively realized that, for the other woman, "it was all an act [hatsaga]." Her intended mother published excerpts from her journal in a national newspaper revealing that she had felt suspicion, doubt, and jealousy toward Sima all along.[43] After reading her intended mother's account, Sima relinquished any last threads of the camaraderie she still felt for her intended mother, telling me that she felt "like a widow." Instead of recounting a narrative of the gift, as other surrogates had, she told me the story of how she had become the couple's commodity from the very beginning: "They thought that I was part of their property. They wanted full control over everything I did." Sima lamented that her gift not only remained unacknowledged after the birth but that the intended father also offended her by implying that she had been an expensive purchase:

> I did not expect them to pay me for what I did in money. . . . I only expected a little more appreciation. No one can pay for such a gift as the one I gave to them in money. The only return is to show the person who did it that you thank them for what they did. After I gave birth, I stayed at home in bed for a week with a high fever. They did not even call to see

if I was okay, even though they knew how hard it was for me. I had done my job, from their point of view, and could now be thrown away. When he finally came to see me, it was only to pay me, and he found it necessary to remind me that he could have gotten another surrogate for five thousand dollars less. . . . "If we were looking today," he said, "there would be thousands lined up at our door."[44]

Sima's narrative of the unreciprocated gift transforms her surrogacy story into a lament over lost property rights to her body-as-commodity and over the loss of a soulmate, evident in her comparison of herself to a "widow." She feels used, discarded, and "othered." Unlike other surrogates, who downplayed the significance of the payment, Sima consistently highlighted the "unfair" financial arrangement, and instead of fantasizing about making her gift truly priceless, as others had, she said, "Today I wouldn't do it for any price in the world."[45] From an article appearing in an Israeli film criticism magazine,[46] Sima found out that the couple had been compensated for the documentary film as well as for the series of journal excerpts that appeared in the newspaper. Angry that her intended mother was about to make another profitable deal to turn her journal into a book, Sima got a court order to prevent the couple from sealing the transaction. From Sima's story, it becomes very clear that when the surrogate's gift is not acknowledged, money takes center stage.

In addition to cases like Sima's, in which the gift is never acknowledged, in some cases the gift is acknowledged and the acknowledgment later retracted. For instance, throughout the pregnancy, Riki acknowledged the contribution of her surrogate, Yelena, as a priceless gift. They were extremely close, and Riki told me midway through the pregnancy that she intended to stay in touch with Yelena after the birth. However, when I visited Riki one week after she had returned home with her twins, she mentioned that there had been an awkward moment in the hospital and that she thought she might have hurt Yelena's feelings:

> Her daughter told me in the hospital that her mommy is sad, because she is going home without a baby. So I told her that her mommy got paid just fine for the work she did, and that she didn't do it for free. I don't know if that was the right thing to say or if I was right in bringing up the money issue, but I felt it was right at that moment.

That day in Riki's kitchen, I had a sinking feeling that this story would not come out well, and I was not surprised to see an article in an Israeli women's magazine soon after featuring an interview with

Yelena.[47] In the interview, Yelena talks about a change in Riki's attitude in the days following the birth that made her uncomfortable. Her retrospective account then centers on the story of how Riki had retracted her acknowledgment of the gift and, then, how Yelena discovered that she had been cheated financially and emotionally betrayed by the couple. She describes a promise she received from Riki of a gift, a bonus payment that Riki would give her after the birth:

> Because I wasn't one hundred percent satisfied with that amount, [she] gave me, with the signing of the contract, a note in her handwriting with an extra amount. She didn't want her husband to know about the note and asked that I keep it. The note read: "You will receive a gift of five thousand shekels, that do not belong to the contract between us. If you do not have a cesarean, you will get an additional five thousand shekels, altogether ten thousand shekels, that I will pay up to six months after the delivery. Good luck and thank you."[48]

On the other side of the note, Riki wrote: "Hi, I wish the both of us lots of luck. That you will, we will, have it easy and good. Amen! Don't worry. You are not alone, and we will do everything to make it good and easy. Keep this note. It is a prayer and a promise."[49] In the interview, Yelena describes the moment when she realized that Riki had not intended to actually give her that gift. A few weeks after she delivered the twins— without a cesarean section—she called Riki and asked her why she had not received the final, major lump-sum payment. Although she had noticed during the pregnancy that her insurance policy had not arrived and that she had not received all of the payments she was owed, she had not worried about it until after delivery "because my relationship with the couple was excellent, I was totally calm."[50] However, after her couple's attitude toward her turned distant, her urgency to see the money grew:

> In my next phone calls with her the tones [of our voices] were already higher. When I reminded her of the personal note, in her own handwriting, she denied it. At one point she bartered with me over the rate of the dollar and demanded that I settle for a rate of four shekels to the dollar. One time she made me hear the crying twins in the phone, and once she yelled: "What are you going to do! Put me in jail!"[51]

Like Sima, Yelena ended up feeling betrayed by Riki's sudden withdrawal from their alliance and by the betrayal of her trust. She too ended up feeling commodified, invaded, fragmented, and as if she had lost part of her personal self in this failed transaction. And because the surrogate sees herself as "giving" not from her detached belly but from her personalized heart and soul, it is her personal self that she sees affected. Fittingly, the emphasized pull quote of the article on Yelena's experience read, "*I gave this couple my soul* and they tricked me and betrayed me. What breaks me is not just the money but their attitude."[52] This highlighted statement represents the core of Yelena's lament, revealing that it is not the child or the money that generated her feelings of disappointment and loss but the notion that she had invested in her couple a part of her personalized self—her soul—and they had not held it safely in a reciprocal relationship. As Rynkiewich notes, the partners in a gift relationship do not feel alienated from their valuables, because those valuables are held safely in a relationship; they know where they are and who has them.[53] Yet when the embodied gift is not cultivated and preserved in a social alliance, the surrogate's detached parts "fall" with the weight of a disembodied commodity.[54] A psychological opinion of Yelena, which was included in the article in which she told her story, dramatically accentuated Yelena's statement, claiming that "the clinical picture that we have before us is of posttraumatic syndrome."[55]

After seeing the article, I spoke to Riki, who told me that she had written out her side of the story and was too angry to speak about it. I then called the former secretary of the approvals committee and asked if she had heard what had happened to this surrogate–intended mother relationship. She answered, "I called Riki when I found out, and I told her that I know that it is not my place to interfere, but why can't you just go to her and apologize, and bring her a gift. That gift! She should never have promised her that gift." Appropriately for a representative of the surrogacy approvals committee, the secretary blames the promise of a gift for troubling the clear contractual boundaries of the commercial arrangement. Gifts, it would seem, only blur the carefully set boundaries that the body politic delineates for commercial surrogacy contracts. If, as the state tries to establish, this were a pure commodity exchange, then technological/consumptive/medically induced separation would preserve clear boundaries of "otherness" between the intended parents and their distanced surrogate-incubator. The confusion and drama are thus perceived as the result of the gifting logic.

GIFTS AND THE NATION

In addition to personal functions, the gift also has implications for the surrogate's national identity. As Titmuss famously argued, the individual act of giving can also be a *collective* social act.[56] In his discussion of anonymous blood transfusions in the United Kingdom, he contends that the altruistic act of giving blood to an "unknown stranger" is a collective act that is carried out within a domain that is paradoxically characterized by commercialization, individualism, and self-interest. Following this idea, I suggest that, by defining her actions as a gift within the explicitly commercial contracted agreement, the surrogate is engaging in a collective social act toward the nation.

Ben-David has studied the gifting of body parts as a collective act in the context of organ donation in Israel.[57] She suggests that death in Israel is culturally graded in terms of three categories: heroic death, usually of soldiers, which incorporates the deceased into the pantheon of heroes in the national collective memory; natural death; and accidental death, for example, as the result of a road accident, which is not considered socially significant. She also suggests that donating the organs of a person whose death is not categorized as heroic transforms this private death into a public one and upgrades the status of the deceased. Moreover, the power of the gift and the cultural veneration of self-sacrifice can move a person whose death is aligned with marginality—such as suicide—within the boundaries of the collective by way of organ donation.

Surrogates are expressly selected by the state for the very attributes that make them marginal: they are single mothers in a society that venerates the "natural," nuclear family, and they are women who are motivated by financial concerns to relinquish a baby in exchange for compensation in a society that expects women to be "responsible, committed and wise" and to raise the children they bear.[58] And while gifts establish relationships, buying and selling is the maximal expression of "otherness."[59] It is thus only by defining surrogacy as a gift that the surrogate can present herself as contributing to the nation and fulfilling her expected duty to "reproduce the nation." By creating families for others and fulfilling her cultural responsibility, she avoids being represented as "other" and marginal. The gift transforms the surrogate's actions into the heroic conduct of a self-sacrificing, brave mother, as she presents herself in part 4; it moves the surrogate from her marginal position into the heart of the collective.

By rejecting the gifting logic, the intended mother not only regards the surrogate as a commodity but also further pushes her to the margins of the collective. Accordingly, when surrogates' gift of life is not acknowledged, they do not narrate the same mythical quest story of surrogates as heroine soldiers, as the women do in part 4. Instead, they draw on an alternative gendered narrative that moves them into the boundaries of the collective and elevates their status to a heroic one.

The narrative then follows the pattern of that reserved for the mothers and wives of fallen military soldiers.

This narrative of self-sacrifice is appropriately retold as a regretful lament to the ears of the nation as a whole: like Sima and Yelena, who sought out journalists to publicly tell their stories, these narratives are voiced in the media to a nation that regularly hears such tales of heroic loss and bereavement. It is also not surprising that, following surrogacy, Sima turned to the National Insurance Institute to receive compensation for the emotional trauma that she convinced them she had sustained during surrogacy; nor was it surprising that she was awarded disability payments. She also contracted a lawyer and sued her couple for the psychological damage she incurred during surrogacy and was awarded two years of psychological counseling for herself and for her son at their expense. She then filed an additional lawsuit, which is still pending, against the surrogacy approvals committee and the state Ministry of Health for outstanding harm and suffering resulting from her surrogacy experience.

When I asked Sima to explain her cause for complaint, she responded, "It is not about the money. It is because they [the committee] should never have found me suitable and allowed me to do this. I am suing to let them know that I have come out of this damaged for life." Sima's campaign for recognition from the state reveals the crucial significance of acknowledgment: if the gift is not acknowledged, then a publicized lament in the national media in which the surrogate describes her self-sacrifice can transform her ordeal into a sacrifice for the nation. And when her unreciprocated gift fails to establish "enduring solidarity" with her couple, this public lament establishes an alternative path for the surrogate into the collective: if not by "making a mother," then by sacrificing a child in war.

Finally, the gifting logic has the power to subversively contest the capitalist framework of the commercial contract by replacing the gendered market economy with a woman-centered, gifting, relational economy. Specifically, as Hyde suggests, when a gift moves across a boundary, it abolishes the boundary.[60] When the surrogate gives her gift, she also opens up a cultural space in which borders and boundaries are crossed and blurred; her relationship with the intended mother involves shifting and merged bodies, enacting different combinations of unity and duality, and even homosocial physical conduct.

When the intended mother acknowledges the surrogate's gift and establishes an ongoing relationship with her surrogate—however mythical it may be—the gift relationship has the potential to lift itself above colonial, capitalist, individualist features and to create something else. The gift keeps the connection between the women symbolically open, in stark contrast to the commercial contract, borders, boundaries, and separations intended by the body politic. When patriarchal commodity exchange is transformed into feminine gift exchange, the surrogacy arrangement has the potential to challenge one of the nation's goals in legalizing surrogacy—clearly defining the boundaries of the family in response to the ambiguity surrogacy creates.[61] When the women speak of themselves as sisters or mother and daughter and form a familial friendship after surrogacy is over, they create a woman-centered "relational economy"[62] that subversively decolonizes the patriarchal commodity economy and state control of surrogacy in Israel.

This feminine gift economy may feature in the women's narratives, and the lasting bond of solidarity may remain in their mythological past, but the capitalist logic of the contracted agreement continues to be central to the surrogacy process itself, because without it, the nation's boundaries would be threatened. As Douglas reminds us, the body and its boundaries are symbolic of the social body,[63] and in a country where there is no express interest in engaging in ongoing exchange with enemy neighbors, and in which body boundaries are policed for the collective's survival, the possibility of ongoing exchange between families is intolerable, because the family is the basic unit of the nation. Thus, just as the body politic ritually enacts the completion of the transaction by assuming temporary guardianship of the child and arbitrating the transfer of custody in a court of law, so, too, the commercial nature of the contract is a necessary divisive measure.

This, in turn, explains why the commercial side of surrogacy was not a central issue of debate in the Israeli Parliament, in contrast to England and some U.S. states, where it was the most important issue considered.[64] In other words, since surrogacy is a cultural anomaly that upsets the categories of motherhood, family, nature, and the bounded body, which, in turn, symbolically stand as foundations of the nation, surrogacy in Israel has to be business. The gift, however, when held in the women's persons in the years following surrogacy, still carries a mark of resistance. To sum up, I borrow from a phone conversation between myself and Sarit, five years after Rinat gave birth to her child. After telling me that she still speaks to Rinat every few weeks and sees her on major Jewish holidays, Sarit told me how the gift triad had a lasting influence on her son:

Sarit: You can see it in him, you know.

Elly: You can see what?

Sarit: You can see in this child all of the love that was around him when he
was in the belly. The love of Rinat towards me and my love for her,
and the love between my husband and me. You know, that connection between all of us during that period. I say, I don't want to have
another child if there won't be that kind of love. I know that it will
be very hard to find another woman like Rinat. No way, our relationship was so special. I look at him and I see the result.

In the next chapter, I examine the role that surrogacy as gift plays
in the surrogate's construction of a quest narrative and in her resultant
process of self-discovery. *Giving* is intricately linked with self-discovery
because, as Hyde notes, gifts have the potential to transform the giver, to
"awaken part of the soul."[65] And if the soul, as we discovered in the surrogate's body map, is representative of the surrogate's personal essence,
then the connection to her personal transformation is clear. I suggest
that when the surrogate's "gift" is acknowledged as such, it leaves her
altered. However, in line with Hyde's argument,[66] when the gift is not
received and reciprocated, she is not able to finish her own process of
transformation or reach catharsis at the completion of her quest.

PART FOUR

Redefining

IN THIS SECTION, I ADDRESS the ultimate question that arises from my data: given circumstances that can easily be cast as nightmarish, alienating, and disempowering, how was it possible for most of the surrogates I interviewed to describe surrogacy as the most meaningful experience of their lives, one from which they emerged empowered and with a renewed sense of self-knowledge and self-worth? In other words, how can we explain the enormous gap between the structure of surrogacy—the constricting contract, the invasiveness of the screening process, and the physical and emotional tensions of the entire process (IVF, pregnancy, and childbirth)—and surrogates' narrated experience? Drawing on Giddens's theory of structuration,[1] I suggest that the structure of surrogacy provides the grounds for women to enact personal agency. I suggest that surrogates perceive the sequential stages of surrogacy as tests of their endurance and their mental and emotional strength. Surrogacy, then, becomes an odyssey in which surrogates learn to depend on their ability to surmount the obstacles thrown in their way by nature, technology, circumstance, and their own bodies. Chapter 8 explores the surrogate's reframing of the challenges of surrogacy as an endurance test. Chapter 9 analyzes her narrative as a "hero's journey."

CHAPTER 8

The Surrogate's Mission

The institutional management of surrogacy until the contract is approved by the state may be likened to a test; prospective surrogates undergo comprehensive institutional screening that is consistent across all cases. The surrogacy law specifies strict criteria governing who can become a surrogate; candidates must provide medical records showing they comply with a long checklist of selection criteria in terms of their physical, mental, and emotional health. They must pass a general medical exam and a gynecological exam, including a pelvic ultrasound, and undergo a battery of blood tests.[1] They must be between the ages of twenty-two and thirty-eight, be at a healthy weight (body mass index [BMI] under 30), and not have delivered more than four children. They must not have had any pregnancy complications in the past—including gestational diabetes (even a borderline case) or miscarriages—and not have had more than one cesarean operation. Applications by women to become surrogates have been rejected by the committee during the past ten years for reasons not specified in the law; women have been denied, for example, for having had cosmetic surgery or surgical weight loss procedures and for past experience with depression or anxiety, including episodes involving temporary use of popular antidepressants. Women have also been disqualified because of past experiences with toxic pregnancy, low-birth-weight infants (under five pounds), and early deliveries (before the thirty-sixth week).

In addition to being physically healthy and fertile, prospective surrogates must undergo comprehensive psychological screening, which lasts up to six hours. The approvals committee carefully interviews all candidates after psychological testing is completed, and, when the woman has a steady boyfriend, the committee usually interviews him as well. Women who pass the psychological tests but have undergone divorce, separation, childbirth, or other loosely defined "trauma" or "stress" are asked to wait before applying to the committee until a year has passed since the incident. Unofficial committee guidelines also prevent women from becoming surrogates if one of their own children is mentally or physically disabled or ill. Original committee guidelines permitted a woman to give birth as a surrogate no more than two times; a recent addition to the committee guidelines now specifies that a woman can only submit an application twice. This means that a potential surrogate can be refused committee approval even if she has twice contracted with couples who pulled out of the agreements for reasons unrelated to her. The stakes, therefore, are very high for a woman to contract with the "right" couple the first time, especially if she plans to be a surrogate twice, as many of the surrogates in this study did.

The testing character of the psychological screening process is revealed in the written assessment that one surrogate permitted me to see.[2] In the report, the psychologist recommended the woman for surrogacy on the basis of his findings that she possessed "a suitable mission-type perspective." He described her conduct as similar to that of a docile soldier, noting that she responded with clarity to the exam instructions, operated strategically to advance her goals, and demonstrated initiative and effective skills for coping with difficulties. The recommendation concluded with the repeated assertion that the candidate was found able to preserve the mission-centered perspective that would carry her through surrogacy. Several other surrogates showed me reports written by the same psychologist revealing that "a mission-type perspective" and "inner strength" were crucial characteristics that he sought in candidates.

The administrators of private surrogacy agencies also subject prospective surrogates to "tests." The owner of the leading private surrogacy agency in Israel told me that she "tests" the women who turn to her agency to see whether they have the qualities of "seriousness, responsibility, and endurance" that she deems necessary—even before she introduces them to a couple: "I check whether they are really serious about it.

For instance, I have them meet me at my office or at a café the first time. I never go to their home for the initial meeting. I want to know if they are going to make that extra effort to get in the car or the bus and come meet me." The agency director also noted that, from the first meeting, she informs the prospective surrogate directly that she must agree to certain requirements to continue through her agency: "I tell them that I expect them to arrive on time, to return my phone calls promptly, to come to the support group meetings, to not be late, and to prove to me that they are serious and that I won't have to worry about them disappearing. The ones that don't return my phone calls, that disappear or don't bring me their documents, I simply don't continue with."

A final structural element of the process that contributes to the view of surrogacy as a test is the long period during which surrogates and their couples wait for their documents to be discussed and approved by the surrogacy approvals committee. Contracts are approved only after much bureaucratic scrutiny, lasting between three and eighteen months. As a result of this complex approval process, a surrogate and couple may be in contact with one another for periods ranging from three months to over a year before receiving the committee's decision. Some triads groom one another during this period, only to have the contract rejected by the committee, and some triads spend additional time contesting the committee's decision, sometimes successfully overturning it. We might consider this lengthy waiting period and the selection process in general as ritualistic "testing" measures to ascertain that only the couples and surrogates who are most determined to have a child by this means will be sanctioned by the state since, in the end, nearly all couples and surrogates who persevere are approved.[3] The former secretary of the approvals committee correspondingly described the lengthy waiting period to me as "a type of endurance test," explaining that "it's not on purpose, but it does sort out those who really want it from those who don't have the patience to wait. Listen, if they can't stand this, then they don't know what is waiting for them later."

Most of the surrogates I met while they were undergoing this waiting period described their frustration with the committee and their loss of patience. Some noted that they might not have chosen to become surrogates had they known how long it would take to begin treatment, especially considering that they do not receive regular payments until they are pregnant and that the entire preapproval period stands between them and their financial goal. However, while surrogates may have been agitated by the lengthy wait that the selection process required, they rarely challenged the necessity of the tests involved. Instead, most of them highlighted how receiving the committee's approval was a personal triumph, as discussed below.

SELECTING SUPERWOMAN

The surrogates tended to interpret the screening process in terms of a "test," an idiom that later informed their understanding of the sequential stages of the process as well. Tamar, for instance, explained, "You want to succeed and not to disappoint, not yourself and not disappoint others. . . . It's like you are going to a test and don't want to fail. You want to pass. . . . It's like anything that you want to succeed in and not to feel disappointed and to say that you succeeded." Other idioms they used to describe surrogacy referenced similar parameters, such as the popular description that surrogacy was a "project" or a "mission." These idioms shared the common theme of a temporary goal that the women are determined to reach but could also fail to achieve. Surrogates viewed passing the committee as the first of many hurdles that they had successfully overcome and as authoritative confirmation of their personal strengths and suitability for difficult "missions." For Sapir, the psychological exams she had undergone seemed mysterious and very selective. She was proud to have "passed" this stage: "I don't know to this day how I passed the test. . . . There are a lot of strong ones that fail. I almost failed. . . . I still don't know which tests I succeeded in and which I didn't."

Just as Sapir saw herself as almost "failing" but ultimately prevailing over other "strong ones" who were not selected, Neta described the medical and psychological evaluations as consecutive obstacles that she had to overcome on the path to being selected: "There is a bit of a strange feeling to it, you know, you feel like you are undergoing tests for entering flight school [in the Air Force]. That you can fall out at any time. Something like you really want to get there, but something horrible can go wrong on the way." She compared the type of woman who could pass the tests to a "superwoman. Yes, superwoman, but not everyone has the personality profile that can really fit it."

Neta's comparison of the tests to those administered to candidates for the Israeli Air Force is telling, since the Air Force is Israel's most elite military unit and the screening process for entry is infamous for its difficulty. Her comparison adds a layer of prestige to her surrogacy in terms of national value, which is compounded by her assertion that

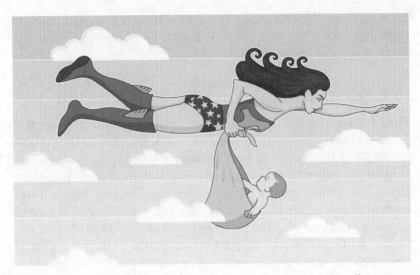

Figure 9. Illustration depicting a surrogate as Superwoman. Originally
appeared in *Haaretz* newspaper. Reproduced with the permission of the artist,
Gila Kaplan.

"not everyone" can become a surrogate and that those who do pass are
"superwomen": the most powerful, strongest, most elite "fighters" of
womankind (see figure 9).

Several surrogates other than Neta described the type of woman
that they thought the surrogacy committee was looking for as "superwoman." Others used military-related descriptors such as "fighter"
[*fighterit*] or "strongwoman" [*jada'it*] to characterize the women who
were "chosen" to be surrogates, implying that the committee could be
compared to a military selection board. Orna described the examiners
both as similar to a selection committee for entering an elite military
unit and like a selection committee for entering university, constructing
her role as a surrogate as equivalent to that of a male combat fighter
and her status as higher than that of people who have achieved a university education:

> The committee takes the opinion of the psychologist, who actually speaks
> to you about everything, from A to Z. Childhood, life history, school, math-
> ematics, history, politics . . . to see who you are, what you are. . . . Do you
> know the verbs, do you know the world. Everything. . . . The Hadassah
> exams and the psychometric exams are nothing [in comparison].[4] To build
> cubes, cube on cube. Psychometric exams, really! Oral, in writing . . . then
> the committee says to you, "You are fit for the mission; you are not fit for

the mission.". . . The three of us sat there. Opposite us was a huge round table, full of doctors, full of gynecologists, full of psychologists . . . a chairman, secretaries, like a court room. "Who are you?" Sentenced to death or not to death. And after an hour or so of questions and hard questions and you really have to know . . . and then they say yes or no . . . they talk for around five minutes between them . . . talking and then, the sentencing . . . "tak tak" [pretends to bang a gavel]. And we are sitting quietly, waiting for the hard questions, and they ask, and we have to answer. And according to the answers . . . like the army . . . the army is nothing [in comparison]!

In the interview, the women are questioned on details of the contract and are asked about how they intend to deal with relinquishment and about their awareness of potential physical and psychological complications. Many of them reported feeling that the interviewers had tried to shake their confidence or disturb their positive outlook by hinting that their participation in surrogacy could potentially be psychologically damaging to their children. Tsila said of this type of tricky testing,

I felt like they were always trying to shake your confidence. I told my friend afterwards that it was like a driving test. I felt like they might fail me for being too confident. Like in a [driving] test, when you know that you know, you know what you are doing, how to drive, you have confidence. But the tester tries to make you doubt yourself.

Shira, who had been interviewed by the committee on the same day as Tsila, overheard her comments to me at the surrogacy support group meeting and joined in, telling the rest of the surrogates who had gathered around the oval table where we were seated that the committee "investigated me, questioned me from all sides. . . . They try to fail you there. . . . I said, 'What is this, a test?' . . . They did test me on my psychological evaluation. . . . In the end, I asked them if I could ask them a question. I asked, 'How was I?' They said, 'You were great.'"

Similar to Shira, who boasted to the other surrogates that the committee had deemed her "great," most of the women I spoke to were proud of having proven themselves by passing the ordeal of the tests. Nearly a year after giving birth to a singleton, Idit recalled her pride at having been approved by the committee and at having been chosen by her couple from among other prospective candidates:

In my head, I achieve. I achieve despite the conditions that are very selective. Because they really select the surrogates. Not everyone who wants to become a surrogate can become a surrogate. . . . First of all, the psychological exams, I passed them fine. They saw that I was right for it. . . . And as you can see, my health is fine. . . . I was chosen from the other twenty

surrogates; they are the ones that chose me. The self-pride was very strong
during the time. . . . The couple contacted me right away. Chose me.

The sense of accomplishment described by Idit is what often led the
women to feel that they had "finished" the process even before they
had actually begun it. Several times, new members of the surrogate
support group introduced themselves by saying that they were "near
the end of the process," when their contracts had not yet even received
committee approval. Even though they still had all of the medical procedures ahead of them, they felt that they had already overcome so
many obstacles along the surrogacy path that the rest of the process was
inconsequential.

THE HURDLES OF IVF

After being approved by the committee, surrogates prepare for the
embryo transfer, which adds to their formulation of surrogacy as a test,
because the success rates for the IVF process are relatively low.[5] IVF
involves a sequence of stages or procedures: the removal of the egg, the
IVF, and the reimplanting of the embryo. The transition between these
stages is not seamless and simple; there are many ways in which each
step can fail.[6] In gestational surrogacy, the stages are divided between
two women's bodies: the egg retrieval from the intended mother's body,
the IVF, and then the embryo transfer into the surrogate's uterus. After
the embryo transfer, the surrogate receives daily injections to help her
body sustain the pregnancy.

These daily injections, administered to the buttocks with a long needle, were reportedly painful. When surrogates did not know how to
self-inject, they had to go to a clinic for the daily injections. Surrogates
received hormone therapy for two weeks following the embryo transfer,
until pregnancy test results were known. If pregnancy occurred, they
continued to receive treatment up through the twelfth week of gestation,
until their body "took over" biologically. If pregnancy did not occur, the
surrogate stopped taking the hormones and began a new round of hormonal preparation for the next embryo transfer attempt.

The hormones caused surrogates to experience many of the same side
effects that infertile women undergoing IVF do, including mood swings,
water retention, weight gain, hair loss, and skin problems. The jury is
still out on the risks of ovarian cancer and other serious side effects of
these hormones, so surrogates may be putting themselves at risk by sub-

jecting themselves to this medical regimen, in addition to the risks associated with pregnancy and childbirth in general. Moreover, chances are that the entire process will have to be repeated in most cases, because, as noted, the IVF process can fail and because initial attempts are usually made with the intended mother's eggs, which are not necessarily of good quality, especially if she is over age forty or if she has never achieved pregnancy.

In some cases, the cycle must be interrupted midway because the surrogate's body or the intended mother's body, which must be simultaneously synchronized to produce the eggs that will be fertilized and implanted in the surrogate's womb, do not respond well to the treatment. In other cases, the surrogate's body reaches optimal conditions for implantation, but the eggs produced by the intended mother do not survive the fertilization process. Even when all logical conditions are met, the technology does not promise immediate success, and most of the surrogates I interviewed did not conceive during the first round of IVF. There are no official statistics, but most of the surrogates I met conceived anywhere from the second to sixth embryo transfer. Unfortunately, clinics and agencies often boast outstanding statistics for marketing purposes, leading surrogates and couples to formulate false hopes of their chances for conceiving on the first attempt.

Even after they have passed the "tests" of the approvals committee, then, surrogates are presented with a new set of difficulties to overcome during the conception stage. Studies of couples undergoing fertility treatment in various countries have shown that infertile couples view the successive stages of the IVF process as a series of "hurdles" or "obstacles" they must overcome.[7] Franklin highlights "the tremendous determination required to undergo IVF, in light of the odds against the women succeeding at the outset" and "the need to acquire the corresponding mindset of a competitor."[8] Whereas surrogacy has been likened to a test, IVF has been described in the popular literature as akin to "lotto" or "Russian roulette."[9] All of these idioms portray a process that requires the endurance and determination of a competitor at each stage, involves an element of chance, and has a high risk of "failure" at each stage.

For the surrogate, the stakes are especially high in this obstacle course, as she can potentially expose herself to the hormones and to a trying medical routine without, in the end, ever profiting from the agreement. Specifically, in a standard contract, the couple and surrogate agree to a limit of six embryo transfers. If conception does not occur after six rounds, the contract is considered void and the surrogate does not receive payment beyond minor reimbursements. Standard contracts entitle the surrogate to the first substantial payment only when a fetal pulse has been detected during the ultrasound in the seventh week of pregnancy. This means that if the surrogate never conceives, the only money she receives for her efforts is a nominal sum payable after the committee approves the contract (three to sixteen months after the initial application to the committee) and a similar payment for each embryo transfer. For the surrogate who does conceive, the payments are dispersed monthly, increasing each trimester, and the final payment is made only after delivery. A surrogate who does not conceive after several embryo transfers or who miscarries early on has undergone this trying medical process for very little reimbursement.

Confident of their fertility given the ease with which they had become pregnant in the past, surrogates are convinced they will become pregnant on the first try. Like the infertile women undergoing IVF who Franklin followed,[10] none of the surrogates had anticipated the complexity of the procedure or the number of things that could go wrong. When IVF failed, the self-knowledge with which they had begun the process was undermined. Surrogates seldom accepted the low statistical chance of conception with the technology as a satisfactory explanation for what they interpreted as their body's own failure to conceive. Belle described her loss of trust in the predictability of her body when the first two embryo transfers failed: "My first two treatments failed for some unknown reason. I was pretty down; I didn't understand why my body was betraying me. I'd had three simple pregnancies. I conceived so easily." After the pregnancy that resulted from her third embryo transfer ended in miscarriage, Belle wrote on the surrogacy forum website, "My personal feeling was that my body had really betrayed me. It was as if it was failing me on purpose! I was angry at it. I didn't expect the [next] treatment to work." When her fourth attempt resulted both in pregnancy and in a long-awaited live birth, she was surprised and wary of this "success."

Experiences like Belle's were fairly frequent among the surrogates I interviewed, as well as among those whose stories I followed through the Internet forum and support group. Often after several failed attempts, tensions begin to arise between the surrogate and the couple, who speculate that the surrogate's behavior or body is at fault. Some couples have told me of their fears that the surrogate is not taking her medication on time or is not resting sufficiently after the embryo transfer. They are suspicious that she is endangering a possible pregnancy by cleaning her house, lifting her children, or in one case, going to the beach the day after an embryo transfer. Similarly, couples question whether the surrogate's uterus is somehow to blame for the failed attempts, and they ask her to undergo additional physical examinations, including invasive and sometimes painful tests such as a uterine X-ray and laparoscopy.

While couples do not usually blame the surrogate directly, they communicate their suspicions implicitly through subtle questions about her behavior and body. This pressure only adds to the surrogate's determination to conceive, to prove to herself that she is fertile and to prove to her couple that she is not at fault. After eight failed embryo transfers, Neta's first couple became increasingly suspicious of her: "They didn't want to blame one another, because they had to stay married. So where did they throw all of the garbage? On me. . . . They didn't blame me to my face. But they give you the feeling that maybe you are not okay. That maybe because you are fat you aren't conceiving. Maybe it's because you didn't rest. . . . What it does is make you think that maybe there really is something wrong with you . . . but on the other hand, I have the best record. I have a kid."

After three long years of repeat negatives, Neta ended the contract and signed a new surrogacy agreement with a different couple. In an interview that took place a few months after she gave birth to a singleton for that couple, Neta reflected on the self-doubt, frustration, and anger she might have been left with if she had not continued surrogacy with a second couple: "What if I had decided not to go for another round? I would have gone on with a feeling of frustration from the surrogacy process." Her persistence and eventual "success" boosted Neta's self-esteem and confidence in her body: "It was also, in some way, winning proof for myself that I am all right. I needed to prove to myself and to come full circle that I am okay . . . [that] I don't have [fertility] problems and everything is all right. It was really important to me. . . . So here is the proof. I'm okay. The ones that are not okay are them."

Like Neta, many other surrogates could reformulate the obstacle as something independent of their own bodies only after they had successfully conceived and delivered a surrogate child. Lihi, for instance, who had been "sure they would put it in and I would be pregnant" on the first try, initially blamed her body for "failing" her. However, after birthing twins for her couple, she retrospectively excused her body from blame, pointing to her couple's infertility and to chancy technology instead: "I had forgotten all of the parameters. That it's not my egg, and that the process isn't natural. That there are all kinds of other factors that come in." From the vantage point of having proved her body fertile and her will strong and determined, Lihi asserts that the challenges incurred along the way made her "victory" even sweeter: "It was like achieving something that is hard to achieve. It's, like, even more joyous. Because when it comes to you easily, then you don't appreciate it. . . . When it is something that is so charged with emotions, even though it isn't actually mine, even if it isn't yours, you are glad. You are glad for them. You are glad for yourself that you succeeded."

Unfortunately, not all of the surrogates I spoke to had the privilege of retrospectively reorganizing these negatives into hurdles on a path to triumph. During my research, I met several surrogates who failed to conceive during the contracted six attempts and thus spent from one-and-a-half to three years of their lives involved in a process in which they expended considerable time, effort, and emotional energy, without profiting in the end. One prospective surrogate, Reli, underwent eleven embryo transfers with two different couples over a period of four years without ever conceiving. During those four years, she "put her life on hold" and refrained from dating. She gained a significant amount of weight and experienced severe mood swings as a consequence of the hormone injections, which also created tension between herself and her children. Like other surrogates whose contracts end without conception, Reli's "fertile" self-perception was "disrupted" by the self-doubt that repeat IVF failures cause in infertile women, as Franklin, Sandelowski, Becker, and others have documented.[11]

Other surrogates I met during my research excitedly discovered that they were pregnant after several failed attempts only to learn that they had ectopic pregnancies or that there was no viable pulse at the eight-week scan. One surrogate I interviewed lost the pregnancy at twenty weeks, and one, tragically, lost the pregnancy at thirty weeks. Interestingly, the women's responses to these reproductive failures, including the miscarriages, contrast sharply with Layne's findings among U.S. women who experienced pregnancy loss at parallel stages.[12] Layne's subjects mourned their loss of an expected child and their loss of the role, status, and identity of mother to that expected child. The surrogates never mentioned the loss of either; their focus was solely on their sense of personal failure at the challenge and their loss of identity as fertile, able-bodied "fighters."

In terms of a "test," surrogacy differentiates between "winners" and "losers," leaving those who have lost the "conception race" with a feel-

ing very close to the one that has been described by infertile women.[13]
They are also left without having attained the monetary goal for which
they initially embarked on the "mission" and with the feeling that they
have disappointed themselves, their couple, and their own children, to
whom they had promised gifts at the end of the process. Metaphorically,
if surrogates who "succeed" in birthing a child for their couple feel as
though they have given "life," then surrogates who "fail" are left to
mourn a symbolic "death."

To work through these feelings and to regain trust in their bodies and
in themselves, several surrogates pursued their own pregnancies after
leaving surrogacy with their goals unfulfilled. Lilach tried to convince
her common-law husband to have a fourth child after her surrogacy
contract ended following four failed embryo transfers. When he did not
agree, she found another "mission" to satisfy her need to regain confidence in her body and her will: she began a cross-country hike on the
Trans-Israel trail. Nevertheless, two years later, she wrote on the surrogacy forum website that she had unexpectedly become pregnant, an
occurrence that she interpreted as a sign that her "natural" fertility was
still intact and that her inability to overcome reproductive challenges
during surrogacy was not her fault.

ANYTHING TO SUCCEED

In light of the assault on their self-identity and bodily confidence that
lack of "success" could produce, surrogates manifested high commitment to achieving a pregnancy at almost any personal cost, including
pain, discomfort, health risks, and more, much as the infertile Israeli
IVF users studied by Rememnick did.[14] Yet surrogates were not partaking in this cultural IVF "obsession"[15] to achieve the role, status, and
identity of motherhood for themselves. They undertook these personal
risks for other reasons: to earn money, to make another woman into a
mother, and most of all, to prove to themselves that they could complete
their "mission" successfully.

Most surrogates found it very hard to admit defeat in their quest.
Few agreed to stop trying until they had completed the contracted
number of attempts, usually six, and several surrogates attempted eight
rounds before "giving up." Each embryo transfer, which represented
another potential failure and another "hurdle on the IVF obstacle
course,"[16] reinforced their image of surrogacy as a test and increased
their determination to overcome the obstacles that they saw working

against them: their bodies, their circumstances, and the statistical odds against conception.

Orna's was the most extreme case I encountered. She viewed each of her first five failed embryo transfers as personal failures: "When I receive a negative answer, then I need to cry. . . . Because it is mourning. . . . It is mourning because I didn't succeed. . . . I wanted to succeed. . . . When you go on a mission, then you do it up till the end." She likened her response to consecutive failures to that of the strategic, unwavering, determined will of a soldier who "sticks to the target": "You need to know how to overcome difficult situations. You need to stay calm under pressure. . . . You don't give up in despair [*lo mitya'ashim*]. You stick to the target [*at dveka bamatara*] and you make it happen." On her sixth and final IVF attempt, she took dangerous measures to force her body to conceive:

> I took, on my own, twice the hormones, twice the injections, and the doctor almost wanted . . . to kill me [because] I took them without asking. Like instead of him telling me to take two pills, I took four pills. And he told me to take two injections—I took four injections. I said [that] this small one [pats her belly], he needs to grow in a bed [*matsa*] of whipped cream. Not just any womb. He needs something special!

Orna excitedly reported how surprised her doctor had been to see her extraordinarily elevated hormone level and how he had scolded her for overmedicating herself. Still, that did not stop Orna from demanding that her doctor endanger her with a multiple pregnancy by implanting four times the conventional number of embryos: "I said to him . . . for the last treatment I want to do the maximum! I want it to be the best it can be. I want twice the amount [of] embryos." Whereas in most cases two to three embryos are transferred, Orna insisted, "I want eight! The doctor said, 'No!' I said, 'Yes! You will do two returns [transfers] for me. . . . I am not interested [I won't hear otherwise]. . . . I want eight. If I have triplets, all the better!' . . . So he said okay. And they returned eight embryos, and from the eight, one remained."

Orna's narrative illuminates the feminist argument that the structural arrangement of surrogacy and the power structure of the IVF technique subject women, often unwillingly, to the external medical control of male doctors.[17] However, Orna perceives the doctor's control of her body as a tool that she can manipulate to force her body to cooperate in furthering her own goals and interests, making it manageable and making it submit to her intentions. She cannot be described as a passive patient, for it is she who effectively "tricks" the doctor into manipulating her body. In this way, Orna's determination and her effort to control the doctor's control of her body end up giving her the opportunity to exercise personal agency through the use of medical technology. Submission to medical procedures thus becomes, as Thompson has observed in the case of other IVF patients,[18] a strategic tactic for making the medically managed, pregnant body a site of female power, directly facilitated by the external medical control of that body.[19]

DOCTORS DON'T KNOW EVERYTHING

Emerging from Orna's case is a theme that has encompassed nearly all of the surrogates' narratives: a simultaneous trust in and admiration for the doctor, together with the realization that the doctor was neither G-d nor a miracle worker, as the doctors themselves and the popular media often promise.[20] Like Orna, other surrogates realized through their private trials and ordeals that "success" was just as dependent on their own determination as on the doctor's expertise. Their discovery that "doctors don't know everything" emerged from their conception stories and from their recollections of other pregnancy events, such as hospitalizations during pregnancy and delivery. This discovery was accompanied by their realization that their own efforts and their faith and determination were more responsible for the live, healthy production of the child than the doctor was.

When Sapir wanted her doctor to induce labor in her thirty-eighth week of gestation, he assured her that he could easily do so. However, the induction failed to bring on labor, and Sapir ended up spending ten days in the hospital. Each day she spent fifteen to sixteen hours in the delivery room, hoping that the induction medication would work. With every day that passed, her faith in her doctor and in the medical system in general dissipated:

> You know, I could already see it in his [the doctor's] eyes, that he is disappointed too. I mean, it was embarrassing [for him]. . . . And they gave me medicines with such a high dosage that the director of the delivery room said that he uses that amount of medicine on the whole delivery room. . . . Nothing! It tickled me one time, gave me a few contractions, but there was an opening of two centimeters and that's it. . . . So I was in the delivery room every day for fourteen, fifteen, sixteen hours, and nothing worked!

Shahar, who carried twins for her couple after birthing her own five children, found herself hospitalized for the last six weeks of the surrogate pregnancy. She contrasted her own confidence in her ability to keep the pregnancy to her doctor's skepticism. She also singled herself out as the one responsible for "holding it in," considering the medications she received to postpone delivery as mere additions to her efforts. Like Orna, she demanded medical control of her body with infusions and medicines as tools to help *her*, and she remained in a supine position so as not to tempt fate:

> I took extra care [*shamarti*]. I saw women walking around. They didn't care. But I didn't walk about. Food in bed. They brought everything to me in bed. . . . Because I said that these were the most critical weeks, and if I walk around I will give birth. I was three fingers dilated already! . . . and I had orderly contractions, you could see really orderly contractions on the monitor as if I was going to give birth any minute. . . . A few times they had already wanted to take me down to the delivery room and I refused. I told them, "No! I will hold it. Give me another infusion." They said, "Fine [in a skeptical tone], hold it." And look, I really did hold it; it's a fact.

When Shahar finally informed the doctor that she was ready to deliver the babies six weeks later, she asked for a cesarean so that she could feel in control of the birth as well. Shahar's birth story illuminates the way that surrogates use intuitive and embodied knowledge to negotiate their positions vis-à-vis the doctor's "authoritative" medical knowledge.[21] While anthropologists of reproduction have shown the many contexts in which birthing women's intuitive and embodied knowledge is dismissed in favor of the doctor's culturally privileged knowledge of the woman's body,[22] surrogates seem to consistently use self-knowledge to play opposite the doctor at the pregnancy game. Idit positioned her knowledge of pregnancy above that of any of the doctors her intended mother consulted:

> If she didn't believe one doctor, she would ask another. And if she didn't believe that doctor, she would go by my suggestion. . . . She trusted me 100 percent. . . . She trusted me more than the doctor, because all of the information was coming from me. . . . I didn't let anything hurt the pregnancy. . . . I controlled everything.

Ye'ara realized during her second surrogacy that her own embodied knowledge was more trustworthy than the doctor's medical-technological authoritative knowledge. After an early episode of heavy bleeding, she was rushed to one of the most respected hospitals in the country. The attending doctor was unable to locate a viable fetus on the ultrasound monitor and sent her to have the pregnancy terminated. Ye'ara insisted on a second ultrasound, but another technician using the same machine was also unable to detect fetal life. Ye'ara still refused the termination procedure and demanded to be administered a third scan on a different machine. When her hunch was confirmed and the other sonogram machine showed a strong and healthy fetal pulse, Ye'ara lost all faith in the medical establishment. She told me,

> In this pregnancy we discovered that as much as we claim that our country is so developed in medicine and especially in fertility and childbirth, the doctors don't know anything about pregnancy and birth.

The common theme of loss of faith in the doctor, who in most cases was one of an elite group of world-renowned gynecology professors, coincided in most narratives with a significant reassessment by the surrogate of her own relative power and of the ultimate will of a higher power. I develop these themes in the following sections.

THE HERO: BRAVERY, STRENGTH, AND ENDURANCE

As they progressed along the surrogacy path, women began to liken themselves to a soldier in a battle in terms of their strength, bravery, and endurance. Masha explained that "not every woman can do it [surrogacy]" and that, to be a surrogate, "a woman has to have a lot of inner strength [kochot nafshiim]." She recommended that a woman who does not have the necessary qualities refrain from becoming a surrogate: "I think that if a surrogate isn't prepared from the very first moment, . . . if she doesn't know herself, if she isn't strong enough of a fighter [lochemet] and isn't sure that she can get past every crisis on the way, . . . then she will crumble [tishaber], and when she falls [nofelet], I don't wish that on any surrogate." Positioning herself as someone who meets these necessary criteria, she professed, "I know myself, I am a strong woman. There are things that I can deal with and overcome better than anyone else."

The characteristics and skills that are seen as "making" or "breaking" a surrogate—having inner strength, being a fighter, having the ability to overcome crisis, knowing oneself, and being mentally prepared—were those that these women may already have known themselves to possess, given that their lives, especially as single mothers, had often been all about overcoming obstacles with their personal strength. Before surrogacy, however, this personal strength went largely unnoticed and did not incur the appreciation and social acknowledgment that it did in surrogacy. The use of militaristic language to articulate strength does not occur among surrogates in India or in the United States, but Franklin found in the British context that the IVF experience, in general, easily gives rise to the militaristically infused language of a "battle" in which "women are warriors, with battle scars attesting to their bravery" in "aggressive pursuit of an elusive goal."[23]

Without specifically referring to militaristic traits, Ragoné reported that the traditional surrogates she interviewed expressed themes of bravery, heroism, and heroic sacrifice.[24] In addition, a story has recently appeared in the U.S. media suggesting that U.S. military wives are being sought after by surrogacy agencies because they are "more regimented" than other women and because of their commendable "sense of discipline, commitment and cooperation."[25] Another story suggests that a military wife can make a good surrogate because she is "organized, disciplined and able to keep up with the grueling schedule of in vitro fertilization" and that military wives are "used to altruism and hardship" and "capable of making the ultimate sacrifice."[26] A surrogate whose husband was deployed in Iraq told *Newsweek,* "In the military, we have that mentality of going to extremes, fighting for your country, risking your life. . . . I think that being married to someone in the military embeds those values in you. I feel I'm taking a risk now, in less of a way than he [her husband] is, but still a risk with my life and body to help someone."[27]

All Jewish-Israelis, men and women, are subject to mandatory draft, so the use of military analogies by Israeli surrogates was not surprising. As a popular cultural script, military language is widely used outside of the military context to narrate success in overcoming physical and mental challenges or to evoke dramatic or heroic effect.[28] Indeed, intended mothers also used militaristic terminology to describe surrogacy, as reflected in Sara's statement that surrogacy was a "military campaign in every sense of the term [*mivtsah tsvaee lekol davar*]" and Yael's assertion that surviving the challenges of surrogacy was a "women's war." The military analogy is an obvious one for surrogates to draw on in articulating their surrogacy experience because of the character of the selection route they undergo, in which they discover that strength and self-mastery are critical. As Ben-Ari notes, Israeli combat soldiers experience much of their military service as a series of tests they must pass, in which they are encouraged to continuously steel and toughen themselves and to display qualities of endurance and control by "mastering" their emotions.[29]

Mostly, however, the military analogy is inviting because its core theme is that of agency,[30] which lies at the center of the surrogate's narrative. As in the military ordeal, the central assumption behind the surrogate's tale is that she acts within a web of agents: the state, the couple, nature, technology, the doctor, and G-d. Moreover, the basic question of the military script that Ben-Ari proposes—"Who will be master of the battle? Situation or person, circumstances or man?"[31]—also encapsulates the core of the surrogate's experience. The stages of the "test" discussed above constitute just that—a battle fought by the surrogate against circumstance and body. The stereotypically masculine cultural script of the male soldier who masters his emotions and his body[32] thus expresses the basic theme of the surrogate's quest narrative: her struggle to avoid being overcome by external controlling forces, to remain in control.

The heroic narrative culminates at that point when even the risk of death becomes worth the reward.[33] The birth is often narrated dramatically as the ultimate heroic event in which the surrogate displays her courageousness and willingness to sacrifice her life for the good of her "mission" (see figure 10). Before turning to these "sacrifice" narratives, I feel it is important to emphasize that the surrogates are not invoking what Kaplan calls "the maternal sacrifice myth."[34] Their narratives of self-sacrifice depart markedly from the paradigm of maternal sacrifice, according to which an ideal mother figure is portrayed as overinvested in her child to the extent of self-negation or self-induced suffering.

Instead of this mother-as-martyr/victim scenario, the surrogates' accounts echo, in many ways, glorious Israeli tales of soldiers in battle, which have been disseminated on a national level through military-associated ritual and myth since the birth of the country.[35] Lihi's surrogacy birth story resonates with such glorified ideals when she describes the way that she faced and conquered her fear of an imminent cesarean section, like a soldier called on to sacrifice her life for her country. When she was told that she would have to undergo a cesarean section under general anesthesia, she panicked: "I was afraid that I wouldn't wake up. . . . I said, 'Wow, just let me return.' I was already afraid." She left notes at home instructing her family of her wishes in case she did not wake up from the surgery: "I prepared the letters and I prepared for the worst." She patriotically described her bravery going into the procedure and her fear of not returning as similar to the emotions of a soldier being sent to the front:

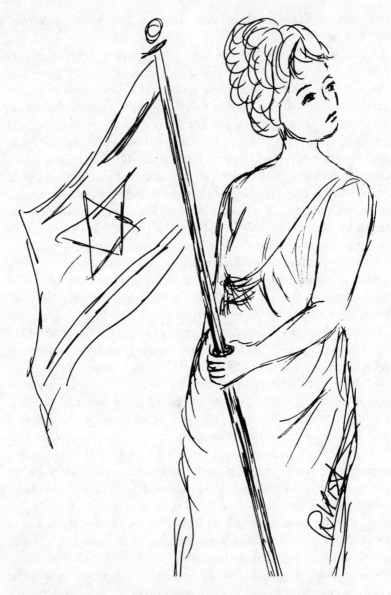

Figure 10. Illustration depicting the surrogate as Israeli national heroine. Reproduced with the permission of the artist, Rhisa Teman.

If let's say something would have happened to me, I wouldn't be sorry, because it is something that I chose consciously. So consciously. I was so confident in myself. . . . I mean, so I died for a good cause. It's like dying in a war. For a good cause. For the country. And at least the children will have money. For university.

From Lihi's narrative, it is evident that she is not passively sacrificing her body for the nation. Instead, like a soldier in battle, she is actively sacrificing her body for two worthy causes: first, for the country, dying a hero's death; and second, for her children, whose future will be financially secured. Likewise, in her birth story, Ye'ara positioned herself as a heroic fighter willing to sacrifice her life for the higher good. Throughout our second interview, Ye'ara's common-law husband participated actively. He repeatedly reminded Ye'ara and me that, when we "reached the birth," he wanted to tell the story himself. Natan's participation in recounting his partner's bravery reinforced her heroic narrative. The birth story began relatively uneventfully, as Ye'ara, Natan, and the intended parents waited in Ye'ara's hospital room for delivery to begin. Suddenly, as Ye'ara dramatically recounted, the night's events took a turn for the worse when her water broke and the fetal pulse dived:

A second after the water broke, suddenly his [the baby's] pulse . . . went to 100, 70, 60, and then we were already on the way to the operating room. She [the doctor] says, "Natan, push the red button!" [hysterically] "Press the button!" [yelling] and suddenly I hear on the loudspeaker, "Code red, code red to room four." And you kind of understand that something isn't [right], something is happening but you don't understand. It's all a matter of seconds. . . . [The doctor] was standing with her hand inside [me] so that he [the baby] wouldn't descend more, trying to push him up as much as possible . . . and from the corner of my eye I saw the [intended] mother and father losing their heads completely [me'abdim et ha'eshtonot lechalutin].

In the midst of all of the hysteria, Ye'ara remained calm and collected, while Natan had a flashback to his own experiences during the first Lebanon war:

At that moment I looked at Ye'ara, and I will never forget that face. I mean, one of the biggest moments of your life is in wars. And I was in the war in Lebanon, and there is that moment when they are shooting at the soldiers. We were shot at. Soldiers go in, five minutes later all of the armored carriers come out with everyone injured, and everyone with that expression. Total shock. And she made that face at me there. . . . I will never forget it.

After describing a scene that she compared to something out of the television drama series *ER*, Ye'ara recalled the moment when the anesthesia wore off and she awoke from the surgery. Her description amplifies the theme of heroism and personal sacrifice in her tale:

> I still remember that when I began to hear people, I was still in that awake-asleep stage. . . . Suddenly I felt my mouth released and I said to them, "Did the baby live? Did the baby live? Where's Natan?" And they [the staff] said that when they heard me first ask about the baby then they all began to cry. Because they couldn't believe that I, the surrogate, who also didn't get nervous . . . they said that other women who are suddenly told that they need to go into surgery get hysterical . . . but my cool demeanor [*kor ruach*] amazed them. That I lay there and let them work. And that afterwards my first question was if the baby had lived amazed them, that I am worried about the baby and not about myself.

Finally, Natan further validated Ye'ara's bravery by contrasting her composure to his own emotional breakdown in the aftermath of the dramatic birth event:

> Those twenty minutes were really difficult. On the one hand, you see this couple falling apart and you see her [Ye'ara] with that face I saw in Lebanon, and they tell you that the umbilical cord was around the neck and all that. . . . I woke up at 5:30 and I started to drive to my parents' house. Suddenly, after twenty kilometers, I started to cry. I couldn't stop it. I tried to speak with my parents, to tell them that I'm on my way . . . and I'm choked up, can't speak. I sat in the car and cried without stopping, without the ability to stop. As if what had happened was beyond my ability to cope. Even today when she was speaking about it, I had tears. . . . Her startled face . . . I see that terrified facial expression [*partsuf mevuhal shel pachad*].

The ultimate example of the heroic narrative appeared in my interview with Rinat. Rinat described proudly how she had waited in the hospital cafeteria during labor for two hours because it was the eve of Independence Day, Israel's fiftieth, and she wanted so much to give birth on the nation's birthday. Rinat said that she knew that if she went upstairs [i.e., to the maternity ward] and the nurse saw how dilated she was, that they would make her go into the delivery room, so she held the baby in until the clock struck twelve, and then she went upstairs. In a video filmed a few hours later as hospital staff wheel Rinat down the hall after delivery, she drowsily lifts her head up from the cot and asks, "Where's the flag?" and then smiles when she sees a small Israeli flag adorning the baby's crib.

Rinat showed me raw footage that was filmed in preparation for a documentary of her surrogacy experience. In the footage, the narrator's voice-over highlights the idea of the new male citizen born on the fiftieth birthday of the country:

> It seems like regular preparations for yet another Jewish ritual in which another Israeli citizen will become a kosher Jew. It seems like another father and mother excited to bring the fruit of his labor and the creation of her belly into the tent of Abraham. But the young and sleepy citizen, that was born two weeks ago, exactly fifty years after the birth of the state, was far from being a regular story of pregnancy, birth and parenthood.

By linking the birth of the surrogate baby to the country's history and development, the documentary imbues Rinat's story with collective importance, rendering surrogacy a national achievement. Watching this documentary with Rinat and two of her children six months after that fateful day, I realized that the heroic narrative and its onscreen retelling affect Rinat's children's respect for their mother. When I asked them what their mother had gained from going through the surrogacy process, her teenage son responded, "My mom has shown everyone what we have always known. That she is a hero." Rinat's preteen daughter then added, "She will be in the history books someday, right, mom?" When Rinat responded positively, I challenged her, "Rinat, how can you be in the history books when your name is not allowed to be reported publicly according to the surrogacy law?" She explained, "It will say in the encyclopedia that, how many? Eight surrogates? Gave birth in 1998. And I will know that I am one of them, and my children will know. That is enough for *me*."

THE BATTLE OF THE GENDERED BODY

Roberts suggests that the U.S. surrogates she interviewed accentuated a strength that could be characterized as feminine in that they emphasized their fertility, ability to give birth, and nurturing empathy for infertile couples.[36] In the Israeli case, the militarized strengths that the surrogates emphasized could be characterized as masculine. Why do surrogates call on a stereotypically masculine script to describe their female bodily experience of conception, pregnancy, and childbirth? I suggest that the answer may lie in the surrogate's assumption that because her personal nature is feminized, she can only "battle the body," "subdue her nature," and manage her emotions and bodily boundaries by aligning herself with a masculine strategic discourse. Reynolds suggests that underlying the concept of "technological progress" is the assumption that masculinized technology can replace feminized "natural" bodies.[37] Since surrogates are involved in a technological process in which they believe they can control "nature," they may intuitively adopt a masculinized jargon.

The female body, particularly the pregnant body, is popularly conceptualized as leaky, seeping, unruly, and threatening to expel matter from inside—menstrual blood, breast milk, and babies.[38] The pregnant body challenges the idea of individualism and the male-gendered image of the controlled, autonomous body with its secure boundaries by threatening to split into two as the human being it contains prepares to cross its boundary.[39] Moreover, the womb, which is the primary module that surrogates detach in their body map work, is conceptualized in gendered technocratic terms as the organ most capable of malfunctioning and the most unpredictable part of the female body.[40] The surrogate's body-mapping order, her strategic boundary and emotion management, and her military rhetoric thus all may be viewed as part of a "battle" she wages against her body and as part of her attempt to control her "faulty female machinery" with male technological control (IVF, cesarean delivery) and masculinized military mastery.[41]

Surrogates can be compared to the anorexics described by Bordo, who were obsessed with suppressing their hunger, conquering the physical urges of the body, and controlling its "unruly forces."[42] Bordo suggests that anorexics constructed the "enemy" they were battling in the body against the feminine stereotypes of hunger and hysteria. The mastery and control they needed to conquer their appetites and enfeebled will were oppositely gendered along the lines of the stereotypically masculine values of strength and resolve. Thus, mastering the body entailed an erasure of feminine characteristics: the anorexics quoted by Bordo were elated when they ceased to menstruate, and they worked to remain as flat-chested as a boy.[43]

Sasson-Levy similarly observed that women soldiers who worked in "masculine" jobs in the Israeli army shaped their identities along the lines of the masculine model of the combat soldier.[44] They would mimic the combat soldiers' bodily and discursive practices; identify themselves with culturally "masculine" traits of will, endurance, determination, and strength; and differentiate themselves from what they understood to be markers of traditional femininity, such as passivity and uncontrollability. This construction of an alternative gender identity also influenced the women's view of their military service as a process of acquiring self-consciousness, self-awareness, and self-confidence during a period of personal growth, empowerment, and autonomy.

In this context, the surrogate's body map can be viewed as a rational, calculated, stereotypically male-gendered strategy for overcoming and conquering resistance to the female bodily order, especially hysteria, emotionality, leakiness, uncontrollability, illness, weakness, hunger, and irrational cravings. For instance, it is the couple's ethnic nature that is assumed responsible for the surrogate's strange cravings and technological artifice that is the specified cause of her illnesses. The surrogate's feminized traits—of caregiving, bonding, connecting, caring—are directed toward her relationship with the intended mother but neutralized vis-à-vis the fetus and the pregnant body, from which she distances herself emotionally.

By associating her body's unpredictable conduct with technological artifice and the intended mother's nature, the surrogate absolves herself from responsibility for that body and deflects any signs of weakness or inability to cope from her personal self. Thus, the surrogate's act of calling on a "masculine," militarized script of strength, courage, and determination reflects a clear gender ideology in which courage, power, and authority are exclusively associated with masculinity.[45] The military analogy is particularly potent in this reproductive context in light of the argument posed by many Israeli feminists that women's gendered citizenship, awarded through reproduction and motherhood, is the symbolic equivalent of men's gendered citizenship through military service.[46] Sered argues that this gendered distinction between men and women in Israeli national discourse stems from the definition of women as reproducers of the nation and therefore in need of protection through military effort.[47] Men are consequently associated with qualities of health, strength, and assertiveness, and even the healthiest and strongest women are assimilated into the category of the weak, vulnerable, sick, and infirm.[48] We can thus argue that this context gives rise to the surrogate's use of masculinized tools of mastery—male military jargon, male body and emotion mastery techniques, and vicarious control of (predominantly male) medical technology—through which she believes she can win her embodied battle.

This leads us to another important question: who really gains from the surrogate's "success" or "failure" at "passing the test" of her quest narrative? Specifically, if her battle to control the body and the emotions is a symbolic one between the stereotypically feminine and the stereotypically masculine, nature and culture, organicism and technology, agency and structure, then when she "wins," is she truly victorious? If the body heeds her instructions and becomes the "docile body"[49] or the "disciplined body"[50] that she tries to shape it into, then the male, medical, technological, capitalist, national side emerges victorious and the surrogate seems like a pawn, or instrument, in carrying out the patriarchal ideologies of the body politic.

Conversely, if the surrogate's body "betrays" her will, then it might be interpreted as the somatic rebellion of her nature against the "artificial" control of medical technology, the commercial provisions of the contract, the foreign "occupation" of her embodied territory, and the harnessing gaze of the doctor, couple, and body politic. The message her so-called failure would thus relay is, ironically, an empowering statement that the female body cannot be completely controlled, just as a technocratic society's attempts to control nature can never be complete.[51]

CHAPTER 9

The Hero's Quest

The surrogate's portrayal of herself as a courageous heroine is a key to understanding an elemental difference between surrogates and intended mothers. It illuminates the surrogacy experience as an initiation for surrogates and intended mothers alike. For both, it involves many of the classic elements of initiation, such as giving and receiving gifts, making sacrifices, overcoming pain or fear, keeping secrets, marking the body symbolically, and so on.[1] However, whereas intended mothers told me about their *initiation rituals* and their rite of passage into their new status, role, and maternal identity, surrogates told me an *initiation story*. Their initiations take the two in different directions: the intended mother undergoes a transition to motherhood, a status change supported by rituals and rites that transform her life. Conversely, the surrogate portrays herself as a mythic heroine who endures hardships on an arduous quest or journey according to a narrative structure that Frank terms "automythology"—a mythical tale of self-reinvention, of not just having survived the quest but of having been reborn.[2] The surrogate's journey does not make her someone else; instead, it takes her inward on a path of self-discovery and deepened self-knowledge.

With these insights in mind, I call on Joseph Campbell's model of "the hero's journey," which he specifically identifies as a common structure of myth across cultures and religions.[3] This structure—the universality of which he ascribes to Jungian unconscious archetypes—consists of three stages: departure, initiation, and return. In the following discussion, I do not ask why surrogates call on mythical elements in their stories or whether these myths are intrinsic to the human psyche. Instead, I simply use the heroic pattern as a template to decipher the common mythic elements and form that the surrogates' narratives employ. I begin with my own retelling of the surrogate's "journey" in this light.

The surrogate, like other mythic heroines, leads a simple life. She usually does not have an exciting career and, as a single mother, faces many hardships in her financial life, family life, and love life. She often feels her life is sedentary and not very interesting; all of that changes when she decides to become a surrogate. In the first stage of the hero's journey—departure—she hears the "the call to adventure" after learning about surrogacy from the broadcast media, the newspaper, or a friend. Her motivations for becoming a surrogate are financial at first, but she soon realizes that there may be more to be gained from the experience. She then seizes the opportunity "as an occasion [for] embarking upon a journey that becomes a quest, even if what is quested for never becomes clear."[4] From this point, the surrogate's experience of the "two worlds" begins: she puts her mundane life on hold and enters into the surrogacy process, a "special" reality that is separate from her everyday life.

She is surrounded by supportive characters who laud her for her success, such as the "oracle" (the nation-state), the "mentor" (the doctor-mediator), and the intended mother, who is her companion throughout. She learns that cohesion with the intended mother is essential to her survival of the process; without the intended mother's appendage of what the surrogate detaches and her shared holding of the pregnancy, the surrogate might not "succeed" in her "mission." Along the way, the surrogate also meets less supportive characters, such as the mythical "shape shifter," represented by the intended father, who is distanced from her with his businesslike focus on their contract.

Like all heroic quests, hers involves the hero's continuing realization of the "mission." This mission is gradually revealed when the surrogate's initial financial motivations are overrun by her motivation to make a family, to make her intended mother into a mother, and in symbolic form, to help this other woman carry out her duty to birth the nation. In the second stage of the hero's journey—initiation or fulfillment—the surrogate details her "road of trials," consisting of several thresholds or challenges she describes as "tests" at which she can "succeed" or "fail" (the surrogacy committee, the embryo transfer). She describes the "meeting with the divinity" when she stands face-to-face with the body politic, as the surrogacy approvals committee judges her worthiness. She bonds with her intended mother in a type of heroic camaraderie that is analogous to "attachment with the father." She then goes on to describe the "temptation away from the true path," in the form of her body's betrayal of her determined will and the moment when she almost gives up.

In the final stage of the hero's journey—return—the surrogate begins to feel ambiguous about her journey's approaching end, in a way that is analogous to the hero's "refusal of the return." Her ambivalence stems from her desire to give birth and end the physical demands of pregnancy; to receive the final, major payment; and to "return to herself" and reassume her regular role in her family. However, she also fears the end of surrogacy because it means the separation from her intended mother, to whom she has become so attached. Separation from the baby, as I have established, is a nonissue to her, even though popular belief holds that it should be her most torturous moment.

The surrogate's heroic journey then turns to "the magic flight," which is represented by the hospital birth. In some cases, this is accompanied by a moment of "rescue from without," in which the surrogate realizes how much the intended mother does, indeed, care about her. This occurs, for example, when the latter makes a symbolic sacrifice for her, such as staying beside her after the birth instead of abandoning her and going immediately to her newborn. The surrogate's journey ends with her "returning to herself" or, in Campbell's terms, "crossing the return threshold."

If her contract ends without her having produced a live birth for her couple, then she becomes the "failed hero." However, if she persists in her quest after "the ultimate boon"—the baby/gift/holy grail—and she shows her "courage," "determination," "heroism," and "inner strength," then she begins to realize that "doctors don't know everything." The surrogate then becomes the "master of the two worlds" when she retells the story of her quest in multiple arenas: to the newspaper reporter, to the television interviewer, to the surrogacy Internet forum, at meetings of the surrogacy support group, in reunions with her couple, and of course, to me, the anthropologist. The hero's quest reaches its climax with what Campbell calls "the freedom to live"; she returns home with what I refer to as the "trophy on her shelf," and the couple return home with the "flesh of their flesh," their "continuing generation," or "a new life."

GIVING LIFE

Most of the surrogates I spoke with saw themselves as having achieved
three significant things: they have helped produce children, a contribution to the continuation of "life"; they have made childless couples into
"families"; and they have made infertile women into "mothers." Many
of the women directly expressed their pride in these achievements. At
a party of surrogates and couples, Nina, then in her seventh month,
described this clearly: "Look, I am not just giving them this baby. I am
giving them a family. I am making this couple into a family. I am making
her [nodding toward her intended mother, standing a few steps away]
into a mother." Like Nina, other surrogates spoke about birthing more
than a baby. Belle wrote proudly on the surrogacy forum website about
her feelings as she went home from the hospital, announcing, "Yes, I did
it and I did it big. I succeeded in making a couple happy, a couple that
would have been unable to share the fruit of their love without me."

Belle's declaration denotes her central role in a family's creation. Only
she could have carried out this sacred quest, for she was the one who
"carried" the couple's fruit/nature/baby/holy grail in her womb. Many
of the women told me that what they were doing was creating a next
generation [dor hemshech] for their couple, a common cultural idiom
that refers not only to a family's personal continuity but also, abstractly,
to the continuity of the Jewish-Israeli nation, which is dependent on its
coming generations.[5] Neta saw herself as "doing a mitzvah . . . it is helping a dynasty, the continuation, it is making life continue. That is the
biggest mitzvah that can be. And especially since it was a son." Neta's
emphasis on the particular social value of a son, who can carry on the
family name and can also be a soldier for the nation, suggests that her
surrogacy also contributed to the continuity of the collective. Her interpretation of her role in surrogacy as "doing a mitzvah" also hints at
the presence of the divine in her understandings: a mitzvah is not just
a good deed, but one that Jews are obligated to perform before G-d.
By equating surrogacy with the mitzvah of making "life" continue, she
elevates her contribution to the highest level of service before G-d.

The particularly intense relationship that surrogates usually had with
their intended mothers led them to see themselves as bestowing "life,"
particularly on the intended mother. In other words, whereas the surrogates with whom I spoke all saw themselves giving the child to both
members of the couple and as creating a family for them, they especially
saw themselves as bestowing the identity-role of mother on their female

partner in the process. Orna saw herself as having given her intended mother "a reason to live":

> It was . . . to give her a reason to live. So that she could get up in the morning and she would have a reason to get up. Because in the end, a child gives you a reason to live. And until you have a child, there is no continuing generation and no reason to live. . . . This couple has no continuing generation, and if they don't have a child, then they will simply be erased from this earth.[6]

As the person who was able to give the intended mother "a reason to live," Orna makes herself into a life-giving deity. Many surrogates described a single moment of epiphany in which they realized what it meant to "give life" to someone else. Sapir described how she realized the significance of her gift when she saw her intended mother suddenly "bloom" like a flower and "sparkle" with life at the moment of birth:

> In the delivery room . . . I saw something in her [the intended mother's] eyes, that in the year that I had known her, I had never sensed that spark. I really didn't sense it. That woman suddenly changed into a daffodil [narkis]. Into an anemone [kalanit]. I don't know how to explain it. Her face shined like a diamond from sheer happiness. Her eyes sparkled like a crown. I do not know how to describe that experience. And then I realized that I had really done something big. That money already really didn't have anything to do with it. Her joy and her mother's joy, I'm telling you. I don't know who cried with whom, I mean, whose tears fell upon me. Hers, her mother's, I don't know. It was really something. . . . You know, when I told my friend afterwards, we both had a kind of shiver [run through] our bodies that you can't explain without feeling it. You can't express it in words. It is not something that you forget quickly. And she will remember it until the day she dies.

The notion that the intended mother was being taken from symbolic *death*—childlessness—to *life* was often described in terms of an organ transplant. Masha explained that her role as a surrogate was similar to that of someone donating an organ, "like in a transplant, which gives you life, which gives you and bestows upon you the experience of parenthood." Lihi also compared her surrogacy role to that of a living organ donor:

> No one knows what it is to give, to give life to someone else. I mean, it is like donating organs while you are still alive. It really is. People donate organs and that's it; they say, "When I die, then they should take my corneas, my heart." . . . But you don't get to see someone else enjoying it. But when you do this [surrogacy], you see it. And the most moving moment was not even after the birth. The most moving was at the *brit* [circumcision

ceremony]. Because at the *brit,* Danit [the intended mother] was so worried, and when they cut him she cried. She was so nervous that she cried, and I also cried. I saw her and then I cried . . . and it was sort of funny, to see both of us crying. [I didn't cry] because he [the baby] was in pain, but because it was hard to see her. It is something that is almost the greatest thing that can be done.

Significantly, the moment that Lihi found most meaningful in her surrogacy experience was when she witnessed her intended mother responding, as a mother, to her infant son. Daniella, who had been a surrogate for her sister, Jenny, and gave birth in England, also described the moment that she realized the power of what she had done in transforming her sister into a mother. After the delivery, Jenny stayed the night in Daniella's hospital room with the baby. Daniella recalled,

We were sort of dozing and I suddenly began to think, it's been quite a long time since he cried. . . . And Jenny got up out of her bed, without us speaking, and went over to him. And it was at that moment that I just thought, "Yeah, she's the mom." It was like magic in a way, the instincts. It was like at that moment that the responsibility was on her shoulders and she had taken it up and it was like, that's it, my duty here is over.

When I asked Daniella what that moment had meant to her, she replied, "It was the most meaningful moment for me, I think. . . . It meant to me that I had passed it on to Jenny and that she was the mom now and she knew what she was doing. . . . Yes, the minute that he was born the mantle was passed to Jenny and she carried on with it."

The sense of having given their couple "life" was described by nearly all of the surrogates. However, it was particularly strong for those whose perceptions were reinforced by their intended mother or by surrogacy forum participants. For instance, Shahar seemed particularly proud of her accomplishment because her intended mother had remained in contact with her in the years following the birth and would often reiterate her appreciation of Shahar's gift. At a face-to-face gathering of the online surrogacy community, Odelya said in front of all who could hear, including Shahar, "She [Shahar] is my daughter for life. She is the one that made me happy. What no one else did for me." Similarly, when I asked Shlomit, an intended mother whose surrogate had born her a son, how she thanked her surrogate, she said, "There is something that I always tell her, the surrogate. I say, 'My mother gave me life the first time, when she gave birth to me. You gave me life the second time, when you gave birth to my son.'" The image of the surrogate as a life-

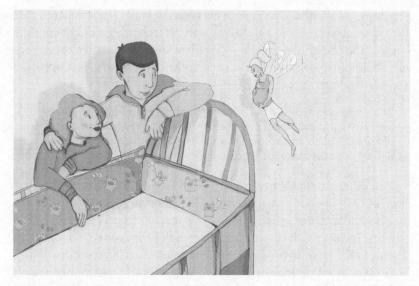

Figure 11. Illustration depicting the surrogate as a pregnant fairy or angel who is flying in to deposit a baby in the empty cradle of the expectant, childless couple. Originally appeared in *Lehiot Mishpacha* magazine. Reproduced with the permission of the artist, Danna Peleg-Segal.

giving deity is reflected in the regular lingo used by intended mothers to describe their surrogates on the forum website. They post messages referring to their surrogate as "my hero," "my angel," and "the amazing woman that gave me my joy." It is also evident in some former surrogates' self-descriptions on the forum, such as Oriya's digital sign-off in all of her messages: "Once an angel, always an angel" (see figure 11).

APOTHEOSIS

Surrogates take most of the credit for the "successful" delivery of the child because they have realized by that point that "doctors don't know everything" and that their own determination to "succeed" enabled the creation of a family that could not have been achieved naturally or supernaturally without their assistance. At a certain point in the surrogate's heroic quest, she undergoes a process that Campbell refers to as "apotheosis," a term that denotes becoming godlike.[7] Surrogates saw themselves as playing a central role within a pantheon of creation in which they were positioned directly under G-d. It was G-d that appointed them as his angels or heavenly messengers and gave them the divine privilege [*zchut*] of taking part in his creation work. They believed that the other players in the pantheon—nature, technology, the doctor, the couple, and the state—could not complete G-d's procreative command-ment without the surrogate's central contribution. Neta described her actions as a surrogate in such terms:

> I feel good about myself and proud of myself. I am telling you, G-d gave me the privilege [*zchut*] that I can give this to someone else. It really is an issue of *zchut*. . . . I am already signed up in heaven. . . . I did my *mitzvah*. . . . I did my good deed [*ma'aseh tov*] in life. I can be regular now.

Reli differentiated between a simple act of giving and the divine priv-ilege of carrying out a mission from G-d: "For me, being a surrogate is a *zchut* and it is not giving [*nitina*]. It is a *zchut* to make a couple into parents. In my eyes, it is something that can't be measured in money. . . . Thank G-d I have two wonderful [children]. And in return for that, I see it as a privilege [*zchut*] and mission [*shlichut*] to help others have children." Reli's positioning of *zchut* and *shlichut* in contradistinction to *giving* is informative. Giving is a personal act originating from within herself; she is not just giving of her own volition, but has been chosen for the honor of carrying out G-d's work. She clarified this, saying,

> G-d gives me the *zchut*. I am a messenger of G-d. But the ones that grant me the means to actualize the *zchut* [*she' m'zache oti*] are the couple. Because they are the ones that are allowing me to give to them, to do what G-d has intended me to do [*ma sh'elokim yi'ed li*]. It is not easy for one woman to allow another woman to do something for her that she can't do herself. Even if it doesn't work out in the end, I believe that G-d has another plan for me. Maybe he is protecting me from something. But for now I am giving my hundred percent.

Most of the surrogates I interviewed and encountered in the support group or web forum described their role in terms of *zchut* and *shlichut*, connoting their positioning as G-d's helper. Tamar wrote in a message to the web forum one week after giving birth to Miri's daughter, "I thank G-d every day that he gave me the *zchut* to be a surrogate, especially to such a great couple. . . . I am proud that I carried such a beautiful treasure in my belly. I feel that G-d chose me to do this *shlichut* and I did it in the best possible way." Responding to Tamar's message, Lihi wrote, "I understand exactly what you are feeling . . . a feeling of whole-ness or perfection [*shlemut*], *zchut*, and in the end comes the feeling of *shlichut*. . . . I remember that in the first period after surrogacy I woke up with a different feeling in the mornings . . . with the strong inner knowledge that 'I did it.' . . . It makes you so happy afterwards. Not just for the parents but also for us!"

Both Tamar and Lihi, who described themselves here as secondary to G-d, also described moments to me when they felt they superseded G-d. For example, when I visited Tamar in the hospital the day after she gave birth to Miri's daughter, she told me that Miri's parents had just visited her: "And her father sat right there, where you are sitting, and he said to me, 'You are G-d.' Can you believe it? He says, 'You are G-d for us.'" When I asked Tamar if she did feel like G-d, she replied, "I don't know. I think that someone like Lihi, when she had twins for her couple and they didn't have any children before that, I think she is G-d. That I can agree with. But Miri already had one daughter; this is the second, so it is less. Maybe I am half-G-d."

Two years later, when I was driving through the streets of Tel Aviv with Tamar on our way to a meeting of the surrogacy support group, I asked if she remembered what Miri's father had said to her right after the birth. She replied, "He told me that I am an angel. That I am their angel who has brought them this girl. . . . He said that I am an angel from G-d." I reminded Tamar that she had told me she had indeed felt godlike that day and asked her if she still felt that way. She responded, "Yes, I feel like I am an angel. That is why I say that I had a *zchut,* that G-d chose me and gave me this *zchut.* G-d intended this for me [*yi'ed li*]. He directed me to go to Dr. Michael, and that's how I got to Miri and David."

Tamar's repositioning of her place in the power hierarchy from G-d to messenger reflects a process of negotiation of her relative position within the web of agents involved in surrogacy. Like Tamar, other surrogates flirted with the idea of being godly but later retracted and positioned themselves one rank below G-d, as angel or divine messenger (see figure 12). Lihi, for instance, whom Tamar mentioned as more godlike than herself, also spoke about her position relative to G-d in our first interview but soon retreated from that position. Six months after she had given birth to twins for her couple, we had the following exchange:

> *Lihi:* It [surrogacy] is something that is almost the biggest thing that one
> can do. I once said to Danit [her intended mother]—I am almost
> sorry that I said it because it is a sentence that it is forbidden to
> utter—but it is like winning against G-d [*linatseach et elohim*]. G-d
> gives and all that, but, I mean, here you can change it. It is forbidden
> to say this, because I believe in G-d, but . . . I guess you could say it's
> like triumphing over nature. Not G-d, because G-d is great.

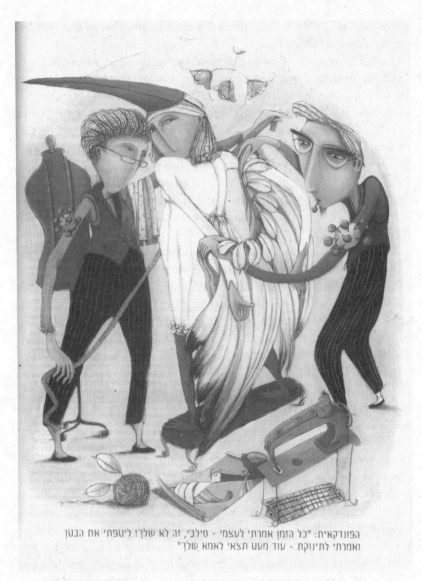

הפונדקאית: "כל הזמן אמרתי לעצמי - סילבי, זה לא שלך! ליטפתי את הבטן
ואמרתי לתינוקת - עוד מעט תצאי לאמא שלך"

Figure 12. Illustration titled "The Training of a Surrogate Mother." The surrogate is being dressed in an angel costume. Originally appeared in *Horim v'Yeladim* magazine. Reproduced with permission of the artist, Danna Shamir.

Elly: Because G-d helped you do it.

Lihi: Yes, exactly, to arrive at this. I didn't word it well. It is to triumph
over nature. . . . Because it wouldn't have [succeeded] if it hadn't
been for the connection [between us] and that sacrifice of the women
toward other people.

Here, Lihi toys with the idea that she and her intended mother, Danit,
were above G-d. To clarify her exact perception, I asked Lihi in a later
phone conversation to explain to me whether she saw herself and Danit
as fooling G-d or fooling nature into making conception happen. She
said, "We're not fooling G-d [*ovdim al elohim*], but we're definitely
fooling nature. Yes, I guess that G-d is the one who helped us find one
another and the doctor, of course—so G-d is helping us fool nature."
Like Tamar, Lihi's assertion of her position over G-d quickly gave way
in this conversation to defining her position as an accomplice of G-d,
together with the doctor and the intended mother, in defying nature.
Her idea, emphasized repeatedly in her description of surrogacy as a
type of *shlichut*, with herself as divine messenger, nevertheless positions
her above nature, technology, and the doctor. None of the surrogates in
this study expressed any problem with defying nature, a theme I shall
return to, but the idea of challenging the will of G-d was another story.
Five weeks after she had become pregnant on her fifth embryo transfer,
Ravit related the following:

I had a dream in which I woke up in the morning and I went outside of my
house and I heard a heavenly voice [*bat kol*] speaking to me. It was G-d.
And he said to me, "Why are you going against nature?" It is five IVFs that
haven't succeeded, maybe it is necessary to back off, and if nature made her
[the intended mother] infertile, then not to try to overcome it. But then the
same week we got word that it had succeeded, so I guess that G-d did want it.

This talk of G-d seems to be related directly to the general Jewish-
Israeli cosmological scheme that informs the women's thinking, since
only two of the surrogates I interviewed were religiously observant.
Thus, the talk of G-d seemed to be more related to their feeling of
involvement in an act of creation than to any religious doctrine. As
Yana put it three months after she gave birth to her couple's child, "You
feel like you are a partner in something that is really creative [*yetsirati
bimyuchad*]. . . . When I saw their faces when their child entered the
world, I saw that I had touched their happiness [*nagati b'osher shela-
hem*]." She described that moment as "the most meaningful moment in
[her] life." This sentiment was particularly evident in Eva's comment

that, after having performed this divine duty, she felt "on a high": "I feel that I am on a high all the time, and that I did a good deed. Part of it is also that everyone has been so supportive all around. I feel like it is a *zchut* that I have been able to contribute [*litrom*] to someone else."

While Eva's description of being "on a high" could literally be interpreted in terms of her height, or elevation, in the surrogacy pantheon, she is using the phrase to describe an extreme thrill or feeling akin to drug-induced or sugar-induced elation. The term "high" is also used in elite Israeli military units to denote soldiers' feeling of excitement at finally prevailing over the enemy in combat situations in which they have faced the possibility of death.[8]

Darash notes, in her discussion of the "high" described by combat soldiers in situations of extreme violence, that the feeling derives from the moment when a person feels total control of his or her body and emotions while breaking the boundary between life and death, and she hypothesizes that an equivalent "thrill" might be expressed by women in control of their own childbirth.[9] Indeed, some of the home-birthing women interviewed by Klassen experienced their self-controlled births as religious experiences.[10] Together, these women's testimonies imply that the term "assisted conception," which suggests that technology is "giving nature a helping hand,"[11] is a misnomer. Instead, the surrogates' testimonies suggest that *assisted conception needs assistance:* they believe that it is only with G-d's will and with the surrogate's determination that the doctor and technology can make conception happen. It is no wonder that the women often describe being transformed by their surrogacy experience.

THE HERO'S RETURN

Frank suggests that quest narratives hold a promissory note for a new life and different future for the protagonist after completion of the quest.[12] When I ask surrogates to tell me how their lives have changed after surrogacy, I often discover that their material circumstances are nearly the same as they were before they became surrogates. In all of the years I have known surrogates, only one of them actually saved all of the money she received ($26,000) and used it as a down payment on a house for herself and her daughter. A few of the women I met used the money to improve their lives by paying for driving lessons, buying a car, or moving to a better flat. One woman took her three children to the United States to visit her sister for a month, and one used the money to pay for a lavish bar mitzvah for her son. However, most of them used up most of what they were paid on living expenses during periods of unemployment or to pay off the debts that had led them to surrogacy in the first place. I have also met surrogates who spent the money they received on plastic surgery, redoing the floors of their rented apartments, or doing other things that did not change their economic status.

From a commodity-centered perspective, it thus seems as though the surrogate has actually failed to attain her goals, because her economic circumstances, employment opportunities, and social status are little changed. However, from the perspective of the quest and the gift, the surrogate's automythological account testifies to how her life has been dramatically altered. Consequently, even if their material situation remained the same, most of the women who had positive relationships with their couple and whose surrogacy experience ended with acknowledgment of their gift described how surrogacy had become an unexpected journey of self-discovery. While none of the surrogates I met claimed to have become someone else entirely, they did see the process as enhancing their self-perception, clarifying their identities and roles, and giving them insight into themselves.[13]

Metaphorically, they knew that they were strong, brave "super-women" all along, but surrogacy gave them the stage and legitimacy to make these qualities known to others and to garner respect and recognition, at least in their immediate spheres, for these qualities. The quest enabled them to structure a new perspective on the surrogate role for their audience. This new perspective counters the popular view that surrogates are poor, forlorn, miserable [*miskenot*] women who rent their wombs out of desperation for money, and portrays them instead through the counterimages of the heroine and the angel, images that are taking root slowly in the public sphere (see figures 9–12). It also reformulates the potentially humiliating selections, interventions, and monitoring a woman goes through during surrogacy as "retrospective necessities,"[14] the kinds of physical and moral challenges that soldiers, heroes, and surrogates must go through on their "missions."

Neta described herself as improving subtly in many ways: "It strengthened me. . . . You could say maybe that I am more assertive, maybe [I have] a little more self-confidence. I have a little more of everything." Neta positions surrogacy as something that she had to go through to become a fuller version of what she was before. She has become an improved model of the person she has always been.[15] The self-discovery process enabled many of the women to realize a sense of personal power that they had never felt before. Daniella, who was a surrogate for her sister, explained that surrogacy gave her "a feeling of power. It's like I finally had the ability to do something to pull my sister out of her predicament. It was like I was able to heal her." She also noted how the support of her family, friends, and even strangers had been empowering: "Also, I must admit that it is also nice to get so much admiration from so many people. It's been good for my self-esteem. . . . Some people really changed the way they speak to me. . . . They are full of admiration."

Much like Daniella, other surrogates derived their sense of empowerment and of self-pride from the support of others, and especially from their own children's admiration for what they had done. One of Masha's two daughters, both of whom were present in Masha's house during a follow-up interview two weeks after she gave birth as a surrogate the first time, told me, "Yes, she has changed. She is much more patient with us. She doesn't yell as much. It [surrogacy] made her calmer, I think. It definitely changed her." Masha added, "I feel full, at peace. I feel whole. I feel better than I ever have." She noted that she has always been "strong," a quality she felt she had inherited from her father, but after surrogacy, others had finally noticed it. When I interviewed her again several years later, after she had birthed twins for the same couple, Masha stressed that surrogacy made her believe in herself and in the power of faith: "Surrogacy really did change the way I see the world. Now I say, believe it and it will happen. . . . You need to stick to that faith, to that positive thinking."

For surrogates who felt that their couple had not acknowledged the value of their gift, this public support helped booster their self-confidence. For instance, when Belle's couple had a falling out with her after the birth, she expressed her disappointment to the surrogacy forum, and the online community lauded her achievement. There, in cyberspace, Belle was called a "hero" and thanked by infertile female members of the community who expressed their wishes that they could find a surrogate "just like you." The manager of the forum even put Belle's surrogacy story, which she had encapsulated in a series of messages, in a special section of the website that was accessible from the home page so that anyone accessing the forum could see it.

The combined effects of the high, the surge of power, and the feeling of having been elevated into the forces of creation left most of the surrogates I spoke to with the desire to engage in the process a second time. Even those who were not able to do so because of governmental regulations made attempts to contest this limit. I have found that, regardless of how much time has passed or whether they are still in contact with their couple, surrogates are happy to speak to me about the experience. They continue to talk about surrogacy whenever they can in the years follow-ing the birth, and several surrogates who gave birth four and five years earlier still attend meetings of the surrogacy support group, participate in the online surrogacy forum, or attend in-person gatherings of the surrogacy community just so that they can relive the experience. Meta-phorically, it seems to me that, in most cases, when I ask a surrogate to tell me her story, she stands up proudly, takes down an old, sometimes dusty trophy from her shelf, wipes it off to a shine, and proceeds to tell me about how she won it.

THE PARADOX

To this point, I have argued that the surrogate's narrative of her heroic journey has the effect of endowing her with increased self-knowledge, self-worth, and a sense of empowerment. I have argued that surrogates transform the constraints of the process into hurdles that they over-come on their journey. The women receive support, encouragement, and acknowledgment of their heroism from the couple, the doctor, the surrogacy community, and even the media. They regard themselves as superhuman conductors of G-d's will, in a position of the highest power and control. In what may appear as a huge gap between the structural, subjugating terms of their circumstances and their debatably contra-dictory agency-centered experiences, their empowerment narratives emerge within an institutionalized, patriarchal, medical-technological framework.

Surrogates embark on their "sacred quest" within a highly struc-tured framework that, arguably, represents the height of medicaliza-tion, commodification, and patriarchal institutional control of women's bodies.[16] Surrogates are necessarily medicalized from the moment they are screened for candidacy for the process. They are necessarily com-modified by the price tag attached in the contract to each stage of the reproductive act. Socially, surrogates are under the constant gaze of their couple and must obey the rules of the contract they have signed. They have little actual control over the events that shape their surrogacy expe-rience. They have no control over the state selection process, in which they are "investigated" by doctors, psychologists, and surrogacy com-mittee representatives. They have no control over conception through the IVF process, with its low statistical rate of success. The process of preparing themselves for the embryo transfer involves their bodily systems being overridden and medically managed to the hilt, controlled by doctors, medicines, and machines. As the surrogates themselves convey in their descriptions of the "artificial body," the hormonal treatments often carry ill effects and the pregnancy is often more difficult for them than their pre-surrogacy pregnancies were.

Taking all of these "harnesses" into consideration, we could view the surrogate through Foucault's theory of discourse as situated at the nexus of power in which institutions, politics, and economics constrain her every move through legal and medical regulatory means.[17] The surrogate is acting within a panopticon, and the means of surveillance are multiply enforced by the doctor, the couple, the body politic, and virtually all parties she comes into contact with. If the terms oppression and subordination refer to the "systematic exclusion from positions of prestige and power, inferior access to valued resources, and cultural valuation as lesser or inferior,"[18] then surrogates are set up by the contracted agreement to be subordinated and oppressed. They are necessarily women who need money. They are single mothers and nonrelatives of a couple that is usually of higher social and economic status. As unmarried women, they can become surrogates for married couples but cannot hire a surrogate themselves; as single mothers in a society where marriage is still the norm, they are more socially marginal than the married couple that contracts their services; and as women in need of money, they are necessarily less financially secure than their couple, who may not be wealthy but who can at least find the means to pay for surrogacy.

How can the surrogate relay such an empowerment narrative while partaking in a process that constrains her autonomy in law, contract, and institutional surveillance and in which she is under the surveillance of the body politic, the medical institution, and the intended couple? How does the experience of empowerment grow out of the contract and a context of extensive subjugation?

I suggest that Giddens's structuration theory might help us understand this apparent paradox.[19] Giddens critiques the conventional sociological approach that sees structure and individual action as opposites. He argues against most structuralists that social order is not merely externally constraining to individuals and that individuals are not just "cleverly programmed automatons."[20] Conversely, he argues against action theorists who tend to ignore the institutional level when they discuss human agency. In response to both camps, Giddens contends that structure is *dual:* structure and agency are mutually dependent, and

structures shape individual practice just as individual practice constitutes and reproduces structures.[21]

In light of Giddens's approach, we can look at the structure of surrogacy
in Israel as a process rather than as a stable, top-down phenomenon.
Surrogates take the restrictive structure of surrogacy and subversively
reinterpret the methods of control into ordeals that they must overcome
on their sacred quest. Each structured hurdle constitutes an opportunity for the enactment of agency. The psychological exams and the state-
appointed selection process become "tests" in which success increases
women's self-worth. Triumphing over the IVF "obstacle course" testifies
to their determination and courage. The medicalization of their bodies
becomes a site in which they subversively control the doctor controlling
their bodies, a tool for directing the pregnancy away from themselves,
and an occasion for dismissing the doctor's "authoritative knowledge"
in favor of their own superior wisdom. The intrusive medical events they
must face, such as emergency cesarean operations, become trials of courage and grounds for shaping a heroic, epic myth of courageous sacrifice.
Finally, the commodity idioms of human incubator and oven become
metaphors of empowerment that they use to emphasize their warmth
and centrality to the process. In this way, much as Bordo suggests occurs
with anorexics,[22] the surrogate may cultivate control-accessing mechanisms that enable her to feel empowered precisely because of her cir-
cumstantial powerlessness. The structural disempowerment becomes the
grounds for these women to exercise agency; they use their subjection
to mechanisms of control to elevate themselves above that control to a
place of power they have never before approached.

ACTORS IN THE FORCES OF CREATION

An alternate explanation for the contradiction may arise from the
mythical nature of the quest narrative and from the women's feeling of
centrality in the creation act: the creation of the child, the mother, and
the family. The surrogate's tale of her heroic quest, like all quest narratives, is recounted with an emphasis on the gains from, rather than the
costs of, the challenges she encounters.[23] As a myth, it "states the salient
contradictions, restates them in more and more modified a fashion, until
in the final statement the contradictions are resolved, or so modified and
masked as to be minimized."[24]

The surrogate narrates the tale of her heroic quest as an ascendance
to a godlike position in which she floats above nature, which did not

enable the intended mother to procreate; transcends technology, which does not live up to its promises of miracles and only works when her own faith and determination force its hand; rises above the doctor, who "doesn't know everything," as his powerful image would seem to promise; and positions herself directly under G-d, where she is handed the privilege [zchut] of carrying out the benevolent act of giving life to her couple. The surrogates' conclusion is that G-d needs surrogates to carry out his divine work and that women are indisputably irreplaceable within the act of creation. It is only women, with their faith, determination, pseudoprocreative rituals, gift relationships, heroic camaraderie, caring, and warmth that can make surrogacy births work.

We must not overlook the lack of opportunities in ordinary life for these women, or any other contemporary Western woman, to feel like they are part of divine creation. Graves suggests that original human society was matriarchal and was grounded on female reproductive power;[25] this goddess tradition was later co-opted by a patriarchal mythology, which reinterpreted power in terms of an absolute male G-d. As feminist scholars have widely noted, the medicalization of childbirth has transformed it from a female domain in which women helped other women of their community give birth at home into a mechanical process in a male, medical establishment.[26] While reproductive technology has led increasingly to conception being crystallized in a language of magic and miracles,[27] women's creative power in this reproductive "miracle" is increasingly demoted in favor of the "helping hand of technology" and the "miracle worker" doctors to the point that conception without technological intervention is now perceived as "miraculous" in itself.[28]

In discussions of reproduction, women do not centralize themselves in the creative act, other than in the rare circumstances of unmedicated home-births.[29] The idea of woman as goddess or creative force is disparaged by doctors, by Western society, and even by childbearing women themselves; contemporary Western women often credit their doctor with producing the child.[30] This is especially true in cases of fertility treatment, in which the doctor is seen not only as "delivering" the baby but also, using technology, as assisting in its conception. Even when women who have conceived after several failed IVFs do speak of themselves as being godlike creators, as in the published accounts that Diepenbrock cites,[31] their feelings of control over creation are interpreted by those writing about them as illusory.

In Israel, in particular, the cultural attitude toward pregnancy "trivializes" the woman's bodily and emotional experience.[32] Ivry found that doctors, husbands, and even those who are pregnant themselves expect women to be as "tough" as African women who mythically give birth while working in the fields; there is no legitimacy to complain about pregnancy fatigue or discomfort, and pregnancy is experienced as a lonely time with little social support. The women Ivry interviewed described making enormous efforts to engage their husbands in the pregnancy and having few opportunities to share and discuss the events of their pregnancies with others. Conversely, the surrogate had the emotional support and attentive ear of her intended mother, who went through the stages of surrogacy with her, accompanying her to every doctor's appointment and sympathizing with bouts of nausea to a degree that surpassed any of the husbands in Ivry's study.

In contrast to their earlier pregnancies, the women's reproductive efforts as surrogates were anything but trivialized. Instead, the surrogate's contribution to creating a mother and a family was commended, the pregnancy itself was celebrated as "miraculous," and the surrogate's efforts were usually acknowledged as generous, brave, and important. Having found little acknowledgment of their bravery in facing the challenges of pregnancy, childbirth, and raising their own children as single mothers, surrogates were usually valorized as "heroines" and as "angels" by the couple and even by the doctor. The women's achievements in surrogacy were also lauded by their friends, family, fellow surrogates attending the support group, and fellow members of the Internet surrogacy forum. Whereas regular medicalized childbirth may remove any notion of achievement from the woman,[33] surrogacy may, paradoxically, reinstate it.

The empowerment narrative is an expression of the women's realization that their actions constitute a meaningful contribution to the world. After realizing the greatness of their contribution, several surrogates quoted above mentioned they would never be forgotten by their couple or even by society as a whole, when they are inscribed in the "history books." Ernest Becker suggested that humans want to believe that their life has a purpose, and they try to attain that meaning through specific beliefs and practices.[34] This is a common explanation for the human desire to procreate and establish a "continuing generation," the desire for fame, the desire to generate enduring works, and the performance of deeds that will be remembered by future generations. The surrogate's quest narrative is an "enacted story of her life"[35] that enables her to recast her surrogacy experience into a tale that she can tell and retell long after it is over to friends, family, and her children; on the Internet, in support groups, and in the media; and even to this anthropologist. She is empowered because she feels she has something unique to say to other women in her situation and perhaps can make a difference to their surrogacy experience, and because she has done something she believes will leave a mark on the world.

As Frank suggests in his examination of illness narratives, the "truth of stories is not in what *was* experienced, but equally what *becomes* experience in the telling and its reception."[36] The "high" that surrogates say they feel at the end of the process can be seen literally as an effect of the heights of power they have reached in their experience of the quest. This high represents the transcendent moment that is produced after the surrogate has disengaged her self from parts of her body, subdued her nature, battled material circumstances, and ascended in the pantheon of creation. She has been joined together with the intended mother in a unity and has passed the tests of her sacred quest by showing courage and bravery. Her "high" is thus an effect of this moment of self-realization, an indescribable moment that may be likened to what Otto termed "the experience of the holy."[37] Consequently, although all signs may point to the surrogate's objectification and victimization, she experiences surrogacy as a liberating process in which she temporarily accesses what was once the feminine domain of creation.

Conclusion

Birthing a Mother has taken us into the world through which Israeli surrogates and intended mothers navigate in their cooperative, but by no means equivalently experienced, endeavor to create both new humans and new kin relations. The women carefully and continuously claim or abdicate the title of mother through individual and interactive cognitive and embodied practices. Through serial moves of embodiment and disembodiment, distancing and appending, giving and reciprocating, the women resolve the anomalies of surrogacy in and among themselves.

DIVIDING, CONNECTING, SEPARATING

Throughout the chapters that make up this volume, we have witnessed a process involving sequential moves of division, connection, and separation.

1. *Dividing:* First, we explored the ways that the surrogate cognitively partitions her body and nature through the careful creation of a body map. This mapping distinguishes between that which represents her personal self in the body and that which can be safely distanced. Body mapping ensures that the surrogate's own maternity remains devoted to her children and that the processes of gestation she embodies facilitate the maternity of the intended mother. Describing themselves as incubators

and ovens, surrogates operationalize the body map to manage their emotions toward the fetus and to safeguard their personal boundaries against intrusion under the constraining circumstances of the contractual agreement.

2. *Connecting*: Second, we explored the ways that intended mothers deployed maternal and kin-claiming practices and materialized their desires to append, encompass, and actualize becoming a mother through their surrogates in a prosthetic process of identity transition. Intended mothers read pregnancy guides, construct pregnant identities, exhibit bodily signs of pseudo-pregnancy, and even engage in couvade-like behaviors during the delivery. These processes are strengthened by interactions in which surrogates engage in caregiving practices toward intended mothers, becoming what I have likened to midwives to other women's motherhood. Progressively, surrogate and intended mother become interlinked and interchangeable, "shift" the pregnant body between them, and merge in a manner that is intimate and exclusive of their husbands and boyfriends both emotionally and sexually. Throughout, doctors and medical staff as well as intended fathers and others support their individual and cooperative projects of the body.

3. *Separating and Redefining*: Lastly, we examined the post-birth process of recategorization and disconnection of the two women into separate, individual bodies and identities. Immediately following delivery, the state and the medical institution begin this classifying process, instilling order and normalizing ideologies to designate only one mother and one family as the end product of this process. Toward the same end, intended mothers partake in ritual actions to finalize their new identities as mothers, while surrogates look toward the contracting couple for signs acknowledging their actions in gifting terms. When acknowledgment is secured, surrogates retrospectively narrate their experiences of the process as a hero's journey with many trials and challenges along a course of self-definition and self-realization. When the gift is denied, surrogates experience a devastating sense of betrayal.

Individual chapter discussions have developed the main theoretical points suggested by the ethnographic material. These relate to a more nuanced approach to questions of exploitation; the concept of nature that emerges from the surrogates' narratives; body mapping as a semiotic mirror of collective values; the shifting body as a type of collaborative body project; gift giving and consumption; and questions of structure, agency, and empowerment. Throughout, we learned of the enormous gap between the theoretical implications of commercial surrogacy and individual experience: the state, market, and medical establishment shape a framework that sets up all of the preconditions for the process to be a humiliating, dehumanizing, and alienating experience for the surrogate through a cold, businesslike relationship with the contracting couple. However, the women in this relationship, together and individually, make surrogacy more about personal agency, gift giving, heroism, and birthing a mother.

THE HIGH STAKES OF MATERNITY

Birthing a Mother conveys that many of the basic cultural scripts that shape the personal experiences of surrogates and intended mothers in Israel have common themes with the scripts that shape reproductive technologies elsewhere. Israeli women struggle with many of the questions that the scholarship emerging from North America and the United Kingdom has conveyed: issues of naturalness, normalcy, and adherence to cultural ideas about appropriate maternal behavior.[1] Moreover, like other recent titles in the anthropology of reproduction—for instance, Paxson's *Making Modern Mothers,* Thompson's *Making Parents,* and Layne's *Motherhood Lost—Birthing a Mother* suggests that reproductive technologies are about more than "elusive embryos," "perfect fetuses," "miracle babies," the "child in mind," and the "child as gift."[2] Instead, these titles convey that reproductive technologies are as much about making particular identities—mothers, fathers, and parents—as they are about making babies.

Yet as one reviewer of *Birthing a Mother* commented, the intensity of the women's investment in preserving and cultivating their maternal identities seems more strongly expressed within this work's pages than in other recent titles .[3] This intensity of feeling could perhaps be ascribed to the Mediterranean character of Israeli society.[4] I would suggest, however, that it may also be understood as a reflection of the cultural importance of motherhood within both Judaism as a religion and Israel as a nation-state. It is in this respect that *Birthing a Mother* shares in the particular relevance of another pair of titles: *Reproducing*

Jews, Kahn's ethnographic account of the influence of Jewish religious law on the practice of reproductive technologies in Israel; and *Birthing the Nation,* Kanaaneh's account of the fertility strategies of Palestinian women in the Galilee.

The careful attention that Israeli surrogates pay to protecting and preserving their own maternity while aiding other women to become mothers, and the lengths to which intended mothers will go to become mothers, reveal how much is at stake in the Israeli case. More than just their personal and social identities as women, mothers, and members of families are at issue; so also are their identities as Jewish women and as gendered citizens of the nation-state. To explain how this comes to affect the women's constructions, we must first understand that, in Israeli society, motherhood historically emerged as a role and symbol that bears major national significance. This is especially meaningful within the context of the Israeli-Palestinian conflict, in which motherhood has been celebrated in the Zionist rhetoric as a "national mission" and in which Jews and Palestinians are depicted as participating in a "demographic race" to birth their respective nations.[5]

Official demographic policy of the Israeli nation-state is often characterized as explicitly pronatalist, and social pressure to have children is very high. Israeli women are depicted in the ethnographic scholarship as participating fully in an ideology of compulsory motherhood, a "cult of fertility," to the extent that they will do anything to have a child.[6] Some feminist commentators have viewed the cultural expectation for Israeli women to become mothers at any cost as oppressive and as a reflection of the patriarchal culture and a Foucauldian control by the body politic.[7] Sered even views this expectation as part of a "patriarchal bricolage" that, in her view, makes Israeli women become sicker and die younger than their counterparts in other Western industrialized nations.[8] Yet these relations are more dynamic and interactive than such top-down theories suggest: consumer demand, through women's campaigns and lawsuits, for legalization and state subsidization of fertility-related services often forces the state into action.[9] This was the case, for instance, with the surrogacy law, which was not initiated as a state venture but rather was a response by the state to the campaigning of infertile couples.[10]

In a country that situates the family as the cornerstone of the nation's construction, women enter into symbolic relations with the state specifically through their roles as wives and mothers.[11] In this way, motherhood also becomes a significant determinant of women's inclusion in the Jewish-Israeli collective and an avenue toward establishing a sense of collective belonging. Kahn has shown, for instance, how unmarried women in Israel use motherhood as a channel of status enhancement, because the stigma against single women in Israel is far greater than that against single mothers.[12] Likewise, Amir and Benjamin have suggested that women who decide to terminate their pregnancies because of personal concerns are symbolically distanced from the collective because they are seen as rejecting their expected national maternal role.[13]

Under these circumstances, going to great lengths to have a child, even by extreme measures such as multiple IVF attempts or surrogacy, is culturally commended and even expected of childless women. Conversely, stopping treatment or remaining childless by choice are labeled deviant.[14] Becker's ethnography of men and women undergoing fertility treatments in the United States bears witness through comparison to the relatively extreme case Israeli society presents in this respect.[15] Becker regards women in her study who had undergone four IVF cycles as "veterans" of fertility treatment; in comparison, several of the women I interviewed turned to surrogacy after twenty-six, twenty-seven, and even thirty-one failed IVF attempts. Becker also discusses the way women who stopped treatment overcame the assault of infertility on their identities as women; the Israeli women I interviewed never viewed giving up as an option.

The only "veteran" of infertility whom I met during this study was Rachel, who affirmatively convinced me that she had relinquished her battle and was coming to terms with childlessness using a "new age" rhetoric after failed IVF, failed surrogacy, menopause, and passing the fifty-year mark in her life. Yet several months after our first interview, in which she professed these sentiments, she called me to say that something in our conversation had stirred up old issues. She said that she had been watching as the space shuttle carrying Israel's first astronaut—a symbol of national hope—exploded in midair.[16] She felt a blow to her stomach, and at that moment she knew that she could not give up. One year later, she text-messaged me as she and her husband got on the plane to go meet their baby girl, whom they adopted from Russia; two years after that, she gave me tips on making homemade baby food as her two-and-a-half-year-old daughter and my baby son played together on the floor.

MOTHER/NATION/STATE

From the perspective of national and religious investment in maternity, family, and reproduction, surrogacy places both the surrogate and the intended mother in unique relations with the nation-state. Intended mothers, viewed publicly and personally as having failed to heed their national calling, call on surrogacy as a medium for fulfilling their national duty and for realizing their gendered citizenship. Conversely, surrogates risk betraying their national duty by agreeing to give birth to a child and then relinquish custody to it in exchange for money. Surrogacy becomes an explosive terrain for the Israeli surrogate to navigate, especially because it is carried out directly under the eyes of the state. In addition, as single mothers in a family-oriented society, women who become surrogates are already in a socially marginal position with limited access to financial resources.[17] In fact, it is precisely their status as unmarried women with children that places them in the stringently defined group of women permitted to be surrogates under Israeli law.

Considering the ideal of national maternal service sheds new light on the women's narratives and practices as documented in the ethnography. When surrogates partake in a procreative process that does not result in their own motherhood, they are forced to realign their role not only with their personal identities but also with national reproductive goals. As a result, when surrogates juggle the meanings of nature, body, family, and maternity, they are also orchestrating their position vis-à-vis the meanings of gender role fulfillment and national belonging. The surrogates' careful body mapping can consequently be seen as a strategy for aligning their actions with cultural understandings of gender and maternity, shaping surrogacy into a status-enhancing experience personally, and dismissing the threat of their further marginalization. By going to such lengths to prove where their own embodied selves end and the surrogate pregnancy begins, they are avoiding the stigma attached to denying their maternal citizenship.[18]

Moreover, by emphasizing how they are birthing another woman as a mother, surrogates align their actions with the reproductive goals of the state.[19] Surrogates establish themselves as conformist Israeli women who have heeded their own national reproductive calling in the past and are now continuing their missions as good national subjects by helping childless women achieve their own national goals. Drawing on military discourse and transforming surrogacy into an act of heroism, they are not acting against Israeli society's interests but rather fulfilling them. One might go so far as to say that the surrogates are literally sacrificing their bodies for the collective, as their disembodied wombs are producing new, state-commissioned citizens. The surrogate's conceptual logic also protects the state's interests because it so vehemently protects maternity's rootedness in nature—an ideological tenet that is in conformity with the patriarchal interests of the state. Ironically, as single women rendering their bodies into fragments to make married women into mothers and married, heterosexual couples into families, they may be seen as reaffirming a patriarchal view of the family that only serves to further marginalize single women.[20]

NATION AND POSTMODERN PROCREATION

This ethnography challenges some of the assumptions that have been voiced about reproductive technologies and some of the predictions that have been made concerning their effects on society. First, given the implications of the nationalist project within the practice of surrogacy in Israel, it challenges the idea that reproductive technologies are leading to the postmodern fragmentation of the nuclear family and to the deconstruction of motherhood.[21] In the Israeli case, it would seem that rather than constituting a threat to the family, surrogacy reaffirms it.[22] Not only have the surrogacy law and approvals committee ensured that only nuclear, heteronormative families can be produced through the surrogacy process, but the ethnography reveals that multiple levels of society are also implicated in the effort to maintain the type of distinctions that protect motherhood and family from dissolution. Rather than fragmenting motherhood, surrogacy in Israel is constructed as a venture with the singular goal of creating only one mother, as institutional policies and the surrogate's and intended mother's individual and collaborative practices convey. The state, the medical institution, and individuals are all revealed as working toward resolving the anomalous connotations of surrogacy and transforming it into an occasion for the nation to extol modern, not postmodern, categories of motherhood and family.

Second, the ethnography challenges the perspective that medical technologies are bringing us closer to "the end of the body" and to the dissolution of the bounded body as a symbol of the nation-state.[23] Van der Ploeg, looking at the construction of the couple as a "hermaphrodite" patient in medical encounters between fertility specialists and couples undergoing infertility treatment, suggests that in vitro fertilization constructs a type of postmodern, hybrid embodiment in which male partners and fetuses are viewed as patients within the woman's body.[24] Yet in the case presented here, even while sharing the body, engaging in practices of interchangeability, merging, clicking, and shifting the body, surrogates retain a strong sense of individual embodied selfhood. This is not the fluidity discussed in some French feminist writings[25] or the anomalous embodiment discussed by Shildrick in the case of conjoined twins.[26] Instead, this is a sharing of the body that is established through careful, self-imposed fragmentation, controlled body mapping, and strategic moves that ensure the maintenance of interpersonal boundaries. If the "end of the body" that Martin envisions[27] involves the commodification and circulation of body parts and the dissolution of the boundaries of the whole body, then the practices of surrogates reify the continued emphasis on boundedness even within practices that engage in extensions, inclusions, and appendages of the embodied self.

Third, the ethnography challenges the speculation that new technologies are bringing an end to "nature" as we know it. Theories within the anthropology of reproduction speculate that the new reproductive technologies are deconstructing the boundaries between nature and artifice and remaking nature into artifice, so that we no longer know which is which.[28] Strathern suggests that reproductive technologies, in particular, may erode the classic analogies that have been used to separate nature from culture,[29] and Rabinow contends that nature will soon be so "operationalized" that it will no longer serve as a central classificatory system.[30] My study confirms that when technologies intervene in human reproduction, the definitions of nature and artifice need to be worked out. However, I would add that the theoretical inferences referenced above may be applicable to certain cultural contexts and not to others. I suggest that in cultures in which nature, as a category, is inextricably entwined in a matrix of other categories that are central to the nation's ongoing construction of itself as a bounded, secure unit, individual bodies and body politics will go far to make sure that these "secure distinctions" are preserved.[31]

Fourth, the ethnography challenges the idea that reproductive technologies are leading to a type of "postmodern procreation."[32] Specifically, surrogacy in Israel presents a case of a "postmodern" medical technology and a type of postmodern embodiment that are being used to achieve highly modern goals of maintaining national boundaries, traditional categories of family, motherhood, and nature, and the bounded body. Surrogates work creatively, using metaphor and cognitive and embodied strategies, to delineate and uphold the core categories of family, motherhood, body, and nature. Even as they engage in such configurations as shared bodies and extended selves that encompass offsite bodily appendages, and as they temporarily lapse into fluid identities, they still stay true to the concept of the modern, individual body and the notion of a "real," core true nature and self within the body. Their oneness and fluidity end; their appendages and distanced parts become reintegrated in a consistent whole, bounded, embodied self.

From this perspective, surrogacy cannot rightly be described in terms of Franklin's "postmodern procreation" because it is so strongly embedded within modernist frames, forms, categories, and goals. Even more, what we are seeing here might actually be described as a postmodern procreative practice used toward "modern" goals that produces what we might call "premodern" ritual practices among the women who use it; they engage in gift exchange, experience pseudopregnancy, exhibit stigmata, and undergo couvade. They believe in miracles, partake in a "virgin birth," and shape surrogacy into a phenomenon I have likened to goddess worship and a return to a mythical matriarchal culture. In this sense, the postmodern, embedded in a modern frame, conjures up premodern cultural scripts.

Lastly, the ethnography challenges the idea that state control of reproduction is always antithetical to women's and children's interests. Indeed, studies of the one-child policy in China have taught us how state intervention in natal issues can result in female infanticide and child abandonment.[33] Likewise, using a Foucauldian perspective, Kligman's study of state-controlled reproduction under Ceausescu in Romania exemplifies how extreme the consequences of such regimens can be.[34] Under an ideology of socialism and goals of demographically achieving a new socialist class of citizenry, the Ceausescu regime banned contraception and abortion and punished doctors who violated the ban, resulting in high maternal morbidity, abandoned children, and an epidemic of AIDS. Kligman ends her ethnography with a warning to other countries to learn from Romania's tragic past and put limits on state control of reproduction.

Still, in the case of surrogate motherhood in Israel, a new perspective on state intervention in natal issues might be forming. Weisberg makes an argument supportive of Israel's exemplary regulation of surrogacy and charges that Israel can be an example to other nations for dealing legislatively with the practice.[35] Surely, the legislation has its drawbacks, including the directive that surrogates must be single women, that gay couples and single persons cannot hire surrogates, and that intended mothers must first have subjected themselves to repeated IVF attempts to prove their candidacy. However, the legislation also protects surrogates, couples, and the resultant child. The government ensures that all parties are diligently screened and that all contracts are valid. Children must be accepted by their intended parents, even if born disabled; surrogates must relinquish the child to the couple; and surrogates are entitled to psychological help for themselves and for their children.[36]

Conversely, most other countries ban commercial surrogacy, and where it is allowed, it is unregulated and offers few protections for those involved. In the United States, where, as Markens notes, hesitancy to allow state intervention in reproductive issues has led to surrogacy being largely unregulated, the practice is vulnerable to market forces and few protections are available.[37] Reputable agencies employ extensive screening procedures and take legal precautions to ensure that contracts are valid and that surrogates have medical insurance during the pregnancy. However, stories of problems resulting from private arrangements or those facilitated by new or less thorough agencies are far from rare. An improperly screened surrogate may physically risk her own health and that of the baby, and improper consideration of insurance carriers and legal statutes may result in the surrogate not being properly insured or the contract being judged invalid.[38] In international surrogacy arrangements, evidence from Japan, India, and Britain has shown that parentage has not always been legally recognized in the intended parents' home country, and citizenship has even been denied their surrogacy-born children.[39] While Israel's intervention into natal issues has been critiqued for various reasons,[40] its approach to surrogacy suggests that, in that arena at least, the benefits of state control outweigh the costs.

POLICY IMPLICATIONS

Finally, I suggest that taking the surrogates' narratives at face value and accepting some of the findings that emerge from the ethnography may have important policy implications. Burfoot reminds us of the danger posed when official reports recommending legislation on reproductive technologies appropriate feminist critiques as the basis for their recommendations, disconnecting the critiques from their political and cultural roots.[41] Likewise, Markens and Andrews warn of the effects of political intervention of religious organizations on such legislation, citing the extent to which lobbying by Catholic organizations impacted the ban on surrogacy in New York.[42] When legislative bodies adopt the social concerns that have been highlighted in the theoretical scholarship on surrogacy or base their policy debates on the cultural anxieties that surrogacy generates, they formulate policies that address issues that are less important rather than on ones the ethnographic data suggest should be addressed.

Policy deliberations often focus on the need to protect the potential surrogate from a choice she may later regret and on the potential for exploitation of a surrogate who is undertaking a risk for financial gain.[43] My study suggests that we must take a more nuanced approach toward the issue of exploitation. Surrogacy does have the potential to exploit women; however, the voices of surrogates counter automatic presumptions of exploitation by showing that a majority achieve a degree of appreciation through surrogacy that they do not get otherwise from partners or from society at large. In a "macho" culture like Israel's, where pregnancy is trivialized and militarism is a prevailing cultural model for emotion management, surrogates experience pregnancy in a new light. Finally, despite—and perhaps because of—the many structural harnesses that surrogacy subjects them to, the surrogates in this study engaged in practices of self-defining and protective boundary policing, and they transformed harnesses into hurdles on a course to heightened self-recognition and self-worth. This result does not appear to be unique to Israel. Comparative ethnographic data suggest that in the United States and even in India, surrogates often experience the process in terms of empowerment.[44]

At the basis of many policy deliberations over surrogacy are concerns over baby selling, the best interests of children, and the impact of separation on a surrogate and a child after prenatal bonding has presumably occurred. The ethnography has shown that surrogates begin a distancing regimen even before they are pregnant. Through their relationships with intended mothers, through an explicit biogenetic frame of thinking about kinship, and through emotion-management practices, they try to help intended mothers bond with the baby while preventing themselves from developing maternal emotions.

If anything, the ethnography speaks to the convincing nature of the cultural expectation that women should and will experience bonding. After the baby is born, surrogates often experience pain because of separation from the couple for whom they birthed the baby, rather than because of separation from the baby. My findings are supported by a significant number of psychosocial studies of surrogacy that aimed to assess the level of bonding surrogates experience toward the baby they carry; none of these studies, to my knowledge, found that surrogates bonded at all.[45] Likewise, statistics, although not exact, speak to the idea that prenatal bonding for surrogates is more of a cultural myth than a reality: it is estimated that less than one-tenth of 1 percent of surrogacies end up in court battles.[46] Finally, studies of the children born through surrogacy have begun to disclose that these children are not harmed by the process and that there are even benefits to being born through a process in which parents made such efforts to bring them into the world.[47]

Policy makers have viewed continuing contact of the surrogate with the intended parents as problematic, assuming that the surrogate has become attached to the newborn and that such contact might remind her of the child she has given up.[48] This ethnography has shown, conversely, that a close relationship develops between surrogates and intended mothers and that, at the end of the surrogacy agreement, surrogates feel grief over the loss of companionship rather than over the loss of the newborn. When contact ceases unexpectedly after the birth, surrogates view it as a betrayal.[49] Contact during the first year after delivery and on special occasions, such as holidays and birthdays, is crucial for the surrogate's recognition that her gift has been acknowledged, and it has repercussions for her ongoing retrospective satisfaction with the agreement.

In addition, the assumption that surrogates struggle primarily with attachment to and relinquishment of the baby leads many policy makers to favor mandatory counseling for the surrogate before, during, and after the pregnancy.[50] However, this ethnography has established that it is the quality of the surrogate's relationship with the contracting couple that largely determines her satisfaction with her experience.[51] The overwhelming majority of surrogates in my study refused to attend counseling sessions, even though they knew that payment for psychological services during and for six months after surrogacy had been set aside in a trust. Few consistently attended voluntary monthly group counseling sessions when they were offered by a surrogacy agency; participation of surrogates in the online support group I observed was also intermittent. Almost all felt they did not need counseling services, as they viewed themselves as coping very well on their own with issues of emotion management toward the baby during pregnancy and relinquishment.

The issues that did become major concerns involved the surrogate's relationship with the couple, especially when misunderstandings arose over control of the surrogate's body; when there were differences in expectations related to level of closeness, respect, and the future of the relationship; and when miscommunication of feelings and needs occurred.[52] Those surrogates who found surrogacy to be a highly negative experience did so because of disrespectful relationships with their couple, feelings of betrayal by the couple after the birth, and the couple's lack of acknowledgment of the importance of their contribution (as exemplified by Sima, Batya, and Yelena). The breakdown of surrogate–intended parent relationships is often the root cause of those few surrogacies that do end up in court battles.[53] In this respect, if mandatory counseling is called for, it should take the form of mediation or group counseling sessions between surrogates and couples—not counseling for surrogates alone—to help them define and maintain interpersonal boundaries and mutual expectations from the relationship.

Finally, informed policy decisions should go beyond paternalistic assumptions that surrogates are denying and deflecting their "true feelings" and instead acknowledge that surrogates do engage in complex cognitive and embodied efforts to manage their emotions, identities, and relationships during surrogacy. Legislation should support surrogates' concerns with preserving their personal identity as "mother" to their own children even as they distance themselves from this title in relation to the surrogate baby. Likewise, it should support intended mothers' concerns with attaining this title singularly for themselves. Currently, policy often presents barriers to these efforts: U.K. surrogacy policy, for example, directs that the surrogate and her husband be registered as the legal parents of the child until a parental order is secured. Some U.S. states have allowed pre-birth custody orders, so that the intended parents' names can be immediately written on the baby's birth certificate; still, other U.S. states require that the parents adopt their own genetic child. In the case of single individuals who hire surrogates or gay male couples who do so, legal issues surrounding recognition of parenthood are even more complicated. A new approach to policy decisions on surrogacy that is based on the perspectives and experiences of those who have been through this process may enable the real core issues to be addressed.

Notes

1. More than fifty articles on surrogacy appeared in the U.S. print media from January to April 2008. See, for instance, coverage of surrogacy in India in *The New York Times* (Amelia Gentlemen, "India Nurtures Business of Surrogate Motherhood," *The New York Times,* March 10, 2008; Judith Warner, "Outsourced Wombs," *The New York Times,* January 3, 2008) and coverage in *Newsweek* of the prevalence of surrogacy among U.S. military wives (Lorraine Ali and Raina Kelley, "Womb for Rent: The Curious Lives of Surrogates," *Newsweek,* April 7, 2008).

2. In Genesis 16:1–2 Sarai says to Abram, "Look, the Lord has kept me from bearing. Consort with my maid; perhaps I shall have a son through her." In Genesis 30:3 Rachel says to Jacob, "Here is my maid Bilhah. Consort with her, that she will bear a child on my knees and through her I too may have children." See also Genesis 30:9: "When Leah saw that she had stopped bearing, she took her maid Zilpah and gave her to Jacob as concubine."

3. Baby M was born to surrogate Mary Beth Whitehead, who refused to relinquish her to the contracting couple, William and Elizabeth Stern. Their dispute turned into an internationally known saga of epic proportions through the widespread media coverage of the legal battle that ensued. A New Jersey courtroom ultimately gave the Sterns legal custody. Whitehead published a bestselling autobiography about her grief-filled experience, and a popular TV movie followed.

4. The incidence of surrogacy is impossible to accurately estimate due to the many informal arrangements that take place. Birth records do not show the

means by which a child was conceived, and clinics and private surrogacy agencies were not asked to release data on surrogacy until 1997, when the Centers for Disease Control (CDC) began collecting statistics. Estimations by surrogacy organizations quoted in the media have suggested that surrogates have given birth to 25,000–28,000 babies in the United States since the mid 1970s (Judy Keen, "Surrogate Relishes Unique Role," *USA Today*, Jan. 23, 2007; Alex Kuczynski, "Her Body, My Baby," *New York Times Magazine*, Nov. 28, 2008). These figures, however, which are based upon reports aggregated by the organizations from clinics, surrogacy agencies, and people involved in informal arrangements, are difficult to accurately verify. Current figures from the CDC report that 571 cycles using nondonor embryos were attempted in 2001 and that the number steadily increased over subsequent years: 548 in 2002, 671 in 2003, 710 in 2004, 1,012 in 2005, and 1,042 in 2006—the most recent year reported—of which a little less than half resulted in live births. These figures, however, do not include traditional surrogacies, those using donor eggs, or those done through clinics not included in the CDC data, so actual figures are probably much higher. The Childlessness Overcome through Surrogacy Organization (COTS), a nonprofit agency that assists surrogates and couples in the United Kingdom, recorded 500 surrogacy births in the United Kingdom as of 2005, and an estimated 350 children have reportedly been born through surrogacy arrangements in Israel as of this writing. It is currently estimated that hundreds of surrogacies are underway in India as well (Gentlemen, "India Nurtures Business").

5. The Society of Assisted Reproductive Technology has reported an increase of 28 percent in surrogacy births in the past five years. Some of the celebrities who have had children with the help of surrogates in recent years include Dennis Quaid, Joan Lunden, Art Garfunkel, Cheryl Tiegs, Angela Bassett, Kelsey Grammer, and Michael Jackson.

6. On ethics, see Anton van Niekerk and Liezl van Zyl, "The Ethics of Surrogacy: Women's Reproductive Labour," *Journal of Medical Ethics* 21 (1995): 345–49, and Rosalie Ber, "Ethical Issues in Gestational Surrogacy," *Theoretical Medicine and Bioethics* 21, no. 2 (2000): 153–69. On radical feminist contentions regarding surrogacy, see Gena Corea, *The Mother Machine: Reproductive Technologies from Artificial Insemination to Artificial Wombs* (New York: Harper & Row, 1985); Dion Farquhar, *The Other Machine: Discourse and Reproductive Technologies* (New York: Routledge, 1996); and Barbara Katz Rothman, *Recreating Motherhood* (New Brunswick, NJ: Rutgers University Press, 2000).

7. Ethnographic exploration of women's reproductive experiences now extends to the study of pregnancy (Lucy Bailey, "Gender Shows: First-Time Mothers and Embodied Selves," *Gender & Society* 15, no. 1 [2001]: 110–29; Sarah Earle, "Bumps and Boobs: Fatness and Women's Experiences of Pregnancy," *Women's Studies International Forum* 26, no. 3 [2003]: 245–52; Tsipy Ivry, *Embodying Culture: Pregnancy in Japan and Israel* [New Brunswick, NJ: Rutgers University Press, 2009]), hospital birth (Robbie Davis-Floyd, *Birth as an American Rite of Passage* [Berkeley: University of California Press, 2003]; Brigitte Jordan, "Authoritative Knowledge and Its Construction," in *Childbirth and Authoritative Knowledge: Cross-Cultural Perspectives*, ed. R. Davis-Floyd

and C.F. Sargent, 55–79 [Berkeley: University of California Press, 1997]; Emily Martin, *The Woman in the Body: A Cultural Analysis of Reproduction* [Boston: Beacon Press, 2001]), home birth (Pamela E. Klassen, *Blessed Events: Religion and Home Birth in America* [Princeton, NJ: Princeton University Press, 2001]), pregnancy loss (Linda L. Layne, *Motherhood Lost: A Feminist Account of Pregnancy Loss in America* [New York: Routledge, 2003]), abortion (Faye D. Ginsburg, *Contested Lives: The Abortion Debate in an American Community* [Berkeley: University of California Press, 1989]), amniocentesis (Rayna Rapp, *Testing Women, Testing the Fetus: The Social Impact of Amniocentesis in America* [New York: Routledge, 1999]), ultrasound (Jan Draper, "'It Was a Real Good Show': The Ultrasound Scan, Fathers and the Power of Visual Knowledge," *Sociology of Health & Illness* 24, no. 6 (2002): 771–95; Lisa Mitchell and Eugenia Georges, "Baby's First Picture: The Cyborg Foetus of Ultrasound Imaging," in *Cyborg Babies, from Techno-Sex to Techno-Tots,* ed. R. Davis-Floyd and J. Dumit, 105–24 [New York: Routledge, 1998]; Margarete Sandelowski, "Separate, but Less Unequal: Fetal Ultrasonography and the Transformation of Expectant Mother/Fatherhood," *Gender and Society* 8, no. 2 (1994): 230–45; Janelle S. Taylor, "Image of Contradiction: Obstetrical Ultrasound in American Culture," in *Reproducing Reproduction: Kinship, Power, and Technological Innovation,* ed. S. Franklin and H. Ragoné, 15–45 [Philadelphia: University of Pennsylvania Press, 1998]), adoption (Christine Ward Gailey, "Ideologies of Motherhood and Kinship in U.S. Adoption," in *Ideologies and Technologies of Motherhood: Race, Class, Sexuality, Nationalism,* ed. H. Ragoné and F.W. Twine, 11–55 [New York: Routledge, 2000]; Judith Modell, *Kinship with Strangers: Adoption and Interpretations of Kinship in American Culture* [Berkeley: University of California Press, 1994]), midwifery (Robbie E. Davis-Floyd and Elizabeth Davis, "Intuition as Authoritative Knowledge in Midwifery and Home Birth," in *Childbirth and Authoritative Knowledge: Cross-Cultural Perspectives,* ed. R.E. Davis-Floyd and C.F. Sargent, 315–49 [Berkeley: University of California Press, 1997]), and infertility (Gay Becker, *The Elusive Embryo: How Women and Men Approach New Reproductive Technologies* [Berkeley: University of California Press, 2000]; Sarah Franklin, *Embodied Progress: A Cultural Account of Assisted Conception* [London: Routledge, 1997]; Marcia Claire Inhorn and Frank van Balen, *Infertility around the Globe: New Thinking on Childlessness, Gender, and Reproductive Technologies* [Berkeley: University of California Press, 2002]), among other topics.

8. Ragoné's ethnography of surrogacy arrangements in the United States in the late 1980s and early 1990s (*Surrogate Motherhood: Conception in the Heart* [Boulder, CO: Westview Press, 1994]) looked at arrangements in which the surrogate was inseminated with the intended father's sperm. The surrogate was both the genetic and the birth mother of the baby she relinquished. Improvements in in vitro fertilization (IVF) technology have sharply changed the face of surrogacy such that, in approximately 95 percent of contemporary arrangements, gestational surrogacy is preferred; that is, a fertilized ovum is implanted in the surrogate's uterus, and she gestates a baby that is not genetically linked to her. The sparse ethnographic research on gestational surrogacy includes Ragoné's analysis of racial and ethnic relations in gestational surrogacy ("Of Likeness and

Difference: How Race Is Being Transfigured by Gestational Surrogacy," in *Ide-ologies and Technologies of Motherhood*), Elizabeth F.S. Roberts's accounts of the experiences of surrogates in California in the early 1990s ("Examining Sur-rogacy Discourses: Between Feminine Power and Exploitation," in *Small Wars: The Cultural Politics of Childhood*, ed. N. Scheper-Hughes and C.F. Sargent, 93–110 [Los Angeles: University of California Press, 1998]; "Native Narratives of Connectedness: Surrogate Motherhood and Technology," in *Cyborg Babies*, 193–211), Gillian M. Goslinga-Roy's study of a specific surrogacy arrangement, which she documented both in film and in writing ("Body Boundaries, Fictions of the Female Self: An Ethnographic Perspective on Power, Feminism and the Reproductive Technologies," *Feminist Studies* 26, no. 1 [2000]: 113–40), and Charis Thompson's study of the techniques used by participants in various forms of surrogacy and egg donation arrangements (*Making Parents: The Ontologi-cal Choreography of Reproductive Technologies* [Cambridge, MA: MIT Press, 2005]). See also my published works on surrogate mothers in Israel (Elly Teman, "Technological Fragmentation and Women's Empowerment: Surrogate Moth-erhood in Israel," *Women's Studies Quarterly* 31, nos. 3&4 [2001]: 11–34; "'Knowing' the Surrogate Body in Israel," in *Surrogate Motherhood: Interna-tional Perspectives*, ed. R. Cook, S.D. Sclater, and F. Kaganas, 261–81 [Oxford, UK: Hart Press, 2003]; "The Medicalization of 'Nature' in the 'Artificial Body': Surrogate Motherhood in Israel," *Medical Anthropology Quarterly* 17, no. 1 [2003]: 78–98; "Bonding with the Field: On Researching Surrogate Motherhood Arrangements in Israel," in *Dispatches from the Field*, ed. A. Gardner and D.M. Hoffman [Long Grove, IL: Waveland, 2006]; "The Social Construction of Surro-gacy Research: An Anthropological Critique of the Psychosocial Scholarship on Surrogate Motherhood," *Social Science and Medicine* 67, no. 7 [2008]: 1104–12; and "Embodying Surrogate Motherhood: Pregnancy as a Dyadic Body Project," *Body and Society* 15, no. 3 [2009]: 47–69).

9. See, for instance, the short item titled "Rent a Womb" on the *New York Post*'s "Page Six" gossip page (Richard Johnson, "Rent a Womb," *New York Post*, Feb. 5, 2008), which asserts that "having a baby without nasty stretch marks is all the rage among rich socialites." See also stories on surrogacy "outsourc-ing" to India in *Marie Claire* (Abigail Haworth, "Surrogate Mothers: Womb for Rent," *Marie Claire*, August 2007) and *The New York Times* (Gentlemen, "India Nurtures Business").

10. The most prevalent reasons for turning to surrogacy reported in the lit-erature are infertility; hysterectomy due to cancer, preceded by the freezing of embryos for surrogacy; damage to the uterus caused by complications during childbirth, miscarriage, or pregnancy termination; Mayer Rokitansky Kuster Hauser (MRKH) syndrome, a condition in which a woman is born without a uterus but often with intact ovaries; inborn uterus malfunction (diethylstil-bestrol, or DES) exposure; intersex spectrum abnormalities; and heart, blood, or immunological conditions endangered by pregnancy (e.g., R. Al-Nasser et al., "Factors Influencing Success in Gestational Surrogacy," *Fertility and Ste-rility* 86, no. 2 [2006]: 132–33). These reasons are consistent with data col-lected by the leading Israeli surrogacy agency based on 100 agreements. In the agency's sample, the intended mothers turned to surrogacy for the following

reasons: female infertility, 36 percent; MRKH syndrome (congenital absence of the uterus), 23 percent; severe health problems endangered by pregnancy, 19 percent; hysterectomy following cancer, 14 percent; hysterectomy after complications from childbirth, 5 percent; and DES, 3 percent. These statistics closely mirror the reasons my informants turned to surrogacy. In the past two years, the same surrogacy center reported an increase in the number of intended mothers with health problems endangered by pregnancy and a decrease in the number of applicants with MRKH syndrome.

11. For a discussion on the effect of media coverage on surrogacy from the 1980s through the early 2000s, see Susan Markens, *Surrogate Motherhood and the Politics of Reproduction* (Berkeley: University of California Press, 2007). Markens also discusses the impact of the media frenzy surrounding the Baby M case on popular opinions about surrogacy. Some of the journalistic coverage of surrogacy has prompted public comments posted online in response, numbering in the hundreds in the case of some of the articles. For instance, Warner's opinion piece in *The New York Times* addressing surrogacy in India ("Womb for Rent") garnered more than 200 public comments in response, representing a full spectrum of opinions on the subject. Kuczynski's controversial personal account of her experiences as an intended mother ("Her Body, My Baby") produced an even more heated online debate in the 400 talkbacks posted in response to her article. Thriller films such as *Final Vendetta* (1996) depict psychologically disturbed surrogate mothers with ulterior motives who terrorize their contracting couples. Dramatic films such as *The Surrogate* (1995) depict the surrogate reneging on the contract, and the recent box office hit *Baby Mama* (2008) portrays a surrogate lying to and fooling the intended mother.

12. See Gentlemen, "India Nurtures Business"; Warner, "Outsourced Wombs"; Ali and Kelley, "Womb for Rent."

13. For a full anthropological critique of the psychosocial studies on surrogacy, see Teman, "The Social Construction of Surrogacy Research."

14. Joan Einwohner ("Who Becomes a Surrogate: Personality Characteristics," in *Gender in Transition: A New Frontier,* ed. J. Offerman-Zuckerberg, 123–33 [New York: Plenum Medical Book Company, 1989]), for instance, found the surrogates in her study to be "intelligent, self-aware, stable adults." Far from psychopathological, Einwohner described surrogates as "down to earth, practical, decent people," who were "optimistic" and "not worriers." H. Baslington ("The Social Organization of Surrogacy: Relinquishing a Baby and the Role of Payment in the Psychological Detachment Process," *Journal of Health Psychology* 7, no. 1 [2002]: 57–71) deemed the surrogates she studied "assertive" and "in control." Betsy Aigen ("Motivations of Surrogate Mothers: Parenthood, Altruism and Self-Actualization," The American Surrogacy Center, 1996, http:// www.surrogacy.com/psychres/article/motivat.html) concluded that the surrogates in her study were "average mothers" and "as 'normal' as anyone else." Hilary Hanafin ("The Surrogate Mother: An Exploratory Study," [PhD diss., California School of Professional Psychology, 1984]) and Ragoné (*Surrogate Motherhood*) both found the majority of surrogates they encountered to be conservative women who subscribed to conventional beliefs about sex roles and motherhood.

15. Lori Andrews (*The Clone Age* [New York: Henry Holt, 1999]) estimates that less than 1 percent of surrogates have changes heart, while others suggest figures as low as 0.25 percent (Chris Taylor, "One Baby Too Many," *Time*, August 27, 2001, http://www.time.com/time/magazine/article/0,9171,1000632,00.html) and 0.1 percent (Keen, "Surrogate Relishes Unique Role"). The British COTS organization estimates that 98 percent of the arrangements in Britain involving their members have "reached successful conclusions" (Childlessness Overcome through Surrogacy (COTS) website, http://www.surrogacy.org.uk). In Israel there has yet to be a case of nonrelinquishment.

16. Janice C. Ciccarelli and Linda J. Beckman, "Navigating Rough Waters: An Overview of Psychological Aspects of Surrogacy," *Journal of Social Issues* 61, no. 1 [2005]: 21–43; Teman, "The Social Construction of Surrogacy Research"; Olga van den Akker, "Psychological Aspects of Surrogate Motherhood," *Human Reproduction* 13, no. 1 (2007): 53–62.

17. Thompson, *Making Parents.*

18. Ragoné (*Surrogate Motherhood*), for instance, mentions in her ethnography of U.S. surrogacy arrangements in the late 1980s and early 1990s that distance and funding limitations forced her to interview many of her informants by phone. Goslinga-Roy ("Body Boundaries") chose to follow only one surrogate-couple triad through their entire surrogacy experience.

19. For discussion of the Jewish-Israeli cult of fertility and discussion of motherhood as a "national mission," see Nitza Berkovitch, "Motherhood as a National Mission: The Construction of Womanhood in the Legal Discourse in Israel," *Women's Studies International Forum* 20, nos. 5–6 (1997): 605–19; Tamar Rapoport and Tamar El-Or, "Cultures of Womanhood in Israel: Social Agencies and Gender Production," *Women's Studies International Forum* 20, nos. 5–6 (1997): 573–80; and Susan Starr Sered, *What Makes Women Sick: Maternity, Modesty and Militarism in Israeli Society* (Hanover, NH: Brandeis University Press: University Press of New England, 2000). On the social repercussions of the local ideology of motherhood, see Delila Amir and Orly Benjamin, "Defining Encounters: Who Are the Women Entitled to Join the Israeli Collective?" *Women's Studies International Forum* 20, nos. 5–6 (1997): 639–50; Orly Benjamin and Hila Ha'elyon, "Rewriting Fertilization: Trust, Pain, and Exit Points," *Women's Studies International Forum* 25, no. 6 (2002): 667–78; and Larissa Remennick, "Childless in the Land of Imperative Motherhood: Stigma and Coping among Infertile Israeli Women," *Sex Roles* 43, nos. 11/12 (2000): 821–41. See Rhoda Ann Kanaaneh, *Birthing the Nation: Strategies of Palestinian Women in Israel* (Berkeley: University of California Press, 2002), for further discussion of Israeli prenatal politics from the perspective of the Arab minority in Israel. See Susan Martha Kahn, *Reproducing Jews: A Cultural Account of Assisted Conception in Israel* (Durham, NC: Duke University Press, 2000), and Yael Hashiloni-Dolev, *A Life (Un)Worthy of Living: Reproductive Genetics in Israel and Germany* (Dordrecht, Netherlands: Springer, 2007), for further discussion of the influence of Jewish law on Israeli politics of reproduction. See Leslie King, "Demographic Trends, Pronatalism, and Nationalist Ideologies in the Late Twentieth Century," *Ethnic and Racial Studies* 25, no. 3 (2002): 367–89, and Gail Kligman, *The Politics of Duplicity: Controlling Reproduction*

in Ceausescu's Romania (Berkeley: University of California Press, 1998), for discussions of pronatalism, more generally; for discussions of Israeli pronatalism, see Helene Goldberg, "The Man in the Sperm" (master's thesis, University of Copenhagen, 2002), and Nira Yuval Davis, "National Reproduction and 'the Demographic Race' in Israel," in *Woman-Nation-State,* ed. N. Yuval Davis and F. Anthias, 92–109 (London: The Macmillan Press, 1989). See Ivry, *Embodying Culture,* for further discussion of Israeli prenatal politics and for her critique of applying the pronatalist label to Israeli reproductive ideologies. See Orna Donath, "Cracks in Pro-Natalism: Choosing a Childfree Life-Style in Israel" (master's thesis, Tel Aviv University, 2007), for a discussion of the experiences of those who choose not to have children in Israel.

20. Kahn, *Reproducing Jews.*

21. These studies were conducted in the United States and in Canada (Ciccarelli and Beckman, "Navigating Rough Waters"; P.C. Dunn, I.J. Ryan, and K. O'Brien, "College Students' Acceptance of Adoption and Five Alternative Fertilization Techniques," *The Journal of Sex Research* 24 [1988]: 282–87; R.J. Edelman, "Surrogacy: The Psychological Issues," *Journal of Reproductive and Infant Psychology* 22, no. 2 [2004]: 123–36; V. Krishnan, "Attitudes toward Surrogate Motherhood in Canada," *Health Care for Women International* 15 [1994]: 333–57; G. Wiess, "Public Attitudes about Surrogate Motherhood," *Michigan Sociological Review* 6 [1992]: 15–27). Similar studies have been conducted to assess attitudes toward surrogacy in Turkey (Baris Bayskal et al., "Opinions of Infertile Turkish Women on Gamete Donation and Gestational Surrogacy," *Fertility and Sterility* 89, no. 4 [2008]: 817–22) and Japan (Kohta Suzuk et al., "Analysis of National Representative Opinion Surveys Concerning Gestational Surrogacy in Japan," *European Journal of Obstetrics and Gynecology* 126, no. 1 [2006]: 39–47) showing low rates of public approval of the practice, even among infertile women. See also note 11.

22. Robbie Davis-Floyd, "The Role of American Obstetrics in the Resolution of Cultural Anomaly," *Social Science and Medicine* 31 (1990): 175–89.

23. Mary Douglas, *Natural Symbols: Explorations in Cosmology* (London: Routledge, 2003).

24. Douglas, *Implicit Meanings: Selected Essays in Anthropology* (London: Routledge, 1999), 257.

25. Davis-Floyd, "Cultural Anomaly."

26. Susan Markens, *Surrogate Motherhood and the Politics of Reproduction* (Berkeley: University of California Press, 2007).

27. David Murray Schneider, *American Kinship: A Cultural Account* (Englewood Cliffs, NJ: Prentice-Hall, 1968).

28. Radhika Rao, "Surrogacy Law in the United States: The Outcome of Ambivalence," in *Surrogate Motherhood: International Perspectives,* ed. R. Cook, S.D. Sclater, and F. Kaganas, 23–35 (Oxford, UK: Hart Press, 2003).

29. Donna Haraway, "The Promises of Monsters: A Regenerative Politics for Inappropriate Others," in *Cultural Studies,* ed. L. Grossberg, C. Nelson, and P. Treichler, 295–337 (New York: Routledge, 1992), 296.

30. Sarah Franklin, Celia Lury, and Jackie Stacey, *Global Nature, Global Culture* (London: Sage, 2000), 21.

31. Sylvia Junko Yanagisako, Carol Lowery Delaney, and American Anthropological Association Meeting, *Naturalizing Power: Essays in Feminist Cultural Analysis* (New York: Routledge, 1995).

32. Davis-Floyd, *Birth as an American Rite of Passage*.

33. Marilyn Strathern, *Reproducing the Future: Anthropology, Kinship and the New Reproductive Technologies* (New York: Routledge, 1992).

34. Emily Martin, "Body Narratives, Body Boundaries," in *Cultural Studies*, ed. L. Grossberg, C. Nelson, and P. A. Treichler, 409–19 (New York: Routledge, 1992), and "The End of the Body?" *American* Ethnologist 19 (1992): 121–38.

35. "Introduction," in *Surrogate Motherhood: International Perspectives*, ed. R. Cook, S. D. Sclater, and F. Kaganas, 1–22 (Oxford, UK: Hart Publishing, 2003), 2.

36. Cook et al., "Introduction."

37. Markens, *Surrogate Motherhood and the Politics of Reproduction*.

38. Lori B. Andrews, *Between Strangers: Surrogate Mothers, Expectant Fathers, and Brave New Babies* (New York: Harper & Row, 1989); Markens, *Surrogate Motherhood and the Politics of Reproduction;* Weisberg, *The Birth of Surrogacy in Israel*, 215.

39. Brenda M. Baker, "A Case for Permitting Altruistic Surrogacy," *Hypatia* 11, no. 2 (1996): 34–48.

40. Emily Jackson, *Regulating Reproduction: Law, Technology, and Autonomy* (Oxford, UK: Hart Publishing, 2001), 262. Cited in Cook et al., "Introduction," 2.

41. Surrogacy is banned in Austria, China, the Czech Republic, Denmark, Egypt, France, Germany, Italy, Jordan, Mexico, Norway, Poland, Portugal, Saudi Arabia, Singapore, Spain, Sweden, Switzerland, Taiwan, Turkey, and some U.S. states. See Cook et al., "Introduction."

42. Debora L. Spar, *The Baby Business: How Money, Science and Politics Drive the Commerce of Conception* (Boston: Harvard Business School Press, 2006), 94; Weisberg, *The Birth of Surrogacy in Israel*, 203.

43. Weisberg, *The Birth of Surrogacy in Israel*.

44. Markens, *Surrogate Motherhood and the Politics of Reproduction*.

45. Spar, *The Baby Business*, 85.

46. Weisberg, *The Birth of Surrogacy in Israel*, 203.

47. *Anna Johnson v. Mark and Crispina Calvert*, California Supreme Court, 5 Cal. 4th 84, 1993.

48. Spar, *The Baby Business*, 86.

49. The recent growth of international surrogacy arrangements in India has become a popular news item in the print and television media; Oprah Winfrey's talk show even devoted an episode to it. Without any regulation, surrogacy clinics have popped up across India. Several press items have suggested that the Indian government is preparing legislation to regulate surrogacy, which may curtail the further development of the practice (see "India Looks to New Laws to Regulate Rent-a-Womb Baby Trade," *FoxNews.com,* March 15, 2008, http://www.foxnews.com/story/0,2933,338139,00.html; Sumit Pande, "Govt Plans New Laws to Curb Rent-a-Womb Rackets," *IBNLive.com,* November 5, 2007, http://ibnlive.in.com/videos/51753/govt-plans-new-lows-to-curb-rentawomb-

rackets.html). For recent ethnographic work on a surrogacy clinic in Anand, India, see Amrita Pande, "'At Least I Am Not Sleeping with Anyone': 'Dirty' Surrogates in India," *Feminist Studies* (forthcoming), and Kalindi Vora, "Indian Transnational Surrogacy and the Commodification of Vital Energy," *Subjectivity* 26, no. 2 (forthcoming).

50. Davis-Floyd, "Cultural Anomaly."

51. See Markens, *Surrogate Motherhood and the Politics of Reproduction.*

52. For a full discussion of the history and workings of the U.S. surrogate market, see Spar, *The Baby Business.*

53. Most of the American surrogacy agency directors I have spoken to estimated that 10–30 percent of their clientele was made up of international couples.

54. Franklin, *Embodied Progress,* 86.

55. Cook et al., "Introduction."

56. See, for example, Katy Hastings, "Surrogate Mother Prepares for Eighth Baby," Telegraph.co.uk., http://www.telegraph.co.uk, Jan. 21, 2008.

57. *The Birth of Surrogacy in Israel,* 4.

58. For further discussion of Israel's "liberal" legislation on reproductive technologies, see Daphna Birenbaum-Carmeli, "'Cheaper Than a Newcomer': On the Social Production of IVF Policy in Israel," *Sociology of Health & Illness* 26, no. 7 (2004): 897–924; Barbara Prainsack, "Negotiating Life: The Regulation of Human Cloning and Embryonic Stem Cell Research in Israel," *Social Studies of Science* 36, no. 2 (2006): 173–205; Teman, "The Last Outpost of the Nuclear Family: A Cultural Critique of Israeli Surrogacy Policy," in *Kin, Gene, Community: Reproductive Technology among Jewish Israelis,* ed. D. Birenbaum-Carmeli and Y. Carmeli (Oxford, UK: Berghahn Books, forthcoming).

59. Teman, "The Last Outpost."

60. Kahn, *Reproducing Jews.*

61. A handful of surrogacy agreements have been signed between immigrants to Israel from the former Soviet Union who were unable to officially qualify as Jews for the purposes of surrogacy, sometimes even after contesting their disqualification in rabbinical courts. As a result, they applied to the surrogacy committee as Christians.

62. According to some rabbis, intrafamilial surrogacy could transgress the religious prohibition on incest by way of a sister hypothetically gestating an embryo created from her brother's sperm. The directive that surrogates must be single, divorced, or widowed relates to issues of adultery and bastardy. Under Jewish law, bastardy can be caused by a married woman becoming impregnated through adulterous relations with a married man. Some rabbis would interpret a married surrogate's gestation of an egg fertilized by a man who is not her husband as adulterous. See Kahn, *Reproducing Jews,* for further explanations of these issues in Jewish law.

63. Other reproductive technologies are generally regulated in Israel with a "liberal hand" (Birenbaum-Carmeli, "'Cheaper Than a Newcomer'") and are subsidized by Israeli national health insurance. Reproductive technologies such as IVF, artificial insemination, and IVF with donated egg and/or sperm are available in Israel to persons of any marital status and sexual preference, merely at the discretion of the medical professionals who administer them. As a measure

of this liberal hand, reproductive technologies that are seen as extremely controversial in other countries are permitted under certain conditions in Israel. These
technologies include stem cell research, preimplantation genetic diagnosis, sex
selection of embryos, and even practices that border on cloning, such as the
transfer of the nucleus from the egg of an infertile woman into the mitochondria
and shell of another woman's egg. Israeli courts have given permission for other
controversial reproductive-related practices, for example, allowing a divorcee
to use embryos created with her ex-husband's sperm despite his refusal (see
D. Kelly Weisberg, *The Birth of Surrogacy in Israel* [Gainesville, FL: University
Press of Florida, 2005]). Formal regulations even allow a bereaved widow to
ask for the removal of sperm from her husband's body immediately after death
(Judy Siegel-Itzkovich, "Israel Allows Removal of Sperm from Dead Men at
Wives' Request," *British Medical Journal* 327, no. 7425 [2003]: 1187), and the
parliament has debated giving parents of combat soldiers the same option to
produce grandchildren posthumously from their dead son's sperm.

64. A single woman wishing to hire a surrogate contested this limitation
of the Israeli Surrogacy Law and lost the case in Israel's highest court in 2002.
Ironically, this means that single women are the only group allowed to become
surrogates in Israel, but they cannot hire surrogates themselves. It also means
that the gay male community in Israel has no access to creating families through
surrogacy within their own country at a time when this community is showing a
growing demand for the practice as a family-building option. As a result, dozens
of gay male couples from Israel have traveled to the United States and India in
recent years to hire surrogates, and some U.S. agencies even market their services to this particular clientele in Israel.

65. Teman, "The Last Outpost."

66. *The Birth of Surrogacy in Israel.*

67. *Reproducing Jews.*

68. Teman, "The Last Outpost."

69. *Surrogate Motherhood and the Politics of Reproduction.*

70. At the time my study began, the majority of couples and surrogates
found one another independent of a matching agency; by 2005, when my fieldwork ended, roughly half used an agency. Today, a sharp rise in the number of
couples pursuing surrogacy—largely because of increased public awareness—
has led the majority of couples to use an agency. The growth in the number
of interested couples has led to a shortage of surrogates who can comply with
the state's restrictive measures for compatibility; many couples thus turn to
an agency because they are unsuccessful in finding a surrogate on their own.
Whereas the leading Israeli agency could once promise a couple that they would
be introduced to a surrogate within six months, the timeline has now shifted to
eight months. While U.S. surrogacy has historically revolved around agencies, it
is estimated that the number of independent surrogacy arrangements is rapidly
growing in the U.S. because of the many Internet sites through which potential
surrogates and parents can now meet.

71. Olga van den Akker, "Organizational Selection and Assessment of
Women Entering a Surrogacy Agreement in the UK," *Human Reproduction* 14,
no. 1 (1999): 262–66.

72. Hastings, "Surrogate Mother Prepares for Eighth Baby."

73. State subsidization of IVF treatment in Israel enables women to afford repeat IVF attempts.

74. Gentlemen, "India Nurtures Business."

75. *The Birth of Surrogacy in Israel.*

76. Ragoné (*Surrogate Motherhood*) and Roberts ("Examining Surrogacy Discourses") were able to contact potential interviewees through U.S. surrogacy agencies. Psychological researchers in the United Kingdom have also been able to contact study participants through the nonprofit COTS organization. Although several agencies appeared in Israel during the years of this research, most agencies disappeared after facilitating only one or two surrogacy agreements. The major surrogacy agency today opened in 2002.

77. The multiple legal sources I gathered included documents and protocols related to court cases, the Aloni commission report, protocols of the Israeli government debates on the law, the text of the law, and the application forms and instructions distributed by the surrogacy approvals committee. I have analyzed these data separately in a cultural critique of the Israeli surrogacy law (Teman, "The Last Outpost").

78. I collected more than 200 newspaper articles and magazine articles from Israeli publications that encompass close to all of the coverage of the surrogacy phenomenon in the Israeli print media from 1990 to 2004. I also took notes on and, when possible, recorded documentary films, interviews, and debates about surrogacy on Israeli television and radio. I used media interviews with lawmakers and other public figures, doctors, surrogates, intended parents, and women who want to become surrogates as supplementary data to the interviews that I conducted.

79. Most interviews lasted an average of two hours, although some lasted up to six. The majority of interviews were recorded and then transcribed verbatim, then translated from Hebrew to English. The few interviews that were not tape-recorded were transcribed by me during the interview. Three interviews (all follow-up interviews) were done with surrogates by telephone, and thirteen interviews (mostly follow-up interviews) with intended mothers were conducted by phone. Typically, the interviews took a narrative form in response to the request to "tell your surrogacy story from wherever it begins." Afterward, I would ask specific questions that had not been covered in the narrative. Such questions dealt with the women's experience with the surrogacy committee, their feelings toward the fetus during pregnancy, their thoughts about their bodies during surrogacy, their relationships with their partners during the process, and their experiences in the period immediately following the birth. I interviewed all but one of the informants myself. Liron Meir, a student in a course that I tutored at Hebrew University, interviewed one intended mother. I instructed Liron in how to conduct the interview. I also attended a four-hour lecture by the same intended mother in which she told her personal story.

80. I was able to follow the progression of ten surrogates from the beginning of the process and three surrogates from their fifth month of gestation. I followed the progression of thirteen intended mothers from the beginning of the process and two intended mothers from the fifth month onward. I maintained

regular contact with the women by phone to get updates and to schedule follow-up interviews with some. I also corresponded with informants by e-mail, read their postings on Internet message boards, and met them at surrogacy support group meetings and at various gatherings. In several cases, I was able to visit the parties in the hospital after the birth and attend baby naming and circumcision ceremonies.

81. Early on in my research, I had hoped to focus on both members of the couple and not exclusively on intended mothers. However, intended mothers were hesitant to have me interview their husbands, and contacting these men directly without their wives' mediation was nearly impossible. As my research progressed, I learned that the majority of surrogacy cases involve the two women in an intense relationship that, by and large, excludes the intended father. For these reasons, my study focuses primarily on the surrogate and intended mother.

82. All forum members were aware that I was an anthropologist studying surrogacy. Created by an intended mother during the early months of her surrogate's pregnancy and still led by her, the forum has approximately twenty active members at any given time, although hundreds of women have posted messages since its inception. The forum is populated by women, roughly half surrogates and half intended mothers, although the presence of the latter is increasing. There are no active male participants. Access to the forum does not seem to be dependent on the members' financial situation but on their technical competency and interest. Members tend to stop active participation in the forum after completing the surrogacy process, and newcomers then take their place as active participants. In their online exchanges, the women write in Hebrew, relaying their personal stories and providing information, advice, and encouragement to one another. Exchanges usually include messages seeking and conveying information and advice on different stages of the process, as well as updates on successful and failed treatments. In addition to these online exchanges, members of the forum meet in person for parties roughly three to four times a year. I have participated in most of these gatherings, which usually include around thirty to fifty individuals, roughly half surrogates and half couples.

83. The support group, initiated by the owner of the leading surrogacy agency in Israel, was formed through the combined efforts of the agency director, myself, and a social psychologist who specializes in "life coaching" and assertiveness training. The monthly meetings, which take place at the agency offices, include ten to twenty surrogates at various stages of the process. Any given meeting includes surrogates who have not yet passed the psychological evaluation, those who have just been approved by the committee and are beginning medical treatment, those who have been through one to six failed attempts, those who are pregnant, and those who completed the process up to two years before. Surrogates who are not contracted through the agency also sometimes attend the meetings. All participants were informed at the beginning of each meeting of my anthropologist role. I did not tape-record the meetings or take active notes during sessions, but I did record field notes after the meetings adjourned.

84. See Ilanit Hayut, "A Womb for Rent or a Good Solution? [*Rehem Lehaskir O' Pitaron Savir*]," *Haaretz Daily,* October 29, 2001, pp. 1, 16); Ruti

Kadosh, "She Is Me and I Am Her: We Are One Body [*He Zo Ani V'ani Zo Hi: Anachnu Guf Echad*]," *Ma'ariv,* July 23, 2001; Siegel-Itzkovich, "Surrogacy: Bearing the Greatest Gift of All," *The Jerusalem Post,* May 27, 2001, p. 17; and Tamara Traubman, "The Surrogates Are Giving Birth Again; The Families Are Having a Second Surrogate Child [*Hapundekaiot Yoldot Ba'shenit, Hamishpachot Kvar Osot Yeled Pundekaut Sheni*]." *Haaretz Daily,* May 25, 2004.

85. Davydd Greenwood and Morten Levin, *Introduction to Action Research* (London: Sage, 1998).

86. Statistical information about Israeli surrogacy births is difficult to come by because no official follow-up by the state has yet been undertaken. In July 2005, the current secretary of the approvals committee informed me that, of 280 applications reviewed by the committee, 230 had been approved. The approvals committee secretary noted that there were no formal statistics on surrogacy births, but she estimated that more than 100 children had been born, and she personally had been informed of the births of 18 sets of twins and one set of triplets. From my estimate, these numbers are much lower than the number of actual births.

87. Critics of the term argue that it ascribes substitute status to the wrong woman and suggest that it is the woman who will raise the child who is the substitute or surrogate for the "real" birth mother (see, e.g., Rita Arditti, Renate Klein, and Shelley Minden, *Test-Tube Women: What Future for Motherhood?* [London: Pandora Press, 1984]; Rothman, *Recreating Motherhood;* Michelle Stanworth, "Reproductive Technologies and the Deconstruction of Motherhood," in *Reproductive Technologies: Gender, Motherhood and Medicine,* ed. M. Stanworth, 10–35 [Cambridge, UK: Polity Press, 1987]). The term is derived from research on nonhuman primates, in which terry cloth dolls have been used as surrogate mothers for young monkeys. The inanimate nature of the surrogate in that research has meant that applying the term to women may be seen as objectifying them and reducing them to their reproductive capabilities. It is also argued that the terminology suggests that the woman who is contracted to birth the child is "somehow less than a mother," and that demoting her to the position of a substitute or stand-in for the "real" mother disparages her efforts. Still others have argued that both the woman who will raise the child and the woman who gives birth are surrogates, because each woman contributes to the continued development of the child, but neither nurtures the child continuously from conception to adulthood.

88. There are two primary definitions of the word *pundekaut.* The first is connected to *pundekai,* a term used in biology to refer to a plant or living organism that carries a parasite or leech (Yossi Ziv, "Surrogacy, the Right to Parenthood and Ethics [*Pundekaut, Hazchut Lehorut v'Musar*]," *Galileo* [magazine], March/April 1997). The second meaning is traced to the word *pundak,* which comes from the Greek *pandokeion,* the Arabic *funduk,* and the Mishnaic Hebrew *pundaki* and refers to a small guesthouse or wayside inn. The female owner of the small *pundak* in Mishnaic texts was the *pundakit*—the innkeeper—who, in Modern Hebrew, has become *pundekait* (Ruth Almagor-Ramon, "Pundak," *A Moment of Hebrew [Rega Shel Ivrit],* Reshet Bet radio station, October 10, 2001). Both terms connote the idea of the surrogate as

carrier or *host* of the pregnancy. The practice was described in terms similar to the English idiom during the 1980s: the surrogate was called a *substitute mother* [*em tachlifit*]. Although no formal documentation of the evolution of the coinage into its current form could be found, Professor Pinhas Shifman of the Hebrew University law faculty, who was one of the earliest Israeli academics to write about surrogacy, told me that he had been "the first person to use that term. It seemed much more fitting."

89. The terminology has received its fair share of criticism. Israeli journalist Yossi Ziv ("Surrogacy") has argued that the word *pundak* evokes images of a place where persons visit for a short period as paying guests, after which they return to their homes. He stresses that guests do not usually form or maintain any uniquely close relationships with the owner of the *pundak*. Rather, they receive services such as room and board from the innkeeper, and both parties go their separate ways without having left any lasting physical or emotional impressions on one another. Ziv argues that the woman who bears a child should be considered the child's mother, and that the term *pundekait* reduces the role of the surrogate to that of providing guest services for the fetus.

90. When I asked surrogates if they had any objections to the terms *surrogate* and *innkeeper*, several commented that what found problematic was being referred to as an "innkeeper mother" [*em pundekait*], because they did not see themselves as an *em*—a mother—at all. In fact, nearly all surrogates referred to themselves simply as the "innkeeper" [*ha'pundekait*] and to their intended mother as the "biological mother" [*ha'em habiyologit*], the "genetic mother" [*ha'em hagenetit*], or simply "the mother" [*ha'ima*].

91. The sociodemographic characteristics that I discuss here refer to the majority of women interviewed for this study. Three intended mothers did surrogacy in California with non-Jewish, American surrogates, and one surrogate–intended mother pair consisted of sisters who did traditional surrogacy. Traditional surrogacy was possible in this case because both were British citizens and because the birth took place in England and did not go through the Israeli legal system.

92. Ragoné, *Surrogate Motherhood*; Roberts, "Examining Surrogacy Discourses."

93. Ragoné, *Surrogate Motherhood*.

94. The surrogacy approvals committee originally allowed women to become surrogates up to age forty; in 2003, the age limit was lowered to thirty-eight.

95. In terms of religiosity, most surrogates and couples ranged somewhere between secular and traditional. Among this majority, three couples were secular to the point of being antireligious. None of the surrogates I interviewed were ultra-Orthodox, and only one of the intended mothers I formally interviewed was ultra-Orthodox, although I have had long conversations and interactions with several other ultra-Orthodox women who had children through surrogacy. Three surrogates and three couples were modern Orthodox.

96. In the wake of cases in which surrogates blackmailed their intended parents, the surrogacy approvals committee has largely denied the applications of completely destitute women to serve as surrogates.

97. Spar, *The Baby Business*.

98. Marcel Mauss, *The Gift: Forms and Functions of Exchange in Archaic Societies* (New York: Norton, 1967).

PART ONE

1. See, e.g., Gailey, "Ideologies of Motherhood and Kinship"; Marcia Claire Inhorn and Frank van Balen, *Infertility around the Globe: New Thinking on Childlessness, Gender, and Reproductive Technologies* (Berkeley: University of California Press, 2002); Heather Paxson, *Making Modern Mothers: Ethics and Family Planning in Urban Greece* (Berkeley: University of California Press, 2005).

2. See Teman, "The Social Construction of Surrogacy Research."

3. Hanafin, "The Surrogate Mother"; Ragoné, *Surrogate Motherhood*.

4. Ragoné, *Surrogate Motherhood*.

5. Berkovitch, "Motherhood as a National Mission"; Rapoport and El-Or, "Cultures of Womanhood."

6. Teman, "The Medicalization of 'Nature' in the 'Artificial Body.'"

7. Teman, "The Social Construction of Surrogacy Research."

8. Christine Overall, Ethics and Human Reproduction: A Feminist Analysis (Boston: Allen and Unwin, 1987), 126–27, cited in Roberts, "Examining Surrogacy Discourses."

9. Edna Lomsky-Feder, "Patterns of Participation in War and the Construction of War in the Life Course: Life Stories of Israeli Veterans from the Yom Kippur War" (PhD diss., Hebrew University, 1994); Lesley A. Sharp, "Organ Transplantation as a Transformative Experience: Anthropological Insights into the Restructuring of the Self," Medical Anthropology Quarterly 9, no. 3 (1995): 357–89, and Strange Harvest: Organ Transplants in America (Berkeley: University of California Press, 2006).

CHAPTER ONE

1. Davis-Floyd, *Birth as an American Rite of Passage;* Martin, *The Woman in the Body.*

2. See, e.g., Arditti et al., *Test-Tube Women;* Corea, *The Mother Machine;* Farquhar, *The Other Machine;* Janice G. Raymond, *Women as Wombs: Reproductive Technologies and the Battle over Women's Freedom* (San Francisco: HarperSanFrancisco, 1993); Rothman, *Recreating Motherhood.*

3. Raymond, *Women as Wombs.*

4. Overall, *Ethics and Human Reproduction,* 126–27, cited in Roberts, "Examining Surrogacy Discourses."

5. Anthropologist Carol Lowery Delaney's work on a Turkish village (*The Seed and the Soil: Gender and Cosmology in Turkish Village Society* [Berkeley: University of California Press, 1991]) and Marcia Claire Inhorn's research on assisted conception in Egypt (*Quest for Conception: Gender, Infertility, and Egyptian Medical Traditions* [Philadelphia: University of Pennsylvania Press, 1994]) have shown how the "seed and the soil" play a central role in the cosmology and conception myths that construct the way the monotheistic peoples

in these two contexts view the world. Kahn (*Reproducing Jews*) alludes to the presence of this imagery in modern-day Israel, citing a rabbi who evokes it to recommend the appropriate use of reproductive technologies.

6. Rothman, *Recreating Motherhood*, 36.

7. Ragoné, *Surrogate Motherhood*; Roberts, "Examining Surrogacy Discourses" and "Native Narratives of Connectedness."

8. Goslinga-Roy, "Body Boundaries"; Roberts, "Native Narratives of Connectedness."

9. Gay Becker, "Metaphors in Disrupted Lives: Infertility and Cultural Constructions of Continuity," *Medical Anthropology Quarterly* 8, no. 4 (1994): 383–410; Sheryl de Lacey, "IVF as Lottery or Investment: Contesting Metaphors in Discourses of Infertility," *Nursing Inquiry* 9, no. 1 (2002): 43–51; Arthur L. Greil, "Infertile Bodies: Medicalization, Metaphor, and Agency," in *Infertility around the Globe: New Thinking on Childlessness, Gender, and Reproductive Technologies*, ed. M.C. Inhorn and F. Van Balen, 101–18 (Berkeley: University of California Press, 2002); Klassen, *Blessed Events*.

10. Laurence J. Kirmayer, "Broken Narratives: Clinical Encounters and the Poetics of Illness Experience," in *Narrative and the Cultural Construction of Illness and Healing*, ed. C. Mattingly and L.C. Garro, 153–81 (Berkeley: University of California Press, 2000).

11. Ibid.

12. Kyra Marie Landzelius, "Charged Artifacts and the Detonation of Liminality: Teddy-Bear Diplomacy in the Newborn Incubator Machine," *Journal of Material Culture* 6, no. 3 (2001): 323–44.

13. For Shahar, not only had the life of the embryos she carried started in an incubator, but the last month of pregnancy was also colored by the constant threat that the babies would be born prematurely and "finished off" in an incubator. Through determination and labor-suppressant drugs, Shahar managed to "hold on" to the fetuses long enough for their lungs to develop fully, so that they did not need an incubator, even though she spent weeks thirty-three to thirty-seven of the pregnancy hospitalized, her cervix dilated to two to three centimeters.

14. The notion of the warm womb is not universal. For instance, in Malaysia, a "cool" state is ideal for pregnancy, and pregnant women should avoid food with "heating" qualities (Laderman, quoted by Davis-Floyd and Georges 1996). In Israel, however, the notion of the warm womb is common, and it recalls the idea expressed by surrogates that they had a "warm heart" and a "warm connection" with their couple in place of a "cold, businesslike" relationship. Couples also frequently divulged to me that the most important characteristic that they had looked for in a surrogate was warmth. The repeated emphasis on the surrogate's warmth alludes to the idea that a fetus should be nurtured in warm surroundings. It also sheds light on the fear of the surrogate becoming a mere "mother machine" and of the assumed coldness of machines replacing the warmth that humanizes pregnancy.

15. For instance, a headline in an Israeli newspaper announced, "Rent the womb to feed the children" (Israel Moskovitz, "I Gave Birth to a Child for Others in Order to Feed My Children [*Yalad'ti Yeled Le'acherim Kedai Le'haachil Et Yeladai*]" *Yediot Aharonot* [newspaper], March 19, 2004).

16. Carole Counihan, *The Anthropology of Food and Body: Gender, Meaning, and Power* (New York: Routledge, 1999).

17. "Native Narratives of Connectedness."

18. Susan Bordo, *Unbearable Weight: Feminism, Western Culture, and the Body* (Berkeley: University of California Press, 1993); Earle, "Bumps and Boobs."

19. Monica Konrad, "Ova Donations and Symbols of Substance: Some Variations on the Theme of Sex, Gender, and the Partible Body," *Journal of the Royal Anthropological Institute* 4, no. 4 (1998): 643–67.

20. Although regimens may vary by doctor, most of the surrogates that I spoke to underwent similar protocols to prepare their wombs to receive the embryos. There were some exceptions; for instance, two surrogates underwent embryo implantation on a "natural" cycle without hormone preparation. However, most of the women received hormone injections, a factor that played a major role in their descriptions of the preparatory phase of the process.

21. "Interview with Orna, a Surrogate Mother," *At Eye Level* [*Be'gova Eynayim*] [radio program], prod. T. Cohen, Jerusalem, 2003.

22. Bonnie Fox and Diana Worts, "Revisiting the Critique of Medicalized Childbirth: A Contribution to the Sociology of Birth," *Gender & Society* 13, no. 3 (1999): 326–46; Greil, "Infertile Bodies"; Margaret M. Lock and Patricia A. Kaufert, *Pragmatic Women and Body Politics* (New York: Cambridge University Press, 1998); Thompson, *Making Parents*.

23. Einwohner, "Who Becomes a Surrogate"; Ragoné, *Surrogate Motherhood.*

24. Forrest D. Tierson, C.L. Olsen, and E.B. Hook, "Nausea and Vomiting of Pregnancy and Its Association with Pregnancy Outcome," *American Journal of Obstetrics and Gynecology* 160 (1989): 518–19.

25. Anne Murcott, "On the Altered Appetites of Pregnancy: Conceptions of Food, Body and Person," *Sociological Review* 36, no. 4 (1988): 733–64.

26. Rita Seiden Miller, "The Social Construction and Reconstruction of Physiological Events: Acquiring the Pregnancy Identity," *Studies in Symbolic Interaction* 1 (1978): 187.

27. Elizabeth Marie Coker, "'Traveling Pains': Embodied Metaphors of Suffering among Southern Sudanese Refugees in Cairo," *Culture, Medicine and Psychiatry* 28 (2004): 26.

28. Janice Patricia Boddy, *Wombs and Alien Spirits: Women, Men, and the Zâar Cult in Northern Sudan* (Madison: University of Wisconsin Press, 1989); Michael Lambeck, *Human Spirits: A Cultural Account of Trance in Mayotte* (Cambridge, UK: Cambridge University Press, 1981).

29. Hilary Graham, "The Social Image of Pregnancy: Pregnancy as Spirit Possession," *Sociological Review* 24, no. 2 (1976): 291–308.

30. Ragoné noted that, among gestational surrogates in the United States, race was sometimes operationalized in a precautionary role to prevent "bonding"; she observed that African-American surrogates preferred to carry the babies of Caucasian couples, because the difference in skin color served as a reminder to the surrogate of her distance from the baby (Ragoné 2000). I did not observe any similar pattern in surrogate-couple matching preferences in

Israel, although, as noted above, ethnic factors sometimes surfaced as a distancing technique.

31. See, e.g., Murcott, "Altered Appetites," 752; Tierson et al., "Nausea and Vomiting."

32. Murcott, "Altered Appetites."

33. Deborah Lupton, *Food, the Body and the Self* (London: Sage, 1996).

34. Graham, "The Social Image of Pregnancy."

35. Renee C. Fox and Judith P. Swazey, *Spare Parts: Organ Replacement in American Society* (Oxford, UK: Oxford University Press, 1992), 43.

36. Sharp, "Organ Transplantation."

37. Fox and Swazey, *Spare Parts.*

38. Judith Modell, "Last Chance Babies: Interpretations of Parenthood in an IVF Program," *Medical Anthropology Quarterly* 3 (1989): 124–38.

39. *Making Parents.*

40. Franklin, *Embodied Progress;* Modell, "Last Chance Babies"; Margarete Sandelowski, *With Child in Mind: Studies of the Personal Encounter with Infertility* (Philadelphia: University of Pennsylvania Press, 1993).

41. Prainsack, "Negotiating Life."

42. Birenbaum-Carmeli, "'Cheaper Than a Newcomer'"; Hashiloni-Dolev, *A Life (Un)Worthy of Living;* Prainsack, "Negotiating Life."

43. Prainsack, "Negotiating Life."

44. Sherry Ortner, "Is Female to Male as Nature Is to Culture?" in *Women, Culture and Society,* ed. M.Z. Rosaldo and L. Lamphere, 67–88 (Stanford, CA: Stanford University Press, 1974).

45. Lois McNay, *Foucault and Feminism* (Cambridge, UK: Polity Press, 1992), 17.

46. Bryan S. Turner, *The Body and Society* (Oxford, UK: Basil Blackwell, 1984).

47. Berkovitch, "Motherhood as a National Mission."

48. *Making Parents.*

49. Rothman, *Recreating Motherhood.*

CHAPTER TWO

1. Catherine Waldby et al., "Blood and Bioidentity: Ideas about Self, Boundaries and Risk among Blood Donors and People Living with Hepatitis C," *Social Science & Medicine* 59 (2004): 1461–71.

2. M.E. English, A. Mechanick-Braverman, and S.L. Corson, "Semantics and Science: The Distinction between Gestational Carrier and Traditional Surrogacy Options," *Women's Health Issues* 1, no. 3 (1991): 155–57.

3. Ivry, *Embodying Culture.*

4. Ragoné, *Surrogate Motherhood;* Roberts, "Examining Surrogacy Discourses."

5. Tsipy Brand, "The Real World behind the News [*Ha'olam Ha'amiti Me'achorei Hachadashot*] [television documentary program], Israel's Channel 10, December 23, 2003.

6. Janet Carsten, *After Kinship* (Cambridge, UK: Cambridge University Press, 2004), 5.

7. For instance, an official ruling of the Israeli High Court of Justice explicitly defined this linkage: "A *pundak* refers to a hostel, a hotel, a guesthouse; a surrogate is the owner of the *pundak,* the owner of the hostel, and the term *pundekaut* is defined by this. . . . The woman who carries the fertilized eggs in her womb has no genetic connection to the fetus that develops from those eggs; she is used as a sort of *pundak* [inn], a sort of guesthouse, for the fertilized eggs and for the fetus, and this is why she is called an innkeeper [*pundekait*]." See *Anonymous v. the Committee,* High Court of Justice 2458/01, 2001, for the approval of embryo-carrying agreements.

8. "Interview with Orna."

9. Paxson, *Making Modern Mothers.*

10. Ivry, *Embodying Culture.*

11. Ibid.

12. Tsipy Ivry and Elly Teman, "Pregnant Metaphors and Surrogate Meanings: Pregnancy and Surrogacy in Israel" (paper presented at the annual conference of the Israeli Anthropological Association, Neve Ilan, Israel, 2002).

13. Paxson, *Making Modern Mothers.*

14. Cook et al., "Introduction"; Ivry and Teman, "Pregnant Metaphors."

15. Shigeo Miyagawa, "Report from Japan: Surrogacy Contracts in the Supreme Court of Japan," *The Court* [newspaper], May 11, 2007.

16. Ragoné, "Of Likeness and Difference."

17. Devorah Shapira, "I Am Convincing Myself That It Is Not My Baby [*Ani Ovedet Al Atzmi She'ze Lo Hatinok Sheli*]." *Maariv Signon* [newspaper], November 20, 1996.

18. Yoram S. Carmeli and Daphna Birenbaum-Carmeli, "Ritualizing the 'Natural Family': Secrecy in Israeli Donor Insemination," *Science as Culture* 9, no. 3 (2000): 301–23; Kahn, *Reproducing Jews;* Michal Nahman, "Materialising Israeliness: Difference and Mixture in Transnational Ova Donation," *Science as Culture* 15, no. 3 (2006): 199–213.

19. Ragoné, "Of Likeness and Difference."

20. Ali and Kelley, "Womb for Rent."

21. Zara Griswold, *Surrogacy Was the Way: Twenty Intended Mothers Tell Their Stories* (Gurnee, IL: Nightengale Press, 2006), 81.

22. *American Kinship.*

23. Marilyn Strathern, *Reproducing the Future: Anthropology, Kinship and the New Reproductive Technologies* (New York: Routledge, 1992).

24. Elly Teman and Tsipy Ivry, "Ultra-Orthodox Women and Prenatal Testing: God Sent Ordeals and Their Discontents" (unpublished manuscript).

25. Kahn, *Reproducing Jews.*

26. Ibid.; Birenbaum-Carmeli, "'Cheaper Than a Newcomer.'"

27. Jean Elson, "Hormonal Hierarchy: Hysterectomy and Stratified Stigma," *Gender & Society* 17, no. 5 (2003): 750–70.

28. *American Kinship.*

29. Coker, "'Traveling Pains'"; Juliet Du Boulay, "The Blood: Symbolic Relationships between Descent, Marriage, Incest Prohibitions, and Spiritual Kinship in Greece," *Man* 19, no. 4 (1984): 533–56.

30. Danny Kaplan, *The Men We Loved: Male Friendship and Nationalism in Israeli Culture* (New York: Berghahn Books, 2006).

31. Etti Samama, "My Womb, Her Baby: Motivations for Surrogate Motherhood as Reflected in Women's Narratives in Israel" (master's thesis, Hebrew University, 2002), 84.

32. Waldby et al., "Blood and Bioidentity."

33. *Natural Symbols.*

34. "Materialising Israeliness."

35. Pande, "'Not Sleeping with Anyone'"; Vora, "Indian Transnational Surrogacy."

36. Ibid.

37. Pande, "'Not Sleeping with Anyone.'"

38. Coker, "'Traveling Pains.'"

39. Byron J. Good, "The Heart of What's the Matter: The Semantics of Illness in Iran," *Culture, Medicine and Psychiatry* 1, no. 1 (1977): 25–28.

40. "'Traveling Pains.'"

41. Fox and Swazey, *Spare Parts;* Sharp, "Organ Transplantation"; Waldby et al., "Blood and Bioidentity."

42. Ibid.

43. Ragoné, *Surrogate Motherhood.*

44. Note that Belle uses masculine pronouns to describe the determination of the surrogate. She consistently used the male form in her writings and in our conversations and interviews.

45. "Interview with Orna."

46. Eyal Ben-Ari, *Mastering Soldiers: Conflict, Emotions and the Enemy in an Israeli Military Unit* (Oxford, UK: Berghahn Books, 1998).

47. Catherine Nash, "Response to Wanda Hurren's 'Living with/in the Lines: Poetic Possibilities or World Writing,'" *Gender, Place and Culture* 6, no. 3 (1999): 273–79.

48. Douglas, *Natural Symbols.*

49. Nash, "Response," 273.

50. Ibid.

51. Veena Das, "Language and Body: Transactions in the Construction of Pain," in *Social Suffering,* ed. A. Kleinman, V. Das, and M.M. Lock, 67–92 (Berkeley: University of California Press, 1997), 85.

52. Kaplan, *The Men We Loved.*

53. Susan Greenhalgh, *Just One Child: Science and Policy in Deng's China* (Berkeley: University of California Press, 2008); Kanaaneh, *Birthing the Nation;* Kligman, *The Politics of Duplicity;* Paxson, *Making Modern Mothers.*

54. Michel Foucault, *Discipline and Punish: The Birth of Prison* (New York: Vintage Books, 1972).

55. Arthur W. Frank, *The Wounded Storyteller: Body, Illness, and Ethics* (Chicago: University of Chicago Press, 1995).

56. Lila Abu-Lughod, "The Romance of Resistance: Tracing Transformations of Power through Bedouin Women," *American Ethnologist* 17, no. 1 (1990): 41–55.

57. Das, "Language and Body," 86.

CHAPTER THREE

1. Arlie Russel Hochschild, *The Managed Heart.* (Berkeley: University of California Press, 1985).

2. Ben-Ari, *Mastering Soldiers.*

3. Draper, "'It Was a Real Good Show'"; Mitchell and Georges, "Baby's First Picture"; Rosalind Pollack Petchesky, "Foetal Images: The Power of Visual Culture in the Politics of Reproduction," in *Reproductive Technologies: Gender, Motherhood and Medicine,* ed. M. Stanworth, 57–80 (Cambridge, UK: Polity Press, 1987); Sandelowski, "Separate, but Less Unequal."

4. Jordan, "Authoritative Knowledge and Its Construction."

5. Sharon Chen, "I Would Do It Again [*Hayiti Osah Et Zeh Shuv*]," *At* [magazine], January 2000, 58–60.

6. Ivry, *Embodying Culture.*

7. The idea of hospital birth as "safer" than home birth is contested by birth activists and in the literature relating to the anthropology of reproduction (see Davis-Floyd, *Birth as an American Rite of Passage;* Klassen, *Blessed Events*).

8. See, e.g., Fox and Worts, "Revisiting the Critique of Medicalized Childbirth."

9. Hochschild, *The Managed Heart.*

10. Rebecca L. Upton and Sallie S. Han, "Maternity and Its Discontents: 'Getting the Body Back' after Pregnancy," *Journal of Contemporary Ethnography* 32, no. 6 (2003): 670–92.

11. Lucy Bailey, "Refracted Selves? A Study of Changes in Self-Identity in the Transition to Motherhood," *Sociology* 33, no. 3 (1999): 335–52.

12. Raymond, *Women as Wombs,* 36.

13. The law does not permit contracts to be discussed publicly; therefore, I describe the contracts I have seen in general terms and do not refer to specifics. There is no standard contract distributed by the state, so contracts differ from lawyer to lawyer. I have seen contracts related to arbitrated and nonarbitrated surrogacy arrangements; those that I refer to as "standard" contracts are those used by a commercial agency that currently arbitrates the majority of Israeli surrogacy arrangements. I have not included a standardized contract here because the agency's lawyer only let me see the contracts on the condition that I not reproduce or distribute them.

14. Rothman, *Recreating Motherhood;* Corea, *The Mother Machine.*

15. Hashiloni-Dolev, *A Life (Un)Worthy of Living;* Ivry, *Embodying Culture.*

16. Amniocentesis is a procedure performed in the sixteenth to eighteenth week of pregnancy in which a large needle is inserted into the woman's uterus and a small amount of amniotic fluid is extracted. The procedure, which is used to detect Down syndrome and other chromosomal anomalies, carries a risk of miscarriage (1 in 200 in Israel). CVS is used to detect fetal anomalies during the

eleventh week of pregnancy. It is riskier than amniocentesis and is used only when the parents are aware that they are carriers of certain genetic anomalies (Rapp, *Testing Women, Testing the Fetus;* Ivry, *Embodying Culture*). In Israel, amniocentesis is usually offered to pregnant women over age thirty-five, but in cases in which the intended mother is over thirty-five and the surrogate is younger, it is the first woman's age that factors into the doctor's recommendation.

17. Anat Shinkman, "This Joy Lasted 27 Weeks [*Ha'osher Hazeh Nimshach 27 Shavuot*]," *Yediot Ahronot* [newspaper], September 17, 1999.

18. James M. Henslin and Mae A. Biggs, "Dramaturgical Desexualization: The Sociology of the Vaginal Examination," in *The Sociology of Sex,* ed. J.M. Henslin, 243–72 (New York: Appleton-Century Crofts, 1971).

19. Nomi Cohen-David, "The Surrogate's Version [*Girsat Hapundekait*]," *Kolbo Haifa* [newspaper], May 8, 1998, 51.

20. Ibid.

21. Ibid.

22. Ibid.

23. Ibid.

24. Ibid.

25. Weisberg, *The Birth of Surrogacy in Israel.*

26. Martin, *The Woman in the Body.*

27. Ibid., 20.

28. Ibid., 21.

29. Ibid., 89.

30. Anne Balsamo, *Technologies of the Gendered Body: Reading Cyborg Women* (Durham, NC: Duke University Press, 1996), 56.

31. Rothman, *Recreating Motherhood.*

32. Ibid., 6.

33. Rothman, *Recreating Motherhood.*

34. *Making Parents.*

35. Ibid.

36. Samantha Warren and Joanna Brewis, "Matter over Mind? Examining the Experiences of Pregnancy," *Sociology* 38, no. 2 (2004): 219–36; Bailey, "Refracted Selves?"; Graham, "The Social Image of Pregnancy."

37. Jordan, "Authoritative Knowledge and Its Construction."

38. See, e.g., Greil, "Infertile Bodies"; Teman, "The Medicalization of 'Nature' in the 'Artificial Body'"; Thompson, *Making Parents.*

39. Eyal Ben-Ari, personal communication, 2004.

PART FOUR

1. *Making Modern Mothers.*

2. See note 10 in notes to Introduction.

3. Much of the scholarship in the anthropology of reproduction reveals how infertility and unwanted childlessness can be experienced as an assault on gender identity, a disruption in the projected life course, and a stigmatizing experience. See, for instance, Becker, *The Elusive Embryo;* Benjamin and Ha'elyon, "Rewriting Fertilization"; Franklin, *Embodied Progress;* Greil, "Infertile Bod-

ies." Birman et al.'s psychological research among Israeli infertility patients ("The Mental and Social Condition of Women Undergoing IVF Treatment," *Society and Welfare* [Hebrew] 12 [1991]: 44–55) suggests that these women may have experienced higher levels of stress than those experienced by the cancer patients with whom they were compared.

4. See, for instance, Elson's ("Hormonal Hierarchy") discussion of women who have undergone hysterectomy and the challenges this posed to their sense of femininity and womanhood.

5. Margarete Sandelowski, "Compelled to Try: The Never-Enough Quality of Conceptive Technology," *Medical Anthropology Quarterly* 5, no. 1 (1991): 29–47.

6. Gagin et al. ("Developing the Role of the Social Worker as Coordinator of Services at the Surrogate Parenting Center," *Social Work in Health Care: The Journal of Health Care Social Work* 40, no. 1 [2005]: 1–14) found that the infertile intended mothers that went through their center had attempted IVF a minimum of eight to ten times before they were declared eligible candidates for surrogacy by the approvals committee.

7. Remennick, "Childless in the Land of Imperative Motherhood."

8. Berkovitch, "Motherhood as a National Mission."

9. Tamar Katriel, *Talking Straight: Dugri Speech in Israeli Sabra Culture* (Cambridge, UK: Cambridge University Press, 1986).

10. Over the years of this study, the surrogacy committee's decisions have been challenged in court in several cases. In one case, a single woman challenged the clause limiting surrogacy to heterosexually paired couples. In a second case, the couple's ages (the intended mother was fifty-two) surpassed the allowable age for surrogacy, and in a third case, the couple already had two biological children. The latter two cases resulted in amendments to committee guidelines, while the first petitioner lost her case (see Teman, "The Last Outpost").

11. In July 2005, the approvals committee coordinator informed me that, in addition to the 280 files that had been reviewed by the committee to that date (230 of those were approved), 100 had been submitted by couples who subsequently withdrew from the process, never having signed a contract. The head social worker at a northern hospital echoed this finding during my interview with her, suggesting that a large number of couples that had begun the process through her hospital-based center had "dropped out" either before or right after securing committee approval. The authors of an article published by this center attribute the high rate of abandonment to "the complexity, hardship and energy input that the process involved" (Gagin et al., "The Role of the Social Worker").

CHAPTER FOUR

1. Margarete Sandelowski, Betty G. Harris, and Diane Holditch-Davis, "'Somewhere out There': Parental Claiming in the Preadoption Waiting Period," *Journal of Contemporary Ethnography* 21, no. 4 (1993): 464–86.

2. Layne, *Motherhood Lost.*

3. Sandelowski, *With Child in Mind.*

4. Becker, "Metaphors in Disrupted Lives."

5. Modell, "Last Chance Babies."

6. Becker, *The Elusive Embryo*; Franklin, *Embodied Progress*.

7. Becker, *The Elusive Embryo*.

8. Emily Martin, "The Egg and the Sperm: How Science Has Created a Romance Based on Stereotypical Male/Female Roles," *Signs* 16, no. 3 (1991): 485–501.

9. Franklin et al., *Global Nature, Global Culture*.

10. Michele Pridmore-Brown, "Reproductive Timing and the Cultural Meaning of Post/Menopausal Motherhood in the U.S." (paper presented at panel on Bio/Politics of Contemporary Motherhood, University of California, Berkeley, December 5, 2007).

11. Gay Becker, "Deciding Whether to Tell Children about Donor Insemination: An Unresolved Question in the United States," in *Infertility around the Globe: New Thinking on Childlessness, Gender, and Reproductive Technologies*, ed. F. Van Balen (Berkeley: University of California Press, 2002); Carmeli and Birenbaum-Carmeli, "Ritualizing the 'Natural Family.'"

12. Corinne P. Hayden, "Gender, Genetics, and Generation: Reformulating Biology in Lesbian Kinship," *Cultural Anthropology* 10, no. 1 (1995): 41–63.

13. Most of the women who used anonymously donated ova did not express ethical concerns about the possibility that the egg donors were probably poor, non-Jewish women in Romania and the Ukraine. There is still no law regulating egg donation in Israel, although a bill addressing the issue passed its preliminary Knesset reading in 2001; most Israeli women who need donor ova use foreign eggs. These eggs are procured by Israeli gynecologists who have set up off-shore egg banks in Romania and in Cypress, to which women from the former U.S.S.R. and other Eastern-bloc nations sell their ova (Nahman, "Materialising Israeliness"; Ran Reznick, "Facing Local Shortage, Israeli Women Go to Romania to Get Eggs Implanted," *Haaretz Daily* [newspaper], September 25, 2000).

14. *The Elusive Embryo*.

15. Sandelowski, "Separate, but Less Unequal."

16. Mitchell and Georges, "Baby's First Picture."

17. Petchesky, "Foetal Images"; Irma van der Ploeg, "Prosthetic Bodies: Female Embodiment in Reproductive Technologies," (PhD diss., University of Amsterdam, 1998), 461.

18. "Separate, but Less Unequal," 230.

19. Petchesky, "Foetal Images."

20. Shinkman, "This Joy Lasted 27 Weeks."

21. Janelle S. Taylor, "Image of Contradiction: Obstetrical Ultrasound in American Culture," in *Reproducing Reproduction: Kinship, Power, and Technological Innovation*, ed. S. Franklin and H. Ragoné, 15–45 (Philadelphia: University of Pennsylvania Press, 1998).

22. Sered, *What Makes Women Sick?* Evil eye beliefs, which are also common in other Mediterranean cultures (see, e.g., Alan Dundes, "Wet and Dry, the Evil Eye: An Essay in Indo-European and Semitic Worldview," in *The Evil Eye: A Folklore Casebook*, ed. Alan Dundes, 257–98 [New York: Garland, 1981]), have historically played a part in Jewish childbirth and life-cycle rituals (see, e.g., Raphael Patai, *On Jewish Folklore* [Detroit: Wayne State University Press, 1983]; Elly Teman, "The Red String: The Cultural History of a Jewish Folk

Symbol," in *Jewishness: Expression, Identity, and Representation,* ed. S. J. Bron-ner, 29–57 [Oxford, UK: Littman Library of Jewish Civilization, 2008]).

23. Landzelius, "Charged Artifacts."

24. Layne, *Motherhood Lost.*

25. Ivry, *Embodying Culture;* Barbara Katz Rothman, *The Tentative Preg-nancy: How Amniocentesis Changes the Experience of Motherhood* (New York: Norton, 1993).

26. Eugenia Georges and Lisa M. Mitchell, "Baby Talk: The Rhetorical Production of Maternal and Fetal Selves," in *Body Talk: Rhetoric, Technology, Reproduction,* ed. M.M. Lay, L.J. Gurak, C. Gravon, and C. Myntti, 184–206. (Madison: University of Wisconsin Press, 2000); Lucy Bailey, "Bridging Home and Work in the Transition to Motherhood," *The European Journal of Women's Studies* 7 (2000): 66.

27. "Baby Talk."

28. Ibid., 187.

29. Susan Starr Sered and Henry Abramovitch, "Pregnant Dreaming: Search for a Typology of a Proposed Dream Genre," *Social Science and Medicine* 34, no. 12 (1992): 1405–11.

30. Ibid.

31. Janelle S. Taylor, Linda L. Layne, and Danielle F. Wozniak, eds., *Con-suming Motherhood* (New Brunswick, NJ: Rutgers University Press, 2004).

32. Griswold, *Surrogacy Was the Way,* 92.

33. Sered, *What Makes Women Sick?*

34. Ivry, *Embodying Culture.*

35. Sandelowski, *With Child in Mind.*

36. Shirley Morah, "I Am Pregnant and Having Fun [*Ani Beherayon V'kef Li*]," *Maariv* [newspaper], May 19, 2006.

37. Ibid.

38. In response, the head of the IVF unit told the press that "dozens of sur-rogacy cases have been treated in our unit without us ever encountering a com-plaint from the biological mother or from the surrogate. Since it is the biological mother who initiates the treatment, meets with the unit physicians multiple times up to the stage that the combined treatment of her and the surrogate begins, it is natural that the doctor/patient relationship that develops is closer with her than between the surrogate and the attending physician. The protocol in our unit before the embryo transfer to the woman's womb is to update the couple of the number of existing embryos, their quality and our suggestions. All of these deliberations occurred while the woman's log with all of its results were open in front of us. Also in this case . . . I turned to the intended mother in the surrogate's presence and explained to her about her embryos. . . . Later I also informed the intended mother that pregnancy had been achieved with the clear knowledge that she would pass on that information to the surrogate." (Morah, "I Am Pregnant"). The surrogate later reported that, at the next meet-ing with the IVF unit staff, for the eight-week ultrasound, a different physician had responded to her wishes to be treated as an equal patient: he wrote both of the women's names on the ultrasound printout and on the referral for further treatment.

39. Jan Draper, "Blurring, Moving and Broken Boundaries: Men's Encounters with the Pregnant Body," *Sociology of Health & Illness* 25, no. 7 (2003): 743–67; Sandelowski, *With Child in Mind,* 83.

40. M.H. Klaus and John H. Kennel, *Maternal-Infant Bonding* (St. Louis: C.V. Mosby Co., 1976); Ivry, *Embodying Culture;* Nancy Scheper-Hughes, *Death without Weeping: The Violence of Everyday Life in Brazil* (Berkeley: University of California Press, 1992); Meira Weiss, *Conditional Love: Parents' Attitudes toward Handicapped Children* (Westport, CT: Bergin & Garvey, 1994).

41. Ivry, *Embodying Culture.*

42. See Rothman, *The Tentative Pregnancy.*

43. See Klein's discussion of the Jewish notion of worry (Michelle Klein, *Not to Worry: Jewish Wisdom and Folklore* [Philadelphia: Jewish Publication Society, 2003]). Sered (*What Makes Women Sick?*) also discusses the image of the worried mother in the context of Jewish-Israeli mothers of combat-soldier sons.

44. Griswold, *Surrogacy Was the Way,* 132.

45. Samama, "My Womb, Her Baby," 69.

46. Ben-Ari, *Mastering Soldiers.*

47. Hochschild, *The Managed Heart.*

48. Carol Gilligan, *In a Different Voice: Psychological Theory and Women's Development* (Cambridge, MA: Harvard University Press, 1993).

49. Shellee Colen, "'Like a Mother to Them': Stratified Reproduction and West Indian Childcare Workers in New York," in *Conceiving the New World Order: The Global Politics of Reproduction,* ed. F.D. Ginsburg and R. Rapp, 78–102 (Berkeley: University of California Press, 1995).

50. Davis-Floyd and Davis, "Intuition as Authoritative Knowledge."

CHAPTER FIVE

1. David H. Knox and Michael J. Sporakowski, "Attitudes of College Students toward Love," *Journal of Marriage and the Family* 30, no. 4 (1968): 638–42.

2. Ragoné, *Surrogate Motherhood.*

3. Robert Rawdon Wilson, "Cyber(Body)Parts: Prosthetic Consciousness," in *Cyberspace, Cyberbodies, Cyberpunk: Cultures of Technological Embodiment,* ed. M. Featherston and R. Burrows, 239–59 (London: Sage, 1995), 242.

4. M. Merleau-Ponty, *Phenomenology of Perception* (London: Routledge and Kegan Paul, 1962), 143.

5. "Body Boundaries."

6. Moshe Zigdon, "I Gave Them the Best Gift in the World [*Natati Lahem Et Hamatana Hachi Tova Bachayim*]" *Zman Ma'aleh* [newspaper], June 8, 2000.

7. Davis-Floyd and Davis, "Intuition as Authoritative Knowledge."

8. Miller, "Acquiring the Pregnancy Identity."

9. Eilat Negev, "Sixty Thousand Dollars and You Have a Child [*Shishim Eleph Dolar V'yesh Lecha Yeled*]" *Maariv* [newspaper], July 1, 1994, 16–18.

10. Griswold, *Surrogacy Was the Way,* 161.

11. Ragoné, *Surrogate Motherhood;* Roberts, "Native Narratives of Connectedness"; Helena Ragoné, personal communication, 2002; Elizabeth F.S. Roberts, personal communication, 2003.

12. See also Bailey, "Gender Shows."

13. Because it convincingly mimics pregnancy, the phenomenon was difficult to detect before the invention of ultrasound. Historically, it could only be detected when a particularly long pregnancy never resulted in a child. This was the case of Mary, Queen of Scots, whose fifteen-month-long pregnancy made the condition famous. The syndrome was also explored in Edward Albee's play *Who's Afraid of Virginia Woolf?*

14. Robert L. Munroe and Ruth H. Munroe, "Psychological Interpretation of Male Initiation Rites: The Case of Male Pregnancy Symptoms," *Ethos* 1, no. 1 (1973): 490–98.

15. Don Handelman, *Models and Mirrors: Towards an Anthropology of Public Events* (New York: Berghahn, 1998).

16. Bordo, *Unbearable Weight;* Judith Butler, *Gender Trouble* (New York: Routledge, 1990).

17. Celia Kitzinger and Jo Willmott, "'The Thief of Womanhood': Women's Experience of Polycystic Ovarian Syndrome," *Social Science & Medicine* 54 (2002): 349–61.

18. Samama, "My Womb, Her Baby," 98.

19. Earle, "Bumps and Boobs."

20. Ibid.

21. Bailey, "Gender Shows."

22. The state offers Riki amniocentesis and genetic counseling because she is over thirty-five, but these options would not ordinarily have been offered to Yelena, who is under thirty-five.

23. Shinkman, "This Joy Lasted 27 Weeks," 69.

24. Orit Harel, "Pressure Cooker: Second Article in the Series 'Womb for Rent' [*Sir Lachatz: Katava Shniya Besidra Rechem Lehaskir*]," *Maariv Weekend* [newspaper], March 27, 1998, 47.

25. Victor W. Turner, *The Ritual Process: Structure and Anti-Structure* (Ithaca, NY: Cornell University Press, 1977), 48.

26. *Uvdah [Fact]*, television documentary program, directed by Mica Limor (Israel's Channel 2, March 8, 1998).

27. Zigdon, "The Best Gift."

28. When I first heard the romantic references in their narratives I wondered whether the women felt the need to bring love and (symbolic) sex into their relationship because the project they were embarking on together was about kinship. Recalling Schneider's (*American Kinship; A Critique of the Study of Kinship* [Ann Arbor: University of Michigan Press, 1984]) famous argument that Euro-American kinship ideology is based on symbols of nature, law, blood ties, love, and sexual intercourse, it seemed fitting that love would play an important role in surrogacy. In terms of Schneider's kinship theory, symbolic sexual union and love might be expected within the surrogate–intended mother relationship because all of the other symbols of kin making are so central to the way the women make sense of their surrogacy experience. Moreover, the symbolic simulation of sexual relations is not foreign to modern medical practice, as Goldberg ("The Man in the Sperm") posits in her study of the ritual handling of semen in Israeli fertility clinics. Therefore, I wondered whether the women were

intuiting through their rhetoric of love that even a high-tech form of kinship creation needed to include all of the symbolic elements of relatedness.

29. The comparison between the surrogate–intended mother relationship and a lesbian courtship is theoretically plausible in terms of the feminist literature on lesbianism. In particular, I refer to Rich's formulation of the "lesbian continuum" (Adrienne Rich, "Compulsory Heterosexuality and Lesbian Existence," *Signs* 5, no. 4 [1980]: 631–60). Distinguishing the lesbian continuum from the sexual component of "lesbian existence," Rich argues that lesbianism should not simply be viewed as an erotic choice but that all support systems and intense interactions among women can be considered degrees of lesbianism. The lesbian continuum is "a range through each woman's life and throughout history of woman-identified experience." It expands the definition of lesbianism "to embrace many more forms of primary intensity between and among women, including the sharing of a rich inner life, the bonding against male tyranny, the giving and receiving of practical and political support" (648–49).

30. A theme that runs through the psychological literature on female homoerotic unions and that, in many ways, parallels the surrogate–intended mother relationship is the "urge to merge," which denotes the symbolic merging of two women into one. The psychological literature employs the concepts of "merging" and "fusion" to describe this phenomenon, which is said to occur among lesbian women involved in "overly close" intimacy, that is, in relationships in which they become embedded or undifferentiated (Kathryn Greene, Vickie Causby, and Diane Helene Miller, "The Nature and Function of Fusion in the Dynamics of Lesbian Relationships," *Affilia Journal of Women and Social Work* 14, no. 1 [1999]: 78–97). This link between the romantic union of two women and the phenomenon of merging sheds important light on the merged body in surrogacy, for both lesbian merging and the "one body" formulation of surrogacy emphasize the same central features—similarity, sameness, and blurred identity boundaries.

31. Jackie Stacey, *Stargazing: Hollywood Cinema and Female Spectatorship* (London: Routledge, 1993).

32. *Uvdah* [Fact].

33. Ibid.

34. Louis Dumont, *Homo Hierarchicus: The Caste System and Its Implications* (Chicago: University of Chicago Press, 1980).

35. R. Hertz, "The Pre-Eminence of the Right Hand: A Study in Religious Polarity," in *Right and Left: Essays on Dual Symbolic Classification*, ed. R. Needham, 3–31 (Chicago: University of Chicago Press, 1973).

36. Robert Parkin, *Louis Dumont and Hierarchical Opposition* (New York: Berghahn Books, 2003).

37. Ibid.

38. Ibid.

39. Zvia Birman and Eliezer Witztum, "Integrative Therapy in Cases of Pregnancy Following Infertility." *Journal of Contemporary Psychotherapy* 30, no. 3 (2000): 273–87.

40. Benjamin and Ha'elyon, "Rewriting Fertilization."

41. Ibid., 676.

42. Orit Harel, "Here Are Our Children: Last Article in the Series 'Womb for Rent' [*Heeneh Hayeladim Shelanu: Katava Achronah Besidra Rechem Lehaskir*]," *Maariv Weekend* [newspaper], April 3, 1998, 75.

43. *Uvdah [Fact]*.

44. Interview with Liron Meir, 1999.

45. Samama, "My Womb, Her Baby," 72.

46. Karen Erickson Paige and Jeffrey M. Paige, *The Politics of Reproductive Ritual* (Berkeley: University of California Press, 1981).

47. Ibid., 189.

48. Karen Middleton, "How Karembola Men Become Mothers," in *Cultures of Relatedness: New Approaches to the Study of Kinship,* ed. J. Carsten, 104–28 (Cambridge, UK: Cambridge University Press, 2000), 115.

49. Paige and Paige, *The Politics of Reproductive Ritual*.

50. Middleton, "Karembola Men," 115.

51. Chris Shilling, *The Body and Social Theory* (London: Sage, 1993).

52. The works of Giddens (Anthony Giddens, *Modernity and Self-Identity: Self and Society in the Late Modern Age* [Cambridge, UK: Polity, 1991]), Shilling (*The Body and Social Theory*), and Turner (*The Body and Society*) have established in different variations how the body has increasingly become a central locus for the construction of social identity in late modernity. Within some of these studies, the concept of self-identity is employed in the sense that Giddens engaged it in his concept of the project of the self in late modernity(*Modernity and Self-Identity,* 224). Giddens regards the project of the self as "the process whereby self-identity is constituted by the reflexive ordering of self-narratives" (ibid., 244).

53. Shilling, *The Body and Social Theory*.

54. Herbert Blumer, *Symbolic Interactionism: Perspective and Method* (Englewood Cliffs, NJ: Prentice Hall, 1969).

55. See also Warren Shapiro and Uli Linke, *Denying Biology: Essays on Gender and Pseudo-Procreation* (Lanham, MD: University Press of America, 1996).

56. Shulamith Firestone, *The Dialectic of Sex: The Case for Feminist Revolution* (New York: Morrow, 1970).

CHAPTER SIX

1. Margrit Shildrick, "'You Are There, Like My Skin': Reconfiguring Relational Economies," in *Thinking through the Skin,* ed. S. Ahmed and J. Stacey, 160–75 (London: Routledge, 2001), 164.

2. Davis-Floyd, "Cultural Anomaly."

3. Orit Brawer Ben-David, *Organ Donation and Transplantation: Body Organs as an Exchangeable Socio-Cultural Resource* (Westport, CT: Greenwood Publishing, 2005); Sharp, *Strange Harvest*.

4. Turner, *The Ritual Process,* 185.

5. Although Turner originally stated that the concept of liminality should only be applied to the analysis of tribal societies, he noted that it could be used metaphorically to interpret complex societies, in which liminal phenomena are not society-wide.

6. Turner, *The Ritual Process*, 95.

7. Ronald L. Grimes, *Deeply into the Bone: Reinventing Rites of Passage* (Berkeley: University of California Press, 2000).

8. Nancy Scheper-Hughes and Margaret M. Lock, "The Mindful Body: A Prolegomenon to Future Work in Medical Anthropology," *Medical Anthropology Quarterly* 1 (1987): 6–41.

9. See Omi Morgenstern-Leissner, "The Israeli Birth Law" (PhD diss., Bar-Ilan University, 2005).

10. Haviva Sharan et al., "Hospitalization for Early Bonding of the Genetic Mother after a Surrogate Pregnancy: Report of Two Cases," *Birth* 28, no. 4 (2001): 272.

11. Ibid.

12. Ibid.

13. Davis-Floyd, *Birth as an American Rite of Passage*.

14. Eric Blyth, "'Not a Primrose Path': Commissioning Parents' Experiences of Surrogacy Arrangements in Britain," *Journal of Reproductive and Infant Psychology* 13, nos. 3–4 (1995): 185–96.

15. See Griswold, *Surrogacy Was the Way*.

16. *Making Parents*.

17. *Strange Harvest*.

18. Meira Weiss, "Bedside Manners: Paradoxes of Physician Behavior in Grand Rounds," *Culture, Medicine and Psychiatry* 17, no. 2 (1993): 235–53.

19. At the time of this writing, no Israeli surrogate has ever challenged the intended parents' custody of the child. However, should this ever occur, it is highly unlikely that the surrogate would receive custody because all surrogacy contracts include the appointment of legal guardians for the child in case of an emergency, such as the death of the intended parents during the pregnancy.

20. Morgenstern-Leissner, "The Israeli Birth Law."

21. Teman, "The Last Outpost."

22. Helena Ragoné, "Surrogate Motherhood, Gamete Donation, and Constructions of Altruism," in *Transformative Motherhood: On Giving and Getting in a Consumer Culture*, ed. L. L. Layne, 65–88 (New York: New York University Press, 1999).

23. Ibid., 72.

24. Turner, *The Ritual Process*, 95.

25. Nissan Rubin, Carmela Shmilovitz, and Meira Weiss, "From Fat to Thin: Informal Rites Affirming Identity Change," *Symbolic Interaction* 16, no. 1 (1993): 1–17.

26. Modell, *Kinship with Strangers*.

27. Eyal Ben-Ari, "Posing, Posturing and Photographic Presences: A Rite of Passage in a Japanese Commuter Village," *Man* 26, no. 1 (1991): 87–104.

28. Mary Boquet, "Making Kinship with an Old Reproductive Technology" in *Relative Values: Reconfiguring Kinship Studies*, ed. S. Franklin and S. McKinnon, 86–114 (Durham, NC: Duke University Press, 2001).

29. Ibid., 111.

30. Susan Sontag, *On Photography* (New York: Farrar, Straus and Giroux, 1977), cited in Boquet, "Making Kinship";

31. Boquet, "Making Kinship," 87.

32. Modell, *Kinship with Strangers;* Sandelowski, *With Child in Mind.*

33. Roger Friedland, "Money, Sex and G-d: The Erotic Logic of Religious Nationalism," *Sociological Theory* 20, no. 3 (2002): 381.

34. Linda L. Layne, ed., *Transformative Motherhood: On Giving and Getting in a Consumer Culture* (New York: New York University Press, 1999); Taylor et al., *Consuming Motherhood.*

CHAPTER SEVEN

1. Ragoné, "Surrogate Motherhood."

2. Rene Almeling, "'Why Do You Want to Be a Donor?': Gender and the Production of Altruism in Egg and Sperm Donation," *New Genetics and Society* 25 (2006): 143–57.

3. Richard V. Grazi and Joel B. Wolowelsky, "Jewish Medical Ethics: Monetary Compensation for Donating Kidneys," *Israel Medical Association Journal* 6, no. 3 (2004): 185–88.

4. Ibid.; Ragoné, "Constructions of Altruism."

5. Linda Renee Block, "Who's Afraid of Being a *Freier?* The Analysis of Communication through a Key Cultural Frame," *Communication Theory* 13, no. 2 (2003): 125–59.

6. Valeri Valerio, "Buying Women but Not Selling Them: Gift and Commodity Exchange in Huaulu Alliance," *Man* 29, no. 1 (1994): 15.

7. Lewis Hyde, *The Gift: Imagination and the Erotic Life of Property* (New York: Vintage Books, 1983).

8. Marilyn Strathern, *The Gender of the Gift: Problems with Women and Problems with Society in Melanesia* (Berkeley: University of California Press, 1988).

9. Fox and Swazey, *Spare Parts.*

10. *Uvdah* [*Fact*].

11. Vered Luvitz, "A Surrogate Mother Who Underwent Two Pregnancy Terminations: 'I Will Continue to Conceive until I Succeed in Giving Them a Child' [*Em Pundekait She'avra Shtei Hapalot: 'Amshich L'hikanes L'herayon Ad Sh'atzliach Latet Lahem Yeled'*]." *Maariv* [newspaper], March 3, 2000.

12. Ibid., 11.

13. Hyde, *The Gift.*

14. Chris Gregory, *Gifts and Commodities* (London: Academic Press, 1982); Strathern, *The Gender of the Gift.*

15. Arjun Appadurai, "Introduction: Commodities and the Politics of Value," in *The Social Life of Things: Commodities in Cultural Perspective,* ed. A. Appadurai, 3–63 (Cambridge, UK: Cambridge University Press, 1986).

16. Ibid.

17. Valerio, "Buying Women but Not Selling Them."

18. Layne, *Transformative Motherhood;* Ragoné, "Constructions of Altruism."

19. Layne, *Transformative Motherhood,* 5–9.

20. Mauss, *The Gift.*

21. Ibid.; Schneider, *American Kinship.*

22. Mauss, *The Gift*, 12.

23. Strathern, *The Gender of the Gift*, 206.

24. Mary Douglas, "Foreword: No Free Gifts," in *The Gift: Form and Reason for Exchange in Archaic Societies*, by Marcel Mauss (New York: Norton, 1990), vii.

25. Mauss, *The Gift*, 20.

26. Hyde, *The Gift*, 70.

27. Ragoné, "Constructions of Altruism."

28. Mauss, *The Gift*, 11.

29. Valerio, "Buying Women but Not Selling Them," 18.

30. Shinkman, "This Joy Lasted 27 Weeks," 76.

31. See Mauss, *The Gift*.

32. Ragoné, "Constructions of Altruism," 72.

33. Ibid.

34. Mauss, *The Gift*.

35. Kaplan, *The Men We Loved*.

36. Ibid.

37. Ben-Ari, *Mastering Soldiers*.

38. Lomsky-Feder, "Patterns of Participation in War."

39. Kaplan, *The Men We Loved*.

40. Strathern, *The Gender of the Gift*, 144.

41. Konrad, "Ova Donations and Symbols of Substance."

42. Kaplan, *The Men We Loved*.

43. Harel, "Between Two Women," "Pressure Cooker."

44. *Uvdah* [*Fact*].

45. Ibid.

46. Roni Dagan and Avner Hofstein, "A Womb and Entertainment [*Rehem V'sha'ashuim*]," *Ha'ayin Hashvi'it* [magazine], May 4, 1998.

47. Nomi Levanon-Kashat, "The Other Side of Surrogacy [*Hatsad Ha'acher Shel Hapundekaut: 'Natati Lazug Hazeh Et Haneshama V'hem Rimu Oti V'bagdu Bi'*]," *Laisha Women's Magazine*, December 10, 1999.

48. Ibid.

49. Ibid.

50. Ibid.

51. Ibid.

52. Ibid.

53. Michael A. Rynkiewich, "The Place That Is Part of It," in *Pacific Places, Pacific Histories: Essays in Honor of Robert C. Kiste*, ed. B.V. Lal, 309–26 (Honolulu: University of Hawai'i Press, 2004).

54. Valerio, "Buying Women but Not Selling Them," 15.

55. Levanon-Kashat, "The Other Side of Surrogacy."

56. Richard Titmuss, *The Gift Relationship: From Human Blood to Social Policy* (New York: New Press, 1997).

57. Orit Ben-David, "Ranking Deaths in Israeli Society: Premature Deaths and Organ Donation," *Mortality* 11, no. 1 (2006): 79–98.

58. Amir and Benjamin, "Defining Encounters."

59. Valerio, "Buying Women but Not Selling Them."

60. Hyde, *The Gift,* 61.
61. Teman, "The Last Outpost."
62. Shildrick, "'You Are There.'"
63. Douglas, *Natural Symbols.*
64. Markens, *Surrogate Motherhood and the Politics of Reproduction.*
65. *The Gift,* 51.
66. Ibid., 45.

PART FOUR

1. Anthony Giddens, *Central Problems in Social Theory: Action, Structure, and Contradiction in Social Analysis* (London: Macmillan Press, 1979).

CHAPTER EIGHT

1. The required blood tests include blood count, Rh factor, creatinine, hepatitis B and C, AIDS, rubella antibodies, syphilis, and an oral glucose tolerance test.
2. As opposed to the policy during the early years of state oversight, in which surrogates did not have access to their evaluations, the current practice of many psychologists is to give the surrogate a copy of the assessment to read and then meet with her to discuss the results.
3. See Amir and Benjamin, "Defining Encounters, for a similar analysis of the ritualistic measures employed by hospital abortion approval committees in Israel.
4. These are standardized exams for high school and college entry comparable to the SAT exams in the United States.
5. In its latest report, the Centers for Disease Control and Prevention (http://www.cdc.gov) found that 28.6 percent of IVF cycles in the United States using non-donor eggs resulted in live births. Within this figure there is variation by age. Statistics reported by the Society for Assisted Reproductive Technology (http://www.sart.org) for 2007 show that 39.9 percent of IVF treatment cycles (using non-donor eggs) in clinics in the United States resulted in live births for women age thirty-five and under. The percentage decreases as age increases: 30.5 percent (thirty-five to thirty-seven), 21.0 percent (thirty-eight to forty), 11.7 percent (forty-one to forty-two). Statistics in Israeli clinics are similar. Live birth rates per cycle are higher for gestational surrogates, although during the years (1998–2005) that many of the women in this study took part in surrogacy, success rates were lower than those for 2007. For instance, the CDC reports 27.0 percent live births per cycle using non-donor eggs in 2001.
6. Franklin, *Embodied Progress.*
7. Becker, *The Elusive Embryo;* de Lacey, "IVF as Lottery or Investment"; Franklin, *Embodied Progress.*
8. *Embodied Progress,* 161.
9. De Lacey, "IVF as Lottery or Investment."
10. *Embodied Progress.*
11. Franklin, *Embodied Progress;* Sandelowski, *With Child in Mind;* Becker, *The Elusive Embryo.*

12. *Motherhood Lost.*

13. De Lacey, "IVF as Lottery or Investment."

14. Remennick, "Childless in the Land of Imperative Motherhood."

15. Carmel Shalev, "*Halakha* and Patriarchal Motherhood: An Anatomy of the Israeli Surrogacy Law," *Israel Law Review* 32, no. 1 (1998): 51–80.

16. Franklin, *Embodied Progress,* 111.

17. Rothman, *Recreating Motherhood.*

18. *Making Parents.*

19. Klassen, *Blessed Events.*

20. Sarah Franklin, "Making Miracles: Scientific Progress and the Facts of Life," in *Reproducing Reproduction: Kinship, Power, and Technological Innovation,* ed. S. Franklin and H. Ragoné, 102–17 (Philadelphia: University of Pennsylvania Press, 1998).

21. Teman, "'Knowing' the Surrogate Body in Israel.'"

22. Jordan, "Authoritative Knowledge and Its Construction."

23. *Embodied Progress,* 162.

24. Ragoné, *Surrogate Motherhood.*

25. Steve Liewer, "Military Wives Find a New Mission with Service as Surrogate Mothers," *San Diego Union-Tribune,* June 29, 2008, 1.

26. Susan Donaldson James, "Baby Carriers: Cold Cash or Warm Heart?" *ABC News* [television program], April 1, 2008.

27. Ali and Kelley, "Womb for Rent."

28. Chaim Noy, "You Must Go Trek There: The Persuasive Genre of Narration among Israeli Backpackers," *Narrative Inquiry* 12, no. 2 (2002): 261–90.

29. Eyal Ben-Ari, "Tests of Soldierhood, Trials of Manhood: Military Service and Male Ideals in Israel," in *Military, State and Society in Israel,* ed. D. Maman, E. Ben-Ari, and Z. Rosenhek, 239–67 (New Brunswick, NJ: Transaction Publishers, 2001).

30. Ben-Ari, *Mastering Soldiers.*

31. Ibid., 44.

32. Ben-Ari, *Mastering Soldiers.*

33. Chloe Diepenbrock, "God Willed It! Gynecology at the Checkout Stand: Reproductive Technology in the Women's Service Magazine, 1977–1996," in *Body Talk: Rhetoric, Technology, Reproduction,* ed. M.M. Lay, L.J. Gurak, C. Gravon, and C. Myntti, 98–124 (Madison: University of Wisconsin Press, 2000), 112.

34. Anne E. Kaplan, *Motherhood and Representation: The Mother in Popular Culture and Melodrama* (London: Routledge, 1992), 77.

35. Reuven Gal, *A Portrait of the Israeli Soldier* (Westport, CT: Greenwood Press, 1986), cited in Ben-Ari, "Tests of Soldierhood, Trials of Manhood."

36. Roberts, "Examining Surrogacy Discourses."

37. Peter C. Reynolds, *Stealing Fire: The Mythology of the Technocracy* (Palo Alto, CA: Iconic Anthropology Press, 1991).

38. Robyn Longhurst, "Breaking Corporeal Boundaries: Pregnant Bodies in Public Places," in *Contested Bodies,* ed. R. Holliday and J. Hassard, 81–94 (London: Routledge, 2001).

39. Iris Marion Young, "Pregnant Embodiment: Subjectivity and Alienation," *Journal of Medicine and Philosophy* 9 (1984): 45–62.

40. Robbie Davis-Floyd, "The Technocratic Body: American Childbirth as Cultural Expression," *Social Science & Medicine* 38, no. 8 (1994): 1125–40.

41. Ben-Ari, *Mastering Soldier.*

42. *Unbearable Weight,* 145.

43. Ibid., 156.

44. Orna Sasson-Levy, "Feminism and Military Gender Practices: Israeli Women Soldiers in 'Masculine' Roles," *Sociological Inquiry* 73, no. 3 (2003): 440–65.

45. Ibid.

46. Rapoport and El-Or 1997, "Cultures of Womanhood."

47. Sered, *What Makes Women Sick?* 5.

48. Ibid., 7.

49. Foucault, *Discipline and Punish.*

50. Arthur W. Frank, "For a Sociology of the Body: An Analytical Review," in *The Body: Social Process and Cultural Theory,* ed. M. Featherston, M. Hepworth, and B. S. Turner, 36–102 (London: Sage, 1991).

51. Davis-Floyd, *Birth as an American Rite of Passage.*

CHAPTER NINE

1. Grimes, *Deeply into the Bone.*

2. Frank, *The Wounded Storyteller,* 122.

3. Joseph Campbell, *The Hero with a Thousand Faces* (London: Fontana Press, 1993).

4. Frank, *The Wounded Storyteller,* 115.

5. Leslie Hazelton, *Israeli Women: The Reality behind the Myths* (New York: Simon & Schuster, 1977).

6. "Interview with Orna."

7. *The Hero with a Thousand Faces.*

8. Neta Bar and Eyal Ben-Ari, "Israeli Snipers in the Al-Aqsa Intifada: Killing, Humanity and Lived Experience," *Third World Quarterly* 26, no. 1 (2005): 133–52; Limor Darash, *Violence, Control and Enjoyment: The Creation of a New Biology. Issues in the Training of the Duvdevan Unit of the Israeli Army* (Jerusalem: Shaine Center for Social Research, Hebrew University, 2005).

9. Darash, *Violence, Control and Enjoyment.*

10. Klassen, *Blessed Events.*

11. Franklin, *Embodied Progress.*

12. Frank, *The Wounded Storyteller,* 129.

13. Steven M. Ortiz, "How Interviewing Became Therapy for Wives of Professional Athletes: Learning from a Serendipitous Experience," *Qualitative Inquiry* 7 (2001): 209.

14. Frank, *The Wounded Storyteller,* 130.

15. Ibid.

16. See Rothman, *Recreating Motherhood.*

17. Michel Foucault, *Madness and Civilization: A History of Insanity in the Age of Reason,* translated by R. Howard (New York: Vintage Books, 1973).

18. Sered, *What Makes Women Sick?* 13.

19. Anthony Giddens, *Central Problems in Social Theory: Action, Structure, and Contradiction in Social Analysis* (London: Macmillan Press, 1979).

20. William H. Sewell, "A Theory of Structure: Duality, Agency and Transformation," *The American Journal of Sociology* 98, no. 1 (1992): 1–29.

21. Ibid.

22. *Unbearable Weight,* 154.

23. Frank, *The Wounded Storyteller,* 128.

24. Douglas, *Implicit Meanings,* 137.

25. Robert Graves, *The White Goddess: A Historical Grammar of Poetic Myth* (New York: Farrar, Strauss and Giroux, 1966).

26. Davis-Floyd, *Birth as an American Rite of Passage;* Klassen, *Blessed Events;* Ann Oakley, *Women Confined: Toward a Sociology of Childbirth* (New York: Schocken, 1980); Rothman, *Recreating Motherhood.*

27. Diepenbrock, "God Willed It!" 108.

28. Franklin, "Making Miracles."

29. Klassen, *Blessed Events.*

30. Martin, *The Woman in the Body.*

31. "God Willed It!"

32. Ivry, *Embodying Culture.*

33. Jordan, "Authoritative Knowledge and Its Construction," 74.

34. Ernest Becker, *The Denial of Death* (New York: Free Press Paperbacks, 1973).

35. Frank, *The Wounded Storyteller,* 116.

36. Frank, *The Wounded Storyteller,* 22.

37. Rudolf Otto, *The Idea of the Holy* (London: Oxford University Press, 1958).

CONCLUSION

1. Becker, *The Elusive Embryo;* Modell, "Last Chance Babies."

2. Becker, *The Elusive Embryo;* Larissa Rememnick, "The Quest after the Perfect Baby: Why Do Israeli Women Seek Prenatal Genetic Testing?" *Sociology of Health & Illness* 28, no. 1 (2006): 21–53; Sarah Franklin, "Postmodern Procreation: A Cultural Account of Assisted Reproduction," in *Conceiving the New World Order: The Global Politics of Reproduction,* ed. F. D. Ginsburg and R. Rapp, 323–45 (Berkeley: University of California Press, 1995); Sandelowski, *With Child in Mind;* Layne, *Transformative Motherhood.*

3. Diane L. Wolf, personal communication, 2007.

4. Mediterranean peoples, such as Greeks, Italians, and Israelis, are often described in popular culture as more emotive than the British or North Americans.

5. Yuval Davis, "National Reproduction."

6. Benjamin and Ha'elyon, "Rewriting Fertilization"; Kahn, *Reproducing Jews;* Remennick, "Childless in the Land of Imperative Motherhood."

7. Sered, *What Makes Women Sick?;* Meira Weiss, *The Chosen Body: The Politics of the Body in Israeli Society* (Stanford, CA: Stanford University Press, 2002).

8. Scrcd, *What Makes Women Sick?*

9. See, e.g., Birenbaum-Carmeli, "'Cheaper Than a Newcomer'"; Ivry, *Embodying Culture.*

10. Teman, "The Last Outpost."

11. Rapoport and El-Or, "Cultures of Womanhood."

12. Kahn, *Reproducing Jews.*

13. "Defining Encounters."

14. Benjamin and Ha'elyon, "Rewriting Fertilization"; Donath, "Cracks in Pro-Natalism."

15. Becker, *The Elusive Embryo.*

16. Ilan Ramon, Israel's first astronaut, became a media hero when he was chosen to represent Israel aboard the U.S. space shuttle *Columbia* in 2003. He took a Torah scroll and an Israeli flag into space. The shuttle disintegrated upon reentry, and Ramon was collectively mourned as a national hero.

17. Kahn, *Reproducing Jews;* Teman, "The Medicalization of 'Nature' in the 'Artificial Body.'"

18. See Paxson, *Making Modern Mothers,* for an account of a completely different approach to taking responsibility for maternal citizenship in Greece. There, despite a similar cultivation of motherhood as a national duty, women choose to delay childbearing so as to be good, responsible mothers.

19. Teman, "The Medicalization of 'Nature' in the 'Artificial Body.'"

20. Kahn, *Reproducing Jews;* Teman, "The Medicalization of 'Nature' in the 'Artificial Body.'"

21. Stanworth, "Reproductive Technologies."

22. Weisberg, *The Birth of Surrogacy in Israel.*

23. Martin, "Body Narratives, Body Boundaries," "The End of the Body?"

24. Irma van der Ploeg, "Hermaphrodite Patients: In Vitro Fertilization and the Transformation of Male Infertility," *Science, Technology and Human Values* 20, no. 4 (1995): 460–81.

25. E.g., Luce Irigaray, "This Sex Which Is Not One," in *Writing on the Body: Female Embodiment and Feminist Theory,* ed. K. Conboy, N. Medina, and S. Stanbury, 248–56 (New York: Columbia University Press, 1997).

26. Shildrick, "'You Are There.'"

27. "The End of the Body?"

28. Franklin, *Embodied Progress;* Kahn, *Reproducing Jews;* Paxson, *Making Modern Mothers;* Marilyn Strathern, *After Nature: English Kinship in the Late Twentieth Century* (Cambridge, UK: Cambridge University Press, 1995).

29. Strathern, *Reproducing the Future.*

30. Paul Z. Rabinow, "Artificiality and Enlightenment: From Sociobiology to Biosociality," in *Incorporations,* ed. J. Crary and S. Kwinter, 234–52 (New York: Zone, 1992),

31. Ibid.

32. Franklin, "Postmodern Procreation."

33. Greenhalgh, *Just One Child.*

34. *The Politics of Duplicity.*

35. *The Birth of Surrogacy in Israel.*

36. See also Weisberg, *The Birth of Surrogacy in Israel.*

37. *Surrogate Motherhood and the Politics of Reproduction.*
38. Weisberg, *The Birth of Surrogacy in Israel.*
39. Miyagawa, "Report from Japan."
40. Hashiloni-Dolev, *A Life (Un)Worthy of Living;* Sered, *What Makes Women Sick?;* Weiss, *The Chosen Body.*
41. Annette Burfoot, "In-Appropriation—A Critique of *Proceed with Care:* Final Report of the Royal Commission on New Reproductive Technologies," *Women's Studies International Forum* 18, no. 4 (1995): 499–506.
42. Markens, *Surrogate Motherhood and the Politics of Reproduction;* Andrews, *Between Strangers.*
43. Edelman, "Surrogacy: The Psychological Issues," 125.
44. Roberts, "Examining Surrogacy Discourses"; Pande, "'Not Sleeping with Anyone.'"
45. See, e.g., Ragoné, *Surrogate Motherhood;* Teman, "The Social Construction of Surrogacy Research"; van den Akker, "Psychological Aspects of Surrogate Motherhood."
46. See "Introduction" note 15.
47. A psychological study found greater well-being and better adaptation to parenthood among mothers and fathers of children born through surrogacy arrangements than among natural-conception parents (Susan Golombok et al., "Families Created through Surrogacy Arrangements: Parent-Child Relationships in the 1st Year of Life," *Developmental Psychology* 40, no. 3 [2004]: 400–411). Medical studies comparing children born by IVF surrogacy and by conventional IVF have shown better developmental outcomes (Paulo Serafini, "Outcome and Follow-up of Children Born after IVF-Surrogacy," *Human Reproduction Update* 7, no. 1 [2001]: 23–27) and lower risks of major malformations (Michael Ludwig and Klaus Diedrich, "Follow-up of Children Born after Assisted Reproductive Technologies," *Reproductive BioMedicine Online* 5, no. 3 [2002]: 317–22) among the surrogacy-born children.
48. Edelman, "Surrogacy: The Psychological Issues."
49. See also Ciccarelli and Beckman, "Navigating Rough Waters"; Ragoné, *Surrogate Motherhood;* Teman, "The Social Construction of Surrogacy Research"; van den Akker, "Psychological Aspects of Surrogate Motherhood."
50. Edelman, "Surrogacy: The Psychological Issues."
51. See also Ragoné, *Surrogate Motherhood;* Teman, "The Social Construction of Surrogacy Research"; van den Akker, "Psychological Aspects of Surrogate Motherhood."
52. See also Ciccarelli and Beckman, "Navigating Rough Waters."
53. E.g., Rebecca Camber, "Couple Launch Custody Battle after Surrogate Mother Decides to Keep Babies," *Daily Mail Online,* http://www.dailymail.co.uk/news/article-431168, Jan. 25, 2007.

Bibliography

Abu-Lughod, Lila. "The Romance of Resistance: Tracing Transformations of Power through Bedouin Women." *American Ethnologist* 17, no. 1 (1990): 41–55.

Aigen, Betsy. "Motivations of Surrogate Mothers: Parenthood, Altruism and Self-Actualization." *The American Surrogacy Center.* http:// www.surrogacy. com/psychres/article/motivat.html.

Al-Nasser, R., et al. "Factors Influencing Success in Gestational Surrogacy." *Fertility and Sterility* 86, no. 2 (2006): 132–33.

Ali, Lorraine, and Raina Kelley. "Womb for Rent: The Curious Lives of Surrogates." *Newsweek,* April 7, 2008.

Almagor-Ramon, Ruth. "Pundak." *A Moment of Hebrew [Rega Shel Ivrit].* Reshet Bet radio station, October 10, 2001.

Almeling, Rene. "'Why Do You Want to Be a Donor?': Gender and the Production of Altruism in Egg and Sperm Donation." *New Genetics and Society* 25 (2006): 143–57.

Amir, Delila, and Orly Benjamin. "Defining Encounters: Who Are the Women Entitled to Join the Israeli Collective?" *Women's Studies International Forum* 20, nos. 5/6 (1997): 639–50.

Andrews, Lori B. *Between Strangers: Surrogate Mothers, Expectant Fathers, and Brave New Babies.* New York: Harper & Row, 1989.

———. *The Clone Age: Adventures in the New World of Reproductive Technology.* New York: Henry Holt, 1999.

Appadurai, Arjun. "Introduction: Commodities and the Politics of Value." In *The Social Life of Things: Commodities in Cultural Perspective,* edited by A. Appadurai, 3–63. Cambridge, UK: Cambridge University Press, 1986.

Arditti, Rita, Renate Klein, and Shelley Minden. *Test-Tube Women: What Future for Motherhood?* London: Pandora Press, 1984.

Bailey, Lucy. "Refracted Selves? A Study of Changes in Self-Identity in the Transition to Motherhood." *Sociology* 33, no. 3 (1999): 335–52.

———. "Bridging Home and Work in the Transition to Motherhood." *The European Journal of Women's Studies* 7 (2000): 53–70.

———. "Gender Shows: First-Time Mothers and Embodied Selves." *Gender & Society* 15, no. 1 (2001): 110–29.

Baker, Brenda M. "A Case for Permitting Altruistic Surrogacy." *Hypatia* 11, no. 2 (1996): 34–48.

Balsamo, Anne. *Technologies of the Gendered Body: Reading Cyborg Women.* Durham, NC: Duke University Press, 1996.

Bar, Neta, and Eyal Ben-Ari. "Israeli Snipers in the Al-Aqsa Intifada: Killing, Humanity and Lived Experience." *Third World Quarterly* 26, no. 1 (2005): 133–52.

Baslington, H. "The Social Organization of Surrogacy: Relinquishing a Baby and the Role of Payment in the Psychological Detachment Process." *Journal of Health Psychology* 7, no. 1 (2002): 57–71.

Bayskal, Baris, et al. "Opinions of Infertile Turkish Women on Gamete Donation and Gestational Surrogacy." *Fertility and Sterility* 89, no. 4 (2008): 817–22.

Becker, Ernest. *The Denial of Death.* New York: Free Press Paperbacks, 1973.

Becker, Gay. "Metaphors in Disrupted Lives: Infertility and Cultural Constructions of Continuity." *Medical Anthropology Quarterly* 8, no. 4 (1994): 383–410.

———. *The Elusive Embryo: How Women and Men Approach New Reproductive Technologies.* Berkeley: University of California Press, 2000.

———. "Deciding Whether to Tell Children about Donor Insemination: An Unresolved Question in the United States." In *Infertility around the Globe: New Thinking on Childlessness, Gender, and Reproductive Technologies,* edited by F. Van Balen. Berkeley: University of California Press, 2002.

Ben-Ari, Eyal. "Posing, Posturing and Photographic Presences: A Rite of Passage in a Japanese Commuter Village." *Man* 26, no. 1 (1991): 87–104.

———. *Mastering Soldiers: Conflict, Emotions and the Enemy in an Israeli Military Unit.* Oxford, UK: Berghahn Books, 1998.

———. "Tests of Soldierhood, Trials of Manhood: Military Service and Male Ideals in Israel." In *Military, State and Society in Israel,* edited by D. Maman, E. Ben-Ari, and Z. Rosenhek, 239–67. New Brunswick, NJ: Transaction Publishers, 2001.

Ben-David, Orit Brawer. *Organ Donation and Transplantation: Body Organs as an Exchangeable Socio-Cultural Resource.* Westport, CT: Greenwood Publishing, 2005.

———. "Ranking Deaths in Israeli Society: Premature Deaths and Organ Donation." *Mortality* 11, no. 1 (2006): 79–98.

Benjamin, Orly, and Hila Ha'elyon. "Rewriting Fertilization: Trust, Pain, and Exit Points." *Women's Studies International Forum* 25, no. 6 (2002): 667–78.

Ber, Rosalie. "Ethical Issues in Gestational Surrogacy." *Theoretical Medicine and Bioethics* 21, no. 2 (2000): 153–69.

Berkovitch, Nitza. "Motherhood as a National Mission: The Construction of Womanhood in the Legal Discourse in Israel." *Women's Studies International Forum* 20, no. 5 (1997): 605–19.

Birenbaum-Carmeli, Daphna. "'Cheaper Than a Newcomer': On the Social Production of IVF Policy in Israel." *Sociology of Health & Illness* 26, no. 7 (2004): 897–924.

Birman, Zvia, et al. "The Mental and Social Condition of Women Undergoing IVF Treatment." *Society and Welfare* [Hebrew] 12 (1991): 44–55.

Birman, Zvia, and Eliezer Witztum. "Integrative Therapy in Cases of Pregnancy Following Infertility." *Journal of Contemporary Psychotherapy* 30, no. 3 (2000): 273–87.

Block, Linda Renee. "Who's Afraid of Being a *Freier*? The Analysis of Communication through a Key Cultural Frame." *Communication Theory* 13, no. 2 (2003): 125–59.

Blumer, Herbert. *Symbolic Interactionism: Perspective and Method.* Englewood Cliffs, NJ: Prentice Hall, 1969.

Blyth, Eric. "'Not a Primrose Path': Commissioning Parents' Experiences of Surrogacy Arrangements in Britain." *Journal of Reproductive and Infant Psychology* 13, nos. 3–4 (1995): 185–96.

Boddy, Janice Patricia. *Wombs and Alien Spirits: Women, Men, and the Zâar Cult in Northern Sudan.* Madison: University of Wisconsin Press, 1989.

Boquet, Mary. "Making Kinship with an Old Reproductive Technology." In *Relative Values: Reconfiguring Kinship Studies,* edited by S. Franklin and S. McKinnon, 86–114. Durham, NC: Duke University Press, 2001.

Bordo, Susan. *Unbearable Weight: Feminism, Western Culture, and the Body.* Berkeley: University of California Press, 1993.

Burfoot, Annette. "In-Appropriation—A Critique of *Proceed with Care:* Final Report of the Royal Commission on New Reproductive Technologies." *Women's Studies International Forum* 18, no. 4 (1995): 499–506.

Butler, Judith. *Gender Trouble.* New York: Routledge, 1990.

Camber, Rebecca. "Couple Launch Custody Battle after Surrogate Mother Decides to Keep Babies." *Daily Mail Online,* January 25, 2007. http://www.dailymail.co.uk/news/article-431168.

Campbell, Joseph. *The Hero with a Thousand Faces.* London: Fontana Press, 1993.

Carmeli, Yoram S., and Daphna Birenbaum-Carmeli. "Ritualizing the 'Natural Family': Secrecy in Israeli Donor Insemination." *Science as Culture* 9, no. 3 (2000): 301–23.

Carsten, Janet. *After Kinship.* Cambridge, UK: Cambridge University Press, 2004.

Chen, Sharon. "I Would Do It Again [*Hayiti Osah Et Zeh Shuv*]." *At* [magazine], January 2000, 58–60.

Childlessness Overcome through Surrogacy (COTS) Website. http://www.surrogacy.org.uk.

Ciccarelli, Janice C., and Linda J. Beckman. "Navigating Rough Waters: An Overview of Psychological Aspects of Surrogacy." *Journal of Social Issues* 61, no. 1 (2005): 21–43.

Cohen-David, Nomi. "The Surrogate's Version [*Girsat Hapundekait*]." *Kolbo Haifa* [newspaper], May 8, 1998.

Coker, Elizabeth Marie. "'Traveling Pains': Embodied Metaphors of Suffering among Southern Sudanese Refugees in Cairo." *Culture, Medicine and Psychiatry* 28 (2004): 15–39.

Colen, Shellee. "'Like a Mother to Them': Stratified Reproduction and West Indian Childcare Workers in New York." In *Conceiving the New World Order: The Global Politics of Reproduction,* edited by F.D. Ginsburg and R. Rapp, 78–102. Berkeley: University of California Press, 1995.

Cook, Rachel, Shelley Day Sclater, and Felicity Kaganas. "Introduction." In *Surrogate Motherhood: International Perspectives,* edited by R. Cook, S.D. Sclater, and F. Kaganas, 1–22. Oxford, UK: Hart Publishing, 2003.

Corea, Gena. *The Mother Machine: Reproductive Technologies from Artificial Insemination to Artificial Wombs.* New York: Harper & Row, 1985.

Counihan, Carole. *The Anthropology of Food and Body: Gender, Meaning, and Power.* New York: Routledge, 1999.

Dagan, Roni, and Avner Hofstein. "A Womb and Entertainment [*Rehem V'sha'ashuim*]." *Ha'ayin Hashvi'it* [magazine], May 4, 1998.

Darash, Limor. *Violence, Control and Enjoyment: The Creation of a New Biology. Issues in the Training of the Duvdevan Unit of the Israeli Army.* Jerusalem: Shaine Center for Social Research, Hebrew University, 2005.

Das, Veena. "Language and Body: Transactions in the Construction of Pain." In *Social Suffering,* edited by A. Kleinman, V. Das, and M.M. Lock, 67–92. Berkeley: University of California Press, 1997.

Davis-Floyd, Robbie. "The Role of American Obstetrics in the Resolution of Cultural Anomaly." *Social Science and Medicine* 31 (1990): 175–89.

——. "The Technocratic Body: American Childbirth as Cultural Expression." *Social Science & Medicine* 38, no. 8 (1994): 1125–40.

——. *Birth as an American Rite of Passage.* Berkeley: University of California Press, 2003.

Davis-Floyd, Robbie E., and Elizabeth Davis. "Intuition as Authoritative Knowledge in Midwifery and Home Birth." In *Childbirth and Authoritative Knowledge: Cross-Cultural Perspectives,* edited by R.E. Davis-Floyd and C.F. Sargent, 315–49. Berkeley: University of California Press, 1997.

de Lacey, Sheryl. "IVF as Lottery or Investment: Contesting Metaphors in Discourses of Infertility." *Nursing Inquiry* 9, no. 1 (2002): 43–51.

Delaney, Carol Lowery. *The Seed and the Soil: Gender and Cosmology in Turkish Village Society.* Berkeley: University of California Press, 1991.

Diepenbrock, Chloe. "God Willed It! Gynecology at the Checkout Stand: Reproductive Technology in the Women's Service Magazine, 1977–1996." In *Body Talk: Rhetoric, Technology, Reproduction,* edited by M.M. Lay, L.J. Gurak, C. Gravon, and C. Myntti, 98–124. Madison: University of Wisconsin Press, 2000.

Donath, Orna. "Cracks in Pro-Natalism: Choosing a Childfree Life-Style in Israel." Master's thesis, Tel Aviv University, 2007.

Douglas, Mary. "Foreword: No Free Gifts." In *The Gift: Form and Reason for Exchange in Archaic Societies*, by Marcel Mauss, vii–xviii. New York: Norton, 1990.

———. *Implicit Meanings: Selected Essays in Anthropology*. London: Routledge, 1999.

———. *Natural Symbols: Explorations in Cosmology*. London: Routledge, 2003.

Draper, Jan. "'It Was a Real Good Show': The Ultrasound Scan, Fathers and the Power of Visual Knowledge." *Sociology of Health & Illness* 24, no. 6 (2002): 771–95.

———. "Blurring, Moving and Broken Boundaries: Men's Encounters with the Pregnant Body." *Sociology of Health & Illness* 25, no. 7 (2003): 743–67.

Du Boulay, Juliet. "The Blood: Symbolic Relationships between Descent, Marriage, Incest Prohibitions, and Spiritual Kinship in Greece." *Man* 19, no. 4 (1984): 533–56.

Dumont, Louis. *Homo Hierarchicus: The Caste System and Its Implications*. Chicago: University of Chicago Press, 1980.

Dundes, Alan. "Wet and Dry, the Evil Eye: An Essay in Indo-European and Semitic Worldview." In *The Evil Eye: A Folklore Casebook*, edited by Alan Dundes, 257–98. New York: Garland, 1981.

Dunn, P.C., I.J. Ryan, and K. O'Brien. "College Students' Acceptance of Adoption and Five Alternative Fertilization Techniques." *The Journal of Sex Research* 24 (1988): 282–87.

Earle, Sarah. "Bumps and Boobs: Fatness and Women's Experiences of Pregnancy." *Women's Studies International Forum* 26, no. 3 (2003): 245–52.

Edelman, R.J. "Surrogacy: The Psychological Issues." *Journal of Reproductive and Infant Psychology* 22, no. 2 (2004): 123–36.

Einwohner, Joan. "Who Becomes a Surrogate: Personality Characteristics." In *Gender in Transition: A New Frontier*, edited by J. Offerman-Zuckerberg, 123–33. New York: Plenum Medical Book Company, 1989.

Elson, Jean. "Hormonal Hierarchy: Hysterectomy and Stratified Stigma." *Gender & Society* 17, no. 5 (2003): 750–70.

English, M.E., A. Mechanick-Braverman, and S.L. Corson. "Semantics and Science: The Distinction between Gestational Carrier and Traditional Surrogacy Options." *Women's Health Issues* 1, no. 3 (1991): 155–57.

Farquhar, Dion. *The Other Machine: Discourse and Reproductive Technologies*. New York: Routledge, 1996.

Firestone, Shulamith. *The Dialectic of Sex: The Case for Feminist Revolution*. New York: Morrow, 1970.

Foucault, Michel. *Discipline and Punish: The Birth of Prison*. New York: Vintage Books, 1972.

———. *Madness and Civilization: A History of Insanity in the Age of Reason*, translated by R. Howard. New York: Vintage Books, 1973.

Fox, Bonnie, and Diana Worts. "Revisiting the Critique of Medicalized Childbirth: A Contribution to the Sociology of Birth." *Gender & Society* 13, no. 3 (1999): 326–46.

Fox, Renee C., and Judith P. Swazey. *Spare Parts: Organ Replacement in American Society.* Oxford, UK: Oxford University Press, 1992.

Frank, Arthur W. "For a Sociology of the Body: An Analytical Review." In *The Body: Social Process and Cultural Theory,* edited by M. Featherston, M. Hepworth, and B.S. Turner, 36–102. London: Sage, 1991.

———. *The Wounded Storyteller: Body, Illness, and Ethics.* Chicago: University of Chicago Press, 1995.

Franklin, Sarah. "Postmodern Procreation: A Cultural Account of Assisted Reproduction." In *Conceiving the New World Order: The Global Politics of Reproduction,* edited by F.D. Ginsburg and R. Rapp, 323–45. Berkeley: University of California Press, 1995.

———. *Embodied Progress: A Cultural Account of Assisted Conception.* London: Routledge, 1997.

———. "Making Miracles: Scientific Progress and the Facts of Life." In *Reproducing Reproduction: Kinship, Power, and Technological Innovation,* edited by S. Franklin and H. Ragoné, 102–17. Philadelphia: University of Pennsylvania Press, 1998.

Franklin, Sarah, Celia Lury, and Jackie Stacey. *Global Nature, Global Culture.* London: Sage, 2000.

Friedland, Roger. "Money, Sex and G-d: The Erotic Logic of Religious Nationalism." *Sociological Theory* 20, no. 3 (2002): 381–425.

Gagin, Roni, et al. "Developing the Role of the Social Worker as Coordinator of Services at the Surrogate Parenting Center." *Social Work in Health Care: The Journal of Health Care Social Work* 40, no. 1 (2005): 1–14.

Gailey, Christine Ward. "Ideologies of Motherhood and Kinship in U.S. Adoption." In *Ideologies and Technologies of Motherhood: Race, Class, Sexuality, Nationalism,* edited by H. Ragoné and F.W. Twine, 11–55. New York: Routledge, 2000.

Gal, Reuven. *A Portrait of the Israeli Soldier.* Westport, CT: Greenwood Press, 1986.

Gentlemen, Amelia. "India Nurtures Business of Surrogate Motherhood." *The New York Times,* March 10, 2008.

Georges, Eugenia, and Lisa M. Mitchell. "Baby Talk: The Rhetorical Production of Maternal and Fetal Selves." In *Body Talk: Rhetoric, Technology, Reproduction,* edited by M.M. Lay, L.J. Gurak, C. Gravon, and C. Myntti, 184–206. Madison: University of Wisconsin Press, 2000.

Giddens, Anthony. *Central Problems in Social Theory: Action, Structure, and Contradiction in Social Analysis.* London: Macmillan Press, 1979.

———. *Modernity and Self-Identity: Self and Society in the Late Modern Age.* Cambridge, UK: Polity, 1991.

Gilligan, Carol. *In a Different Voice: Psychological Theory and Women's Development.* Cambridge, MA: Harvard University Press, 1993.

Ginsburg, Faye D. *Contested Lives: The Abortion Debate in an American Community.* Berkeley: University of California Press, 1989.

Goldberg, Helene. "The Man in the Sperm." Master's thesis, University of Copenhagen, 2002.

Golombok, Susan, et al. "Families Created through Surrogacy Arrangements: Parent-Child Relationships in the 1st Year of Life." *Developmental Psychology* 40, no. 3 (2004): 400–411.

Good, Byron J. "The Heart of What's the Matter: The Semantics of Illness in Iran." *Culture, Medicine and Psychiatry* 1, no. 1 (1977): 25–28.

Goslinga-Roy, Gillian M. "Body Boundaries, Fictions of the Female Self: An Ethnographic Perspective on Power, Feminism and the Reproductive Technologies." *Feminist Studies* 26, no. 1 (2000): 113–40.

Graham, Hilary. "The Social Image of Pregnancy: Pregnancy as Spirit Possession." *Sociological Review* 24, no. 2 (1976): 291–308.

Graves, Robert. *The White Goddess: A Historical Grammar of Poetic Myth.* New York: Farrar, Strauss and Giroux, 1966.

Grazi, Richard V., and Joel B. Wolowelsky. "Jewish Medical Ethics: Monetary Compensation for Donating Kidneys," *Israel Medical Association Journal* 6, no. 3 (2004): 185–88.

Greene, Kathryn, Vickie Causby, and Diane Helene Miller. "The Nature and Function of Fusion in the Dynamics of Lesbian Relationships." *Affilia Journal of Women and Social Work* 14, no. 1 (1999): 78–97.

Greenhalgh, Susan. *Just One Child: Science and Policy in Deng's China.* Berkeley: University of California Press, 2008.

Greenwood, Davydd, and Morten Levin. *Introduction to Action Research.* London: Sage, 1998.

Gregory, Chris. *Gifts and Commodities.* London: Academic Press, 1982.

Greil, Arthur L. "Infertile Bodies: Medicalization, Metaphor, and Agency." In *Infertility around the Globe: New Thinking on Childlessness, Gender, and Reproductive Technologies,* edited by M.C. Inhorn and F. Van Balen, 101–18. Berkeley: University of California Press, 2002.

Grimes, Ronald L. *Deeply into the Bone: Reinventing Rites of Passage.* Berkeley: University of California Press, 2000.

Griswold, Zara. *Surrogacy Was the Way: Twenty Intended Mothers Tell Their Stories.* Gurnee, IL: Nightengale Press, 2006.

Hanafin, Hilary. "The Surrogate Mother: An Exploratory Study." PhD diss., California School of Professional Psychology, 1984.

Handelman, Don. *Models and Mirrors: Towards an Anthropology of Public Events.* New York: Berghahn, 1998.

Haraway, Donna. "The Promises of Monsters: A Regenerative Politics for Inappropriated Others." In *Cultural Studies,* edited by L. Grossberg, C. Nelson, and P. Treichler, 295–337. New York: Routledge, 1992.

Harel, Orit. "Pressure Cooker: Second Article in the Series 'Womb for Rent' [*Sir Lachatz: Katava Shniya Besidra Rechem Lehaskir*]." *Maariv Weekend* [newspaper], March 27, 1998.

———. "Here Are Our Children: Last Article in the Series 'Womb for Rent' [*Heeneh Hayeladim Shelanu: Katava Achronah Besidra Rechem Lehaskir*]." *Maariv Weekend* [newspaper], April 3, 1998.

Hashiloni-Dolev, Yael. *A Life (Un)Worthy of Living: Reproductive Genetics in Israel and Germany.* Dordrecht, Netherlands: Springer, 2007.

Hastings, Katy. "Surrogate Mother Prepares for Eighth Baby." *Telegraph.co .uk,* January 21, 2008. http://www.telegraph.co.uk/news/uknews/1576150/ Surrogate-mother-prepares-for-eighth-baby.html.

Haworth, Abigail. "Surrogate Mothers: Womb for Rent." *Marie Claire,* August 2008.

Hayden, Corinne P. "Gender, Genetics, and Generation: Reformulating Biology in Lesbian Kinship." *Cultural Anthropology* 10, no. 1 (1995): 41–63.

Hayut, Ilanit. "A Womb for Rent or a Good Solution? [*Rehem Lehaskir O' Pitaron Savir*]." *Haaretz Daily* [newspaper], October 29, 2001.

Hazelton, Leslie. *Israeli Women: The Reality behind the Myths.* New York: Simon & Schuster, 1977.

Henslin, James M., and Mae A. Biggs. "Dramaturgical Desexualization: The Sociology of the Vaginal Examination." In *The Sociology of Sex,* edited by J.M. Henslin, 243–72. New York: Appleton-Century Crofts, 1971.

Hertz, R. "The Pre-Eminence of the Right Hand: A Study in Religious Polarity." In *Right and Left: Essays on Dual Symbolic Classification,* edited by R. Needham, 3–31. Chicago: University of Chicago Press, 1973.

Hochschild, Arlie Russel. *The Managed Heart.* Berkeley: University of California Press, 1985.

Hyde, Lewis. *The Gift: Imagination and the Erotic Life of Property.* New York: Vintage Books, 1983.

"India Looks to New Laws to Regulate Rent-a-Womb Baby Trade." *FoxNews. com,* March 15, 2008. http://www.foxnews.com/story/0,2933,338139,00 .html.

Inhorn, Marcia Claire. *Quest for Conception: Gender, Infertility, and Egyptian Medical Traditions.* Philadelphia: University of Pennsylvania Press, 1994.

Inhorn, Marcia Claire, and Frank van Balen. *Infertility around the Globe: New Thinking on Childlessness, Gender, and Reproductive Technologies.* Berkeley: University of California Press, 2002.

"Interview with Orna, a Surrogate Mother." *At Eye Level* [*Be'gova Eynayim*] [radio program], prod. by T. Cohen, Jerusalem, 2003.

Irigaray, Luce. "This Sex Which Is Not One." In *Writing on the Body: Female Embodiment and Feminist Theory,* edited by K. Conboy, N. Medina, and S. Stanbury, 248–56. New York: Columbia University Press, 1997.

Ivry, Tsipy. *Embodying Culture: Pregnancy in Japan and Israel.* New Brunswick, NJ: Rutgers University Press, 2009.

Ivry, Tsipy, and Elly Teman. "Pregnant Metaphors and Surrogate Meanings: Pregnancy and Surrogacy in Israel." Paper presented at the annual conference of the Israeli Anthropological Association, Neve Ilan, Israel, 2002.

———. "Expectant Israeli Fathers and the Medicalized Pregnancy: Power, Pragmatism and Resistance." *Culture, Medicine and Psychiatry* 32, no. 3 (2008): 358–85.

Jackson, Emily. *Regulating Reproduction: Law, Technology, and Autonomy.* Oxford, UK: Hart Publishing, 2001.

James, Susan Donaldson. "Baby Carriers: Cold Cash or Warm Heart?" *ABC News* [television program], April 1, 2008.

Johnson, Richard. "Rent a Womb." *New York Post,* February 5, 2008.

Jordan, Brigitte. "Authoritative Knowledge and Its Construction." In *Child-birth and Authoritative Knowledge: Cross-Cultural Perspectives,* edited by R. Davis-Floyd and C.F. Sargent, 55–79. Berkeley: University of California Press, 1997.

Kadosh, Ruti. "She Is Me and I Am Her: We Are One Body [*He Zo Ani V'ani Zo Hi: Anachnu Guf Echad*]." *Maariv* [newspaper], July 23, 2001.

Kahn, Susan Martha. *Reproducing Jews: A Cultural Account of Assisted Conception in Israel.* Durham, NC: Duke University Press, 2000.

Kanaaneh, Rhoda Ann. *Birthing the Nation: Strategies of Palestinian Women in Israel.* Berkeley: University of California Press, 2002.

Kaplan, Anne E. *Motherhood and Representation: The Mother in Popular Culture and Melodrama.* London: Routledge, 1992.

Kaplan, Danny. *The Men We Loved: Male Friendship and Nationalism in Israeli Culture.* New York: Berghahn Books, 2006.

Katriel, Tamar. *Talking Straight: Dugri Speech in Israeli Sabra Culture.* Cambridge, UK: Cambridge University Press, 1986.

Keen, Judy. "Surrogate Relishes Unique Role." *USA Today,* January 23, 2007.

King, Leslie. "Demographic Trends, Pronatalism, and Nationalist Ideologies in the Late Twentieth Century." *Ethnic and Racial Studies* 25, no. 3 (2002): 367–89.

Kirmayer, Laurence J. "Broken Narratives: Clinical Encounters and the Poetics of Illness Experience." In *Narrative and the Cultural Construction of Illness and Healing,* edited by C.Mattingly and L.C. Garro, 153–81. Berkeley: University of California Press, 2000.

Kitzinger, Celia, and Jo Willmott. "'The Thief of Womanhood': Women's Experience of Polycystic Ovarian Syndrome." *Social Science & Medicine* 54 (2002): 349–61.

Klassen, Pamela E. *Blessed Events: Religion and Home Birth in America.* Princeton, NJ: Princeton University Press, 2001.

Klaus, M.H., and John H. Kennel. *Maternal-Infant Bonding.* St. Louis: C.V. Mosby Co., 1976.

Klein, Michelle. *Not to Worry: Jewish Wisdom and Folklore.* Philadelphia: Jewish Publication Society, 2003.

Kligman, Gail. *The Politics of Duplicity: Controlling Reproduction in Ceausescu's Romania.* Berkeley: University of California Press, 1998.

Knox, David H., and Michael J. Sporakowski. "Attitudes of College Students toward Love." *Journal of Marriage and the Family* 30, no. 4 (1968): 638–42.

Konrad, Monica. "Ova Donations and Symbols of Substance: Some Variations on the Theme of Sex, Gender, and the Partible Body." *Journal of the Royal Anthropological Institute* 4, no. 4 (1998): 643–67.

Krishnan, V. "Attitudes toward Surrogate Motherhood in Canada." *Health Care for Women International* 15 (1994): 333–57.

Kuczynski, Alex. "Her Body, My Baby." *New York Times Magazine,* November 28, 2008.

Lambeck, Michael. *Human Spirits: A Cultural Account of Trance in Mayotte.* Cambridge, UK: Cambridge University Press, 1981.

Landzelius, Kyra Marie. "Charged Artifacts and the Detonation of Liminality: Teddy-Bear Diplomacy in the Newborn Incubator Machine." *Journal of
Material Culture* 6, no. 3 (2001): 323–44.

Layne, Linda L., ed. *Transformative Motherhood: On Giving and Getting in a
Consumer Culture.* New York: New York University Press, 1999.

———. *Motherhood Lost: A Feminist Account of Pregnancy Loss in America.*
New York: Routledge, 2003.

Levanon-Kashat, Nomi. "The Other Side of Surrogacy [*Hatsad Ha'acher
She Hapundekaut: 'Natati Lazug Hazeh Et Haneshama V'hem Rimu Oti
V'bagdu Bi'*]." *Laisha Women's Magazine,* December 10, 1999.

Liewer, Steve. "Military Wives Find a New Mission with Service as Surrogate
Mothers." *San Diego Union-Tribune,* June 29, 2008.

Lock, Margaret M., and Patricia A. Kaufert. *Pragmatic Women and Body Politics.* New York: Cambridge University Press, 1998.

Lomsky-Feder, Edna. "Patterns of Participation in War and the Construction of
War in the Life Course: Life Stories of Israeli Veterans from the Yom Kippur
War." PhD diss., Hebrew University, 1994.

———. "The Meaning of War through Veterans' Eyes: A Phenomenological
Analysis of Life Stories." In *Military, State, and Society in Israel,* edited by
D. Maman, E. Ben-Ari, and Z. Rosenhek, 269–94. New Brunswick, NJ:
Transaction Publishers, 2001.

Longhurst, Robyn. "Breaking Corporeal Boundaries: Pregnant Bodies in Public
Places." In *Contested Bodies,* edited by R. Holliday and J. Hassard, 81–94.
London: Routledge, 2001.

Ludwig, Michael, and Klaus Diedrich. "Follow-up of Children Born after
Assisted Reproductive Technologies." *Reproductive BioMedicine Online* 5,
no. 3 (2002): 317–22.

Lupton, Deborah. *Food, the Body and the Self.* London: Sage, 1996.

Luvitz, Vered. "A Surrogate Mother Who Underwent Two Pregnancy Termina-
tions: 'I Will Continue to Conceive until I Succeed in Giving Them a Child'
[*Em Pundekait She'avra Shtei Hapalot: 'Amshich L'hikanes L'herayon Ad
Sh'atzliach Latet Lahem Yeled'*]." *Maariv* [newspaper], March 3, 2000.

Markens, Susan. *Surrogate Motherhood and the Politics of Reproduction.*
Berkeley: University of California Press, 2007.

Martin, Emily. "The Egg and the Sperm: How Science Has Created a Romance
Based on Stereotypical Male/Female Roles." *Signs* 16, no. 3 (1991): 485–501.

———. "Body Narratives, Body Boundaries." In *Cultural Studies,* edited by
L. Grossberg, C. Nelson, and P.A. Treichler, 409–19. New York: Routledge,
1992.

———. "The End of the Body?" *American Ethnologist* 19 (1992): 121–38.

———. *The Woman in the Body: A Cultural Analysis of Reproduction.* Boston:
Beacon Press, 2001.

Mauss, Marcel. *The Gift: Forms and Functions of Exchange in Archaic Societies.* New York: Norton, 1967.

McNay, Lois. *Foucault and Feminism.* Cambridge, UK: Polity Press, 1992.

Merleau-Ponty, M. *Phenomenology of Perception.* London: Routledge and
Kegan Paul, 1962.

Middleton, Karen. "How Karembola Men Become Mothers." In *Cultures of Relatedness: New Approaches to the Study of Kinship,* edited by J. Carsten, 104–28. Cambridge, UK: Cambridge University Press, 2000.

Miller, Rita Seiden. "The Social Construction and Reconstruction of Physiological Events: Acquiring the Pregnancy Identity." *Studies in Symbolic Interaction* 1 (1978): 181–204.

Mitchell, Lisa, and Eugenia Georges. "Baby's First Picture: The Cyborg Foetus of Ultrasound Imaging." In *Cyborg Babies, from Techno-Sex to Techno-Tots,* edited by R. Davis-Floyd and J. Dumit, 105–24. New York: Routledge, 1998.

Miyagawa, Shigeo. "Report from Japan: Surrogacy Contracts in the Supreme Court of Japan." *The Court* [newspaper], May 11, 2007.

Modell, Judith. "Last Chance Babies: Interpretations of Parenthood in an IVF Program." *Medical Anthropology Quarterly* 3 (1989): 124–38.

———. *Kinship with Strangers: Adoption and Interpretations of Kinship in American Culture.* Berkeley: University of California Press, 1994.

Morah, Shirley. "I Am Pregnant and Having Fun [*Ani Beherayon V'kef Li*]." *Maariv* [newspaper], May 19, 2006.

Morgenstern-Leissner, Omi. "The Israeli Birth Law." PhD diss., Bar-Ilan University, 2005.

Moskovitz, Israel. "I Gave Birth to a Child for Others in Order to Feed My Children [*Yalad'ti Yeled Le'acherim Kedai Le'haachil Et Yeladai*]." *Yediot Aharonot* [newspaper], March 19, 2004.

Munroe, Robert L., and Ruth H. Munroe. "Psychological Interpretation of Male Initiation Rites: The Case of Male Pregnancy Symptoms." *Ethos* 1, no. 1 (1973): 490–98.

Murcott, Anne. "On the Altered Appetites of Pregnancy: Conceptions of Food, Body and Person." *Sociological Review* 36, no. 4 (1988): 733–64.

Nahman, Michal. "Materialising Israeliness: Difference and Mixture in Transnational Ova Donation." *Science as Culture* 15, no. 3 (2006): 199–213.

Nash, Catherine. "Response to Wanda Hurren's 'Living with/in the Lines: Poetic Possibilities or World Writing.'" *Gender, Place and Culture* 6, no. 3 (1999): 273–79.

Negev, Eilat. "Sixty Thousand Dollars and You Have a Child [*Shishim Eleph Dolar V'yesh Lecha Yeled*]." *Maariv* [newspaper], July 1, 1994.

Noy, Chaim. "You Must Go Trek There: The Persuasive Genre of Narration among Israeli Backpackers." *Narrative Inquiry* 12, no. 2 (2002): 261–90.

Oakley, Ann. *Women Confined: Toward a Sociology of Childbirth.* New York: Schocken, 1980.

Ortiz, Steven M. "How Interviewing Became Therapy for Wives of Professional Athletes: Learning from a Serendipitous Experience." *Qualitative Inquiry* 7 (2001): 192–220.

Ortner, Sherry. "Is Female to Male as Nature Is to Culture?" In *Women, Culture and Society,* edited by M. Z. Rosaldo and L. Lamphere, 67–88. Stanford, CA: Stanford University Press, 1974.

Otto, Rudolf. *The Idea of the Holy.* London: Oxford University Press, 1958.

Overall, Christine. *Ethics and Human Reproduction: A Feminist Analysis.* Boston: Allen and Unwin, 1987.

Paige, Karen Erickson, and Jeffrey M. Paige. *The Politics of Reproductive Ritual*. Berkeley: University of California Press, 1981.

Pande, Amrita. "'At Least I Am Not Sleeping with Anyone': 'Dirty' Surrogates in India." *Feminist Studies* (forthcoming).

Pande, Sumit. "Govt Plans New Laws to Curb Rent-a-Womb Rackets." *IBN-Live.com*, November 5, 2007. http://ibnlive.in.com/videos/51753/govt-plans-new-lows-to-curb-rentawomb-rackets.html.

Parkin, Robert. *Louis Dumont and Hierarchical Opposition*. New York: Berghahn Books, 2003.

Patai, Raphael. *On Jewish Folklore*. Detroit: Wayne State University Press, 1983.

Paxson, Heather. *Making Modern Mothers: Ethics and Family Planning in Urban Greece*. Berkeley: University of California Press, 2005.

Petchesky, Rosalind Pollack. "Foetal Images: The Power of Visual Culture in the Politics of Reproduction." In *Reproductive Technologies: Gender, Motherhood and Medicine*, edited by M. Stanworth, 57–80. Cambridge, UK: Polity Press, 1987.

Prainsack, Barbara. "Negotiating Life: The Regulation of Human Cloning and Embryonic Stem Cell Research in Israel." *Social Studies of Science* 36, no. 2 (2006): 173–205.

Pridmore-Brown, Michele. "Reproductive Timing and the Cultural Meaning of Post/Menopausal Motherhood in the U.S." Paper presented at panel on Bio/Politics of Contemporary Motherhood held at the University of California, Berkeley, December 5, 2007.

Rabinow, Paul Z. "Artificiality and Enlightenment: From Sociobiology to Biosociality." In *Incorporations*, edited by J. Crary and S. Kwinter, 234–52. New York: Zone, 1992.

Ragoné, Helena. *Surrogate Motherhood: Conception in the Heart*. Boulder, CO: Westview Press, 1994.

——. "Surrogate Motherhood, Gamete Donation, and Constructions of Altruism." In *Transformative Motherhood: On Giving and Getting in a Consumer Culture*, edited by L.L. Layne, 65–88. New York: New York University Press, 1999.

——. "Of Likeness and Difference: How Race Is Being Transfigured by Gestational Surrogacy." In *Ideologies and Technologies of Motherhood: Race, Class, Sexuality, Nationalism*, edited by H. Ragoné and F.W. Twine, 56–75. New York: Routledge, 2000.

Rao, Radhika. "Surrogacy Law in the United States: The Outcome of Ambivalence." In *Surrogate Motherhood: International Perspectives*, edited by R. Cook, S.D. Sclater, and F. Kaganas, 23–35. Oxford, UK: Hart Press, 2003.

Rapoport, Tamar, and Tamar El-Or. "Cultures of Womanhood." *Women's Studies International Forum* 20, nos. 5–6 (1997): 573–80.

Rapp, Rayna. *Testing Women, Testing the Fetus: The Social Impact of Amniocentesis in America*. New York: Routledge, 1999.

Raymond, Janice G. *Women as Wombs: Reproductive Technologies and the Battle over Women's Freedom*. San Francisco: HarperSanFrancisco, 1993.

Remennick, Larissa. "Childless in the Land of Imperative Motherhood: Stigma and Coping among Infertile Israeli Women." *Sex Roles* 43, nos. 11/12 (2000): 821–41.

——. "The Quest after the Perfect Baby: Why Do Israeli Women Seek Prenatal Genetic Testing?" *Sociology of Health & Illness* 28, no. 1 (2006): 21–53.

Reynolds, Peter C. *Stealing Fire: The Mythology of the Technocracy.* Palo Alto, CA: Iconic Anthropology Press, 1991.

Reznick, Ran. "Facing Local Shortage, Israeli Women Go to Romania to Get Eggs Implanted." *Haaretz Daily* [newspaper], September 25, 2000.

Rich, Adrienne. "Compulsory Heterosexuality and Lesbian Existence." *Signs* 5, no. 4 (1980): 631–60.

Roberts, Elizabeth F.S. "Examining Surrogacy Discourses: Between Feminine Power and Exploitation." In *Small Wars: The Cultural Politics of Childhood,* edited by N. Scheper-Hughes and C.F. Sargent, 93–110. Los Angeles: University of California Press, 1998.

——. "Native Narratives of Connectedness: Surrogate Motherhood and Technology." In *Cyborg Babies: From Techno-Sex to Techno-Tots,* edited by R. Davis-Floyd and J. Dumit, 193–211. New York: Routledge, 1998.

Rothman, Barbara Katz. *The Tentative Pregnancy: How Amniocentesis Changes the Experience of Motherhood.* New York: Norton, 1993.

——. *Recreating Motherhood.* New Brunswick, NJ: Rutgers University Press, 2000.

Rubin, Nissan, Carmela Shmilovitz, and Meira Weiss. "From Fat to Thin: Informal Rites Affirming Identity Change." *Symbolic Interaction* 16, no. 1 (1993): 1–17.

Rynkiewich, Michael A. "The Place That Is Part of It." In *Pacific Places, Pacific Histories: Essays in Honor of Robert C. Kiste,* edited by B.V. Lal, 309–26. Honolulu: University of Hawai'i Press, 2004.

Samama, Etti. "My Womb, Her Baby: Motivations for Surrogate Motherhood as Reflected in Women's Narratives in Israel." Master's thesis, Hebrew University, 2002.

Sandelowski, Margarete. "Compelled to Try: The Never-Enough Quality of Conceptive Technology." *Medical Anthropology Quarterly* 5, no. 1 (1991): 29–47.

——. *With Child in Mind: Studies of the Personal Encounter with Infertility.* Philadelphia: University of Pennsylvania Press, 1993.

——. "Separate, but Less Unequal: Fetal Ultrasonography and the Transformation of Expectant Mother/Fatherhood." *Gender and Society* 8, no. 2 (1994): 230–45.

Sandelowski, Margarete, Betty G. Harris, and Diane Holditch-Davis. "'Somewhere out There': Parental Claiming in the Preadoption Waiting Period." *Journal of Contemporary Ethnography* 21, no. 4 (1993): 464–86.

Sasson-Levy, Orna. "Feminism and Military Gender Practices: Israeli Women Soldiers in 'Masculine' Roles." *Sociological Inquiry* 73, no. 3 (2003): 440–65.

Scheper-Hughes, Nancy. *Death without Weeping: The Violence of Everyday Life in Brazil.* Berkeley: University of California Press, 1992.

Scheper-Hughes, Nancy, and Margaret M. Lock. "The Mindful Body: A Prolegomenon to Future Work in Medical Anthropology." *Medical Anthropology Quarterly* 1 (1987): 6–41.

Schneider, David Murray. *American Kinship: A Cultural Account.* Englewood Cliffs, NJ: Prentice-Hall, 1968.

———. *A Critique of the Study of Kinship.* Ann Arbor: University of Michigan Press, 1984.

Serafini, Paulo. "Outcome and Follow-up of Children Born after IVF-Surrogacy." *Human Reproduction Update* 7, no. 1 (2001): 23–27.

Sered, Susan Starr. *What Makes Women Sick?: Maternity, Modesty and Militarism in Israeli Society.* Hanover, NH: Brandeis University Press, University Press of New England, 2000.

Sered, Susan Starr, and Henry Abramovitch. "Pregnant Dreaming: Search for a Typology of a Proposed Dream Genre." *Social Science and Medicine* 34, no. 12 (1992): 1405–11.

Sewell, William H. "A Theory of Structure: Duality, Agency and Transformation." *The American Journal of Sociology* 98, no. 1 (1992): 1–29.

Shalev, Carmel. "*Halakha* and Patriarchal Motherhood: An Anatomy of the Israeli Surrogacy Law." *Israel Law Review* 32, no. 1 (1998): 51–80.

Shapira, Devorah. "I Am Convincing Myself That It Is Not My Baby [*Ani Ovedet Al Atzmi She'ze Lo Hatinok Sheli*]." *Maariv Signon* [newspaper], November 20, 1996.

Shapiro, Warren, and Uli Linke. *Denying Biology: Essays on Gender and Pseudo-Procreation.* Lanham, MD: University Press of America, 1996.

Sharan, Haviva, et al. "Hospitalization for Early Bonding of the Genetic Mother after a Surrogate Pregnancy: Report of Two Cases." *Birth* 28, no. 4 (2001): 270–73.

Sharp, Lesley A. "Organ Transplantation as a Transformative Experience: Anthropological Insights into the Restructuring of the Self." *Medical Anthropology Quarterly* 9, no. 3 (1995): 357–89.

———. *Strange Harvest: Organ Transplants in America.* Berkeley: University of California Press, 2006.

Shildrick, Margrit. "'You Are There, Like My Skin': Reconfiguring Relational Economies." In *Thinking through the Skin,* edited by S. Ahmed and J. Stacey, 160–75. London: Routledge, 2001.

Shilling, Chris. *The Body and Social Theory.* London: Sage, 1993.

Shinkman, Anat. "This Joy Lasted 27 Weeks [*Ha'osher Hazeh Nimshach 27 Shavuot*]." *Yediot Ahronot* [newspaper], September 17, 1999.

Siegel-Itzkovich, Judy. "Surrogacy: Bearing the Greatest Gift of All." *The Jerusalem Post,* May 27, 2001.

———. "Israel Allows Removal of Sperm from Dead Men at Wives' Request." *British Medical Journal* 327, no. 7425 (2003): 1187.

Sontag, Susan. *On Photography.* New York: Farrar, Straus and Giroux, 1977.

Spar, Debora L. *The Baby Business: How Money, Science, and Politics Drive the Commerce of Conception.* Boston: Harvard Business School Press, 2006.

Stacey, Jackie. *Stargazing: Hollywood Cinema and Female Spectatorship.* London: Routledge, 1993.

Stanworth, Michelle. "Reproductive Technologies and the Deconstruction of Motherhood." In *Reproductive Technologies: Gender, Motherhood and Medicine,* edited by M. Stanworth, 10–35. Cambridge, UK: Polity Press, 1987.

Strathern, Marilyn. *The Gender of the Gift: Problems with Women and Problems with Society in Melanesia.* Berkeley: University of California Press, 1988.

———. *Reproducing the Future: Anthropology, Kinship and the New Reproductive Technologies.* New York: Routledge, 1992.

———. *After Nature: English Kinship in the Late Twentieth Century.* Cambridge, UK: Cambridge University Press, 1995.

Suzuki, Kohta, et al. "Analysis of National Representative Opinion Surveys Concerning Gestational Surrogacy in Japan." *European Journal of Obstetrics and Gynecology* 126, no. 1 (2006): 39–47.

Taylor, Chris. "One Baby Too Many." *Time,* August 27, 2001. http://www.time.com/time/magazine/article/0,9171,1000632,00.html.

Taylor, Janelle S. "Image of Contradiction: Obstetrical Ultrasound in American Culture." In *Reproducing Reproduction: Kinship, Power, and Technological Innovation,* edited by S. Franklin and H. Ragoné, 15–45. Philadelphia: University of Pennsylvania Press, 1998.

Taylor, Janelle S., Linda L. Layne, and Danielle F. Wozniak, eds. *Consuming Motherhood.* New Brunswick, NJ: Rutgers University Press, 2004.

Teman, Elly. "Technological Fragmentation and Women's Empowerment: Surrogate Motherhood in Israel." *Women's Studies Quarterly* 31, nos. 3 & 4 (2001): 11–34.

———. "'Knowing' the Surrogate Body in Israel." In *Surrogate Motherhood: International Perspectives,* edited by R. Cook, S.D. Sclater, and F. Kaganas, 261–81. Oxford, UK: Hart Press, 2003.

———. "The Medicalization of 'Nature' in the 'Artificial Body': Surrogate Motherhood in Israel." *Medical Anthropology Quarterly* 17, no. 1 (2003): 78–98.

———. "Bonding with the Field: On Researching Surrogate Motherhood Arrangements in Israel." In *Dispatches from the Field,* edited by A. Gardner and D.M. Hoffman. Long Grove, IL: Waveland, 2006.

———. "The Red String: The Cultural History of a Jewish Folk Symbol." In *Jewishness: Expression, Identity, and Representation,* edited by S.J. Bronner, 29–57. Oxford, UK: Littman Library of Jewish Civilization, 2008.

———. "The Social Construction of Surrogacy Research: An Anthropological Critique of the Psychosocial Scholarship on Surrogate Motherhood." *Social Science and Medicine* 67, no. 7 (2008): 1104–12.

———. "Embodying Surrogate Motherhood: Pregnancy as a Dyadic Body Project." *Body and Society* 15, no. 3 (2009): 47–69.

———. "The Last Outpost of the Nuclear Family: A Cultural Critique of Israeli Surrogacy Policy." In *Kin, Gene, Community: Reproductive Technology among Jewish Israelis,* edited by D. Birenbaum-Carmeli and Y. Carmeli. Oxford, UK: Berghahn Books, forthcoming.

Teman, Elly, and Tsipy Ivry. Ultra-Orthodox Women and Prenatal Testing: God Sent Ordeals and Their Discontents. Unpublished manuscript, n.d.

Thompson, Charis. *Making Parents: The Ontological Choreography of Reproductive Technologies.* Cambridge, MA: MIT Press, 2005.

Tierson, Forrest D., C.L. Olsen, and E.B. Hook. "Nausea and Vomiting of Pregnancy and Its Association with Pregnancy Outcome." *American Journal of Obstetrics and Gynecology* 160 (1989): 518–19.

Titmuss, Richard. *The Gift Relationship: From Human Blood to Social Policy.* New York: New Press, 1997.

Traubman, Tamara. "The Surrogates Are Giving Birth Again; The Families Are Having a Second Surrogate Child [*Hapundekaiot Yoldot Ba'shenit, Hamishpachot Kvar Osot Yeled Pundekaut Sheni*]." *Haaretz Daily* [newspaper], May 25, 2004.

Turner, Bryan S. *The Body and Society.* Oxford, UK: Basil Blackwell, 1984.

Turner, Victor W. *The Ritual Process: Structure and Anti-Structure.* Ithaca, NY: Cornell University Press, 1977.

Upton, Rebecca L., and Sallie S. Han. "Maternity and Its Discontents: 'Getting the Body Back' after Pregnancy." *Journal of Contemporary Ethnography* 32, no. 6 (2003): 670–92.

Uvdah [Fact]. Television documentary program. Directed by Mica Limor. Israel's Channel 2, March 8 and April 5, 1998.

Valerio, Valeri. "Buying Women but Not Selling Them: Gift and Commodity Exchange in Huaulu Alliance." *Man* 29, no. 1 (1994): 1–24.

van den Akker, Olga. "Organizational Selection and Assessment of Women Entering a Surrogacy Agreement in the UK." *Human Reproduction* 14, no. 1 (1999): 262–66.

———. "Psychological Aspects of Surrogate Motherhood." *Human Reproduction* 13, no. 1 (2007): 53–62.

van der Ploeg, Irma. "Hermaphrodite Patients: In Vitro Fertilization and the Transformation of Male Infertility." *Science, Technology and Human Values* 20, no. 4 (1995): 460–81.

———. "Prosthetic Bodies: Female Embodiment in Reproductive Technologies." PhD diss., University of Amsterdam, 1998.

van Niekerk, Anton, and Liezl van Zyl. "The Ethics of Surrogacy: Women's Reproductive Labour." *Journal of Medical Ethics* 21 (1995): 345–49.

Vora, Kalindi. "Indian Transnational Surrogacy and the Commodification of Vital Energy." *Subjectivity* 26, no. 2 (forthcoming).

Waldby, Catherine, et al. "Blood and Bioidentity: Ideas about Self, Boundaries and Risk among Blood Donors and People Living with Hepatitis C." *Social Science & Medicine* 59 (2004): 1461–71.

Warner, Judith. "Outsourced Wombs." *The New York Times,* January 3, 2008.

Warren, Samantha, and Joanna Brewis. "Matter over Mind? Examining the Experiences of Pregnancy." *Sociology* 38, no. 2 (2004): 219–36.

Weisberg, D. Kelly. *The Birth of Surrogacy in Israel.* Gainesville, FL: University Press of Florida, 2005.

Weiss, Meira. "Bedside Manners: Paradoxes of Physician Behavior in Grand Rounds." *Culture, Medicine and Psychiatry* 17, no. 2 (1993): 235–53.

———. *Conditional Love: Parents' Attitudes toward Handicapped Children.* Westport, CT: Bergin & Garvey, 1994.

———. *The Chosen Body: The Politics of the Body in Israeli Society.* Stanford, CA: Stanford University Press, 2002.

Wiess, G. "Public Attitudes about Surrogate Motherhood." *Michigan Sociological Review* 6 (1992): 15–27.

Wilson, Robert Rawdon. "Cyber(Body)Parts: Prosthetic Consciousness." In *Cyberspace, Cyberbodies, Cyberpunk: Cultures of Technological Embodiment,* edited by M. Featherston and R. Burrows, 239–59. London: Sage, 1995.

Yanagisako, Sylvia Junko, Carol Lowery Delaney, and American Anthropological Association Meeting. *Naturalizing Power: Essays in Feminist Cultural Analysis.* New York: Routledge, 1995.

Young, Iris Marion. "Pregnant Embodiment: Subjectivity and Alienation." *Journal of Medicine and Philosophy* 9 (1984): 45–62.

Yuval Davis, Nira. "National Reproduction and 'the Demographic Race' in Israel." In *Woman-Nation-State,* edited by N. Yuval Davis and F. Anthias, 92–109. London: The Macmillan Press, 1989.

Zigdon, Moshe. "I Gave Them the Best Gift in the World [*Natati Lahem Et Hamatana Hachi Tova Bachayim*]." *Zman Ma'aleh* [newspaper], June 8, 2000.

Ziv, Yossi. "Surrogacy, the Right to Parenthood and Ethics [*Pundekaut, Hazchut Lehorut v'Musar*]" *Galileo* [magazine], March/April 1997.

Index

abortion, 9, 12, 291, 329n3
abstinence, 163. *See also* sexual
  intercourse
Abu-Lughod, Lila, 73
acknowledgment, 215–21. *See also* gifts;
  debt of life
  and enduring solidarity, 221–23,
    294–95
  not received, 225–29, 231, 233, 276,
    284
  of surrogate efforts, 26, 56, 100, 212–
    14, 275, 277, 281, 284
adoption, 13, 66, 199, 202, 295
  vs. surrogacy, 2, 110–12, 140–41
adultery, 13, 176, 305n62
agencies, 10–11, 24–25, 125, 306n70. *See
    also* contract
  Israeli surrogacy law, 12
  matching, 15, 108
  and military wives, 22, 254
  and same-sex couples, 11, 131, 306n64
  screening process, 15–16, 23, 208,
    239–40, 292
  statistics, 245, 297–98n4, 305n53
agency, 40, 53, 102, 104, 279
  personal, 31, 37, 126, 237, 277–78,
    285
    body mapping, 30, 73
  and technologies, 41, 251
agents, web of, 255, 271
Almeling, Rene, 207
amniocentesis, 16, 87, 157–58, 163

anomalies
  cultural, 6–7, 185–86, 232,
    289–90
  fetal, 87, 92, 116, 123, 318n16
  of surrogacy, 178, 185, 283
anthropological studies, 2, 4, 68, 107,
    113, 127, 176
anthropologists, xx, 3, 5–6, 52, 176, 252
appendage, 116, 213. *See also* prosthetic
    consciousness
  belly, 139, 141–42, 146, 149, 171
  surrogate, 25, 140, 165–68, 264,
    283–84, 290–91
artificial body, 38–46, 278. *See also*
    technology
attachment. *See* bonding
Atwood, Margaret, 174
authoritative knowledge, 77, 252, 279
automythology, 263, 275

beten, 71
Baby M, 1, 3, 297n3, 301n11
babysitter idiom, 55–57, 132. *See also*
    caregiver idiom
Bailey, Lucy, 84, 156
Baird, Patricia, 9
Balsamo, Anne, 101
bans on surrogacy, 9–10, 292,
    304n41
Becker, Ernest, 281
Becker, Gay, 114, 248, 287
bed rest, 88

Text: 10/13 Sabon
Display: Sabon
Compositor: BookComp, Inc.
Indexer: Alissa Surges